Domestic Violence

D0025541

Domestic Violence

A Multi-Professional Approach for Healthcare Practitioners

June Keeling and Tom Mason

TOURO COLLEGE LIBRARY
2002 Ave. J.

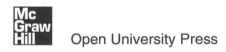

Open University Press

BP45

Open University Press
McGraw-Hill Education
McGraw-Hill House
Shoppenhangers Road
Maidenhead
Berkshire
England
SL6 2QL

email: enquiries@openup.co.uk
world wide web: www.openup.co.uk

and Two Penn Plaza, New York, NY 10121—2289, USA

First published 2008

Copyright © June Keeling and Tom Mason 2008

All rights reserved. Except for the quotation of short passages for the purpose of criticism and review, no part of this publication may be reproduced, stored in a retrieval system, or transmitted, in any form or by any means, electronic, mechanical, photocopying, recording or otherwise, without the prior written permission of the publisher or a licence from the Copyright Licensing Agency Limited. Details of such licences (for reprographic reproduction) may be obtained from the Copyright Licensing Agency Ltd of Saffron House, 6–10 Kirby Street, London, EC1N 8TS.

A catalogue record of this book is available from the British Library

ISBN-10: 0-33-522281-1 (pb) 0-33-522282-X (hb)
ISBN-13: 978-0-33-522281-0 (pb) 978-0-33-522282-7 (hb)

Library of Congress Cataloging-in-Publication Data
CIP data applied for

Typeset by Kerrypress Ltd, Luton, Bedfordshire
Printed in the UK by Bell & Bain Ltd, Glasgow

Fictitious names of companies, products, people, characters and/or data that may be used herein (in case studies or in examples) are not intended to represent any real individual, company, product or event.

The McGraw·Hill Companies

3/06/09

Contents

Part two: Reaction

Part three: Involvement

Part four: Outcome

The editors

June Keeling, MEd, BSc (Hons), RM, RGN, is a senior lecturer at the Faculty of Health and Social Care, University of Chester, UK. June has been in nursing for over 20 years and has been in clinical practice for 15 of those, predominantly relating to women's health issues. Her main research interest is in the field of family violence and professionalism in nursing. She is currently undertaking her PhD in the area of childbirth as a catalyst for disassociation from intimate partner violence.

Tom Mason, PhD, BSc (Hons), RMN, RNMH, RGN, is Professor of Mental Health and Learning Disability at the Faculty of Health and Social Care, University of Chester, UK. Tom has been in nursing for over 30 years, 17 in clinical practice and the remainder in academic posts. He is the co-author and co-editor of 12 books and has published over 70 journal articles on mental health and learning disability issues.

The contributors

Farah Ahmad, PhD, is a post-doctoral fellow at the Centre for Research on Inner City Health, funded by the Canadian Institutes of Health Research. She has training in medicine (Punjab University) and public health (Harvard University). Her research achievements include over 20 peer-reviewed papers and reports along with several scientific and invited presentations. Currently, Dr Ahmad's research is examining the effectiveness and feasibility of computer-assisted screening for increasing detection of intimate partner violence in a family practice setting.

Jeanne L. Alhusen, MSN, BSN, is a doctoral student at the Johns Hopkins University School of Nursing, USA. Her research interests include the impact of intimate partner violence on children who witness the violence and maternal perceptions related to the stressors of parenting. She volunteers at the House of Ruth of Maryland as a family nurse practitioner. She received a pre-doctoral fellowship in violence research through the National Institute of Mental Health Institutional NRSA from 2006–8.

Georgia J. Anetzberger, PhD, ACSW, LISW, is Assistant Professor for Health Care Administration at Cleveland State University, USA. She has spent over 25 years addressing the problem of elder abuse and was the 2005 recipient of the Rosalie Wolf Memorial Elder Abuse Prevention Award – National Category. Dr Anetzberger has authored more than 30 publications on elder abuse. She was the architect of Ohio's protective services law for adults and various subsequent amendments, and established the Ohio Coalition for Adult Protective Services and Consortium Against Adult Abuse as well as the Greater Cleveland Elder Abuse/Domestic Violence Roundtable. She served as principal investigator for the project 'A Model Intervention for Elder Abuse and Dementia', which won the American Society on Ageing 2000 Best Practice in Human Resources and Ageing Award.

Marguerite L. Baty, MSN, BSN, BA, is a doctoral student at the Johns Hopkins University School of Nursing, USA. She received a pre-doctoral fellowship in violence research through the National Institute of Mental Health Institutional NRSA from 2005–7. She also received the Isabel McIsaac Memorial Award from the Nurses' Educational Fund in 2005, and the Betty Cuthbert Award for leadership and service in 2004. She was inducted to the Sigma Theta Tau International Honor Society of Nursing in 2004.

Jacquelyn C. Campbell, PhD, MSN, BSN, is Anna D. Wolf Chair and Professor at the Johns Hopkins University School of Nursing, USA. Dr Campbell has been the principal investigator for ten major national institutes of health, national institutes of justice and CDC research grants, and published more than 150 articles and seven books on violence against women. She is an elected member of the Institute of

Medicine and the American Academy of Nursing, was a member of the Congression-ally Appointed Task Force on Domestic Violence in the military, received the 2005 Vollmer Award from the American Society of Criminology and the 2006 Pathfinder Award from the Friends of the National Institute of Nursing Research. She has worked with domestic violence shelters and advocacy organizations for 25 years

Senator Anne Cools, BA, is an Ontario conservative senator representing Toronto-Centre-York, Canada. She was summoned to the Senate in January 1984 by His Excellency Governor General Edward Schreyer and was the first black person appointed to the Senate of Canada and the first black female senator in North America. Prior to the Senate, Senator Cools was a social worker in innovative social services in Toronto. In 1974, she founded one of Canada's first women's shelters, Women in Transition Inc., serving as its executive director. She co-organized Canada's first domestic violence conference, 'Couples in Conflict'. Senator Cools has received many awards including an Honourary Doctor of Laws Degree (2004) from the Canada Christian College, Toronto, and the Woman of Excellence Leadership Award 2004 from National Center for Strategic Nonprofit Planning and Community Leadership, Washington, DC.

Ajitha Cyriac is a PhD student at the University of Toronto, pursuing a degree in public health. Her research focuses on the intersections of intimate partner violence and HIV, with a particular emphasis on the health of immigrant and refugee populations. She works directly with the South Asian community on issues of HIV and violence in Toronto and is a member of the board of directors for the YWCA. In 2006 she was awarded a Canadian Doctoral Research Award from the Canadian Institutes for Health Research. She received her MSc degree from Columbia University. She has been involved in women's health research for over ten years and plans on continuing to research in this field, for the rest of her career.

Dana DeHart, PhD, is Principal Investigator at South Carolina's Department of Health and Human Services, USA. She was project director for the National Institute of Justice's *Victimization Experiences of Incarcerated Women* study. Dr DeHart serves as evaluator for the Office for Victims of Crime's (OVC) 'Collaborative Response to Crime Victims in Urban Areas', an effort to link faith-based and secular services in five US cities. She was project director for OVC's National Victim Assistance Standards Consortium, as well as principal investigator on related projects including the *Ethics in Victim Services* CD-ROM curriculum .

Laura Dugan is Assistant Professor in the Department of Criminology and Criminal Justice, University of Maryland, College Park, USA. She is an active member of the National Consortium on Violence Research, the Maryland Population Research Center, and the National Center for the Study of Terrorism and the Response to Terrorism. Her research examines the consequences of criminal victimization and the efficacy of victimization prevention policy and practice. In her recent work, she has also examined the root causes of, and policy responses to, terrorism. Finally, she designs methodological strategies to overcome data limitations inherent in the social sciences.

Aaron T. Goetz, MA, BA, is currently a PhD candidate in evolutionary psychology at Florida Atlantic University. His research interests include men's anti-cuckoldry tactics and sexual coercion in intimate relationships.

Iona Heath, FRCGP, MRCP, is a general practitioner (GP) at the Caversham Group, London, UK. Iona has been working as an inner-city GP at this practice in Kentish Town since 1975. She has been a nationally elected member of the Council of the Royal College of General Practitioners since 1989 and chaired the Health Inequalities Standing Group from 1997 to 2003, and the Committee on Medical Ethics from 1998 to 2004. She is currently chairing the Ethics Committee of the *British Medical Journal*.

Richard E. Heyman, PhD, is Research Professor at the State University of New York, Stony Brook, USA. He has been principal investigator or co-principal investigator on 25 grants/contracts from US federal funders, including the National Institute of Mental Health, the National Institute of Child Health and Human Development, the Centers for Disease Control and Prevention, and the Department of Defense. He is the author of over 60 publications in scientific journals and scientific books that focus predominantly on the etiology, assessment and treatment of family maltreatment and relationship dysfunction. He developed the most widely used active coding system for couple interaction (the Rapid Marital Interaction Coding System) and has published extensively on couples' observational research.

Poco Kernsmith, PhD, MSW, is Assistant Professor in the School of Social Work at Wayne State University, Detroit, Michigan, USA, and has been working in the area of family and sexual violence as a research activist and practitioner for more than 15 years. In 2002, Dr Kernsmith received her PhD in social welfare from the University of California, Los Angeles. Her research areas include domestic and dating violence, sexual coercion and assault, stalking, treatment of sex offenders and the impact of childhood trauma and violence victimization.

Michael S. Kimmel is Professor of Sociology at the State University of New York, Stony Brook, USA. His books include *Changing Men* (1987), *Men Confront Pornography* (1990), *Against the Tide: Profeminist Men in the United States, 1776–1990* (1992), *The Politics of Manhood* (1996), *Manhood: A Cultural History* (2nd edn, 1996), *Men's Lives* (6th edn, 2003) and *The Gendered Society* (2nd edn, 2003). He co-edited *The Encyclopedia on Men and Masculinities* (2004) and the *Handbook of Studies on Men and Masculinities* (2004). He is the spokesperson for the National Organization for Men Against Sexism (NOMAS) and lectures extensively at corporations and on campuses in the US and abroad.

Karel Kurst-Swanger, PhD, MSEd, BS, is Associate Professor in the Department of Public Justice at the State University of New York, Oswego, USA. She serves as a planning consultant for numerous organizations and has served as the executive director of the Crime Victim Assistance Center, Inc. of Broome County, NY, and the Victim Services Coordinator of the Rochester City Police Department in Rochester, NY.

Marybeth J. Mattingly is a postdoctoral research fellow at the University of New Hampshire's Family Research Laboratory, USA. Her research interests span gender issues within the family and she has studied differences in men's and women's activity patterns, parenting styles and contributions to family income. Her current research examines women's and children's lives following violent victimization and she is particularly interested in examining what policies and interventions are most beneficial.

Danielle M. Mitnick (née Provenzano) is a graduate student in the PhD programme in clinical psychology at State University of New York, Stony Brook, USA. She is interested in couple communication and processes.

Christopher M. Murphy, PhD, is an associate professor of psychology at the University of Maryland, Baltimore County, USA. He also directs the New Behaviors Program at the Domestic Violence Center of Howard County, Maryland – a clinical service, training, and research program focused on perpetrators of intimate partner violence. Dr Murphy's research focuses on cognitive-behavioural and motivational treatments for abusive behaviour in intimate adult relationships, factors that predict successful response to partner violence treatment, emotional abuse in relationships, and the links between intimate partner violence and the use of alcohol and drugs.

Patricia O'Campo, PhD, is director at the Inner City Health Research Unit, St Michael's Hospital, and Professor of Public Health Sciences at the University of Toronto, Canada. She has been conducting research on the social determinants of health and well-being among women and children for over 15 years. She pioneered the application of multi-level modelling in the field of maternal and child health in the early 1990s. She has conducted a number of clinic and community-based evaluations of programmes concerning smoking cessation, prevention of perinatal transmission of HIV and prevention of infant mortality. She has also focused on methods development as part of her research, including the application of multi-level modelling to understand residential and workplace contexts on health and development.

Jay Peters, PhD, worked as a clinical social worker in New York City, USA, for eight years. During that time he worked primarily with chronic trauma survivors and, for the last four years, in an agency providing integrated mental health, crisis and social services support for domestic violence, rape and homicide survivors. Currently, when not teaching social work or conducting research related to violence against women, Jay can be found sailing among the islands of Maine with his wife, Imi Ganz.

Albert R. Roberts has over 30 years of full-time university teaching experience, both in criminal justice and social work. He has over 200 publications to his credit, including 32 books and numerous peer-reviewed journal articles and book chapters. Dr Roberts and Dr Gina Robertiello are currently completing a national organizational study of 170 shelters for battered women and their children. Dr Roberts is also currently completing the third national organizational survey of the structure and functions of suicide prevention agencies and crisis intervention units at community mental health centres.

Julie A. Schumacher, PhD, is Assistant Professor of Psychiatry and Human Behavior at the University of Mississippi Medical Center, USA. She received her PhD in clinical psychology from the State University of New York at Stony Brook. She went on to complete a National Institute on Alcohol Abuse and Alcoholism postdoctoral training fellowship in alcohol etiology and treatment at the University at Buffalo's Research Institute on Addictions (RIA), and then remained at RIA briefly as a research scientist. Dr Schumacher is a National Institutes of Health-funded researcher with primary research interests in the areas of drug and alcohol abuse and violent behaviour, particularly intimate partner violence.

Todd K. Shackelford, PhD, is Associate Professor of Psychology at Florida Atlantic University and chair of the Evolutionary Psychology Area. His current research interests include conflict between the sexes, particularly sexual conflict.

Phyllis W. Sharps, PhD, RN, CNE, FAAN, is an Associate Professor at the Johns Hopkins University School of Nursing, USA. She is an advanced nurse educator and in addition to her teaching responsibilities is the coordinator of a nurse-managed clinic for residents of a shelter for abused women. In February 2006 she received a five-year, $3.5 million research grant funded by the National Institute of Nursing Research to test a public health home nurse intervention to reduce the effects of intimate partner violence among pregnant women and their newborns.

Melanie Shepard is a professor of social work at the University of Minnesota, Duluth, USA. She has published numerous works in the field of domestic violence, including co-editing the book, *Coordinating Community Responses to Domestic Violence: Lessons from Duluth and Beyond* (1999). She has been an evaluator for many domestic violence projects and a group facilitator for both men's and women's groups. Currently, she is writing a manual for groups of battered women who have been arrested for domestic violence.

Adrian Sutton FCRC Psychiatry, MB, BS, BSc (Hons), is a UKCP registered psycho-analytic psychotherapist at the Winnicott Centre, Central Manchester & Manchester Children's University Hospitals NHS Trust, UK. As the Director of Studies at Manchester Medical School, he has a specific remit to develop the undergraduate teaching of ethics and law. He has extensive clinical experience in the field of child abuse and the impact of violence on children. Previously he was vice-chair of the UK Department of Constitutional Affairs North West Court Circuit Domestic Violence Group. He is currently a member of the Greater Manchester Family Justice Council.

Katherine van Wormer is Professor of Social Work at the University of Northern Iowa, USA, and is the author or co-author of nine books in the fields of women and criminal justice, addictions treatment, social welfare in a global perspective and confronting oppression.

Christina G. Watlington, PhD, is a clinical psychologist at the VA Maryland Healthcare System. She provides treatment and outreach services to veterans returning from overseas and training to organizations and clinicians in the community who work with returning veterans. Her research has focused on mental health consequences of partner violence exposure, bi-directional violence, and ways in which women cope with domestic violence.

Marianne R. Yoshioka, PhD, MSW is Associate Professor of Professional Practice at the Columbia University School of Social Work, USA. Her professional and research interests include domestic violence among immigrant populations, HIV prevention and the design of culturally appropriate interventions. She has received funding from the National Institute of Mental Health (NIMH) and private foundations to conduct research in these areas.

Preface

The inspiration for this book originated a few years ago while working as a domestic violence coordinator/researcher in a large general hospital in the UK. Having previously worked as a nurse and then as a midwife for some 15 years prior to this role, I developed a long-standing interest in the field of domestic violence. To be a midwife was a privilege, sharing a most intimate moment of childbirth and empowering a woman to metamorphose from a woman to a mother. For some women, however, this unique extraordinary life event lay in a shadow as a result of cruel and insidious abuse from their partner. Worse still, perhaps, were all the women I had cared for, oblivious of the dynamics of intimate partner abuse, whose violent lives I had missed, believing the responses given by the perpetrating partner. Thus, the role of domestic violence coordinator was one I developed and took forward to improve the responses given by health professionals, simultaneously improving the outcomes for survivors who disclosed their abuse. I have been fortunate to work with many wonderfully supportive and empathic professionals, all working in some capacity within the arena of domestic violence.

June Keeling
Chester, UK
2007

There are two main motivations for my involvement in this book. The first is that I have had a long-standing professional interest in the area of violence, particularly in mental health settings but also in many other areas of health care. In fact, it is the stark reality of violence perpetrated against vulnerable groups that has caused the greatest unease in my clinical practice and my research endeavours. This disquiet lies at the heart of being human in the face of aggression and violence. The second reason for my involvement was a chance encounter with my co-editor, June, whose early research produced such distressing results on the use of violence by males on females in intimate partnerships. These results were all the more alarming given the fact they were produced in what otherwise were perceived as warm and loving relationships. This led to a working partnership on this book which is based on a passionate endeavour to attempt to understand the complexities of this most disquieting event.

Tom Mason
Chester, UK
2007

Acknowledgements

We would like to express our deep gratitude to all those who contributed chapters to this book. Without their knowledge, expertise and motivation this project would never have come to fruition. We would also like to thank all those at Open University Press, and in particular Rachel Crookes, for their patience and guidance during the construction of this work. Finally, we give thanks to our families who gave us time and space to undertake this editing role and for their understanding in difficult times.

1   Introduction

June Keeling and Tom Mason

Violence is central to the historical development of mankind, or at least aggression is, for without this we would not have striven above the others in our animal kingdom. Aggression was originally required to protect ourselves from being eaten by other animals or killed by other clans and tribes. It may have been necessary in order to fight others for the right to mate, with an inherent drive to pass on the genes. It would certainly have been required to kill animals for the supply of food. In any event, whatever the prehistoric motivation, what we can say is that in contemporary times violence is still a major aspect of the human condition (Mason and Chandley 1999). So much so, that even though we may expect it to be repressed and channelled through appropriate outlets, and sublimated to activities such as sports and pursuits, if someone is perceived as not having the minimum amount of aggression we consider them in need of assertiveness training. Thus, it would seem that the long scale from the extremes of violence seen in wars and certain heinous crimes to the basic assertiveness required in order to maintain one's position in a queue is a complex one indeed. Where these boundaries lie is difficult to locate, how the definitions are constructed is individually, socially, culturally and politically determined, and how the values, norms and standards within each parameter are operationalized differs around the world. While the extremes of assertiveness and violence are obvious, what is acceptable or unacceptable in the grey middle ground is less so. However, this is not to say that we cannot make statements regarding this acceptability – or not, as the case may be. In fact, this book is replete with such statements.

It is often said that our contemporary society is more aggressive, more violent, than any previous generation. However, this is not necessarily the case (Marsh 1986).

One only has to think about the marauding Ghengis Khan, or the Vikings, to imagine what daily life was like in those times. Or we can cite the more historically recent 'ethnic cleansing' wars involving Adolf Hitler, Pol Pot and Idi Amin, and those wars in Bosnia and Africa. Furthermore, in the UK, we are fond of claiming that each successive generation is becoming more violent, with statements such as 'it wasn't like that when I was young', but once again history does not bear this out (Marsh 1986). For example, football hooliganism is said to be a modern phenomenon but its roots go back to the 1920s, 'steaming' (gangs of youths running down the street snatching bags and purses) is merely modern-day pillage, and mugging goes back as far as the history of man does. Certainly the Victorians had a particular problem with the 'garrotters' of London (muggers who would garrotte their victim first) (Marsh

1986). Thus, although we may feel that we live in violent times, and we most certainly do, this is not a new phenomenon, and neither is the *fear* of violence (Boran 2002).

It would appear that it is within the realms of violent action and the fear of violence that the roots of unacceptability grow. If a society is living in fear of violence then this violence must surely be unacceptable, and similarly if an individual is living in fear of violence then that action itself must be unacceptable. We note the abhorrence that is felt when faced with media images of, say, an elderly person who has been severely battered for a few pounds or a young child bruised and burnt by an adult – often a parent. These are clearly unacceptable actions on two of the most vulnerable groups in our society. But, as we will see, there are more, less visible, vulnerable groups that are abused in contemporary times. It is our intention in this book to focus on violent action and the fear of violence that is situated in the domestic setting. This in itself is a complex dynamic that has many vagaries that require unravelling in our quest to understand and assist those trapped in the cycle of abuse.

Historically, intimate partner violence (IPV) had been afforded privacy, being a subject that was not spoken about nor brought into the public domain. IPV remained 'behind doors', being spoken of in whispers and 'gossiped' about by neighbours. Minimal support was offered to those who experienced abuse as the general public alienated them and their problems. Perpetrators often perceived the legal system and law enforcement agencies as condoning their behaviour as long as it remained a private issue and a third party was not involved. However, late in the previous century the feminist movement demonstrated a proactive stance towards IPV. Concurrent with this development was the formation of the refuge movement which provided a safe haven for women and their children to escape violence at home, and simultaneously an understanding of some of the dynamics of abusive relationships began to emerge. Perhaps as a result of these organizations educating and informing the general public about partner abuse, albeit with a gender bias, a transition occurred from partner abuse being a private issue to one that lay in the public domain.

IPV pervades through all socioeconomic, gender and cultural boundaries. It is insidious and may intensify over time, involving financial control, physical violence, sexual assault and psychological intimidation. Universally, the results of such abuse have a devastating impact on the lives of the survivors, and their families, the survivors often remaining in a violent relationship for years, living in fear and pain. An underpinning love for their partner and hope that it was just a 'bad patch' in their relationship may have negated any desire to leave when the abuse began. Experiences of such abuse are often affected by recall bias, some experiences being too traumatic to recall, and some not perceived as being controlling or abusive. Many survivors minimize their injuries, either due to fear of persecution or accepting their treatment as a 'cultural norm'. The use of alcohol and drugs may confound the abusive relationship. However, for those being abused and contemplating disclosure there are a plethora of issues that influence the decision to disclose and to whom. Throughout the chapters of this book many of these issues are explored.

Research has informed us of the deleterious effects that IPV has on the health of survivors, the long-term and devastating effects on children and the financial cost both to employers and to the health service. For women, pregnancy may be a catalystic event for the abuse, which may begin and then escalate during the pregnancy, posing a significant threat to the health and well-being of both the woman and her unborn child (Keeling and Birch 2004). This abuse may then continue into the post-partum period, putting both lives at significant risk of injury or death. Indeed, from the moment of conception the foetus may experience abuse *in utero*, and then it may continue throughout childhood, having a devastating impact on the infant's psychological and physical development.

Structure of the book

The book is divided into four parts: 'Recognition', comprising Chapters 2–8; 'Reaction', comprising Chapters 9–13; 'Involvement', comprising Chapters14–18; and 'Outcome', comprising Chapters 19–22. A logical and coherent flow between the four sections enables the reader to be guided through each as it explores IPV from differing perspectives.

The sequential order of the chapters follows a systematic approach commencing with 'Recognition', which explores IPV from a personal perspective through the age continuum. Contextualizing the violence within a family – the development of strategies by which the family can keep the problem of IPV invisible to others and remain loyal to those involved in the violence – is discussed. Historically, IPV has been considered a gender-based crime. Thus this section of the book also discusses gender-based violence and its subtleties, exploring both factual and fictional anecdotes.

In 'Reaction' the wider perspective of IPV is reflected within the chapters, acknowledging cultural complexities and abuse, and the political and societal interfaces for both victims and perpetrators. This part of the book addresses the contiguous challenges involved in the management of IPV in a broader sense, exploring the roles of agencies in the provision of support for victims and perpetrators. The genre of support for victims is discussed and juxtaposed with the recognition and detection of abuse within the health sector. There are contributions from both voluntary and statutory agencies, ensuring the reader will enhance their knowledge base of the issues surrounding domestic abuse and the longer-term processes in addressing the problem. This theme is continued with a discussion about the challenges facing a multi-disciplinary working team. The wider perspective on the intimacies of IPV gives the reader a broader understanding of its complexities and of the myths that continue to propel the inappropriate responses received by so many victims.

The emphasis of 'Involvement' lies within the exploration of provision of appropriate support for the victim and perpetrator, in particular in terms of family health. The involvement of the family as a unit rather than as individuals is recognized. The discussion surrounding the interface between victim and perpetrator, examining perpetrators' experiences and also a conjoined approach to therapy, has created a balanced viewpoint.

Finally, the book is completed by 'Outcome', which projects the reader forward into an understanding of how abusive relationships may end, with the finality of homicide or a change in the dynamics of the violent relationship. Several considerations regarding victim and perpetrator behaviours are challenged and explored.

The chapters therefore weave their way from an individual perspective on IPV to a wider approach, with the authors contributing their own expertise in each area discussed. The book is drawn to a close with a discussion of the concluding stages of an abusive relationship, and also identifies how response to IPV has a direct impact on further assaults.

The specific chapters are as follows. Abuse of the elderly is a growing international concern and is particularly problematic due, in part, to the subtleties by which it can be enacted. Georgia Anetzberger, in Chapter 2, gives us a clear insight into many of the overlapping methods by which elderly abuse can occur. From the overt signs of physical abuse and neglect to the more covert threats of abandonment and the forging of their signatures, the methods of abuse of the elderly are diverse. It is a sad and startling fact that not only is abuse of the elderly on the increase but also the manner in which it is undertaken reflects the deviousness of the human imagination.

In Chapter 3 the major debate regarding gender symmetry in domestic violence is given a sharp focus. Michael Kimmel draws on many sources to bring into sharp relief the depth and breadth of issues that serve to confuse and confound both professional and lay workers in this area. These complexities within gender symmetry studies are teased out and crafted into a convincing argument that underscores the pivotal perspective that perpetrators of violence are overwhelmingly male.

In Chapter 4 Marguerite Baty, Jeanne Alhusen, Jacquelyn Campbell and Phyllis Sharps provide a succinct yet comprehensive overview of IPV. The picture painted here is both alarming and at the same time depressing as the ravages of this abuse are starkly revealed. The frequency of IPV around the globe is worrying, and the increasing rates are of great concern with the health consequences being so diverse and damaging. These authors highlight the wide range of corollaries to IPV and provide a factual account that cannot fail to stir the reader into a state of concern.

The complexity of domestic violence, not only in terms of its dynamic directly between perpetrator and victim, but also in the social sphere of adult family and friends, is well established. However, we often fail to appreciate or understand how this domestic violence impacts on young children who witness it, perceive it and 'deal' with it within the family sphere. In Chapter 5 Adrian Sutton brings a clarity to the notion that this adult domestic violence can be understood as a form of child abuse. He argues that children can manifest an array of dysfunctional traits in response to witnessing violence between parents. The children are caught in a 'web' of interpersonal feelings involving a cauldron of inner angst, creating the potential for severe psychological trauma.

In Chapter 6 Poco Kernsmith deals with the thorny and sensitive nature of sexual coercion within marriage, as a form of domestic violence. Historically seen as a taboo area, for law or science, the sanctity of marriage is now no longer a veil for any form of domestic violence, including sexual coercion. Kernsmith deals bluntly with this issue by employing the term 'marital rape' to hit home the point that, irrespective of the social forms of marriage, sexual relations require the consent of adults. Although relationships within (and without) marriage are complex, Kernsmith opens up this debate to establish a 'lens' of opportunity into this dark domain.

In Chapter 7 Aaron Goetz and Todd Shackelford outline an evolutionary psychological perspective on men's violence against intimate partners. In this revealing chapter, inherent motivations driving violence and sexual aggression toward females are seen in relation to emotional and sexual infidelity. This is then juxtaposed to the animal kingdom in which competition for genetic dominance gives us glimpses into the darker elements of our contemporary human souls.

In Chapter 8 June Keeling argues for an educational strategy, not only to inform about the problem of domestic violence but also to contribute towards prevention. She develops a convincing argument for an educational package which ought to be based on sound academic rigour and validated by professional bodies. Keeling bases her educational framework in multi-professional collaboration, without which, she argues, a disparate approach will lead to isolation and a lack of prevention. Waiting for further debate is not an option and Keeling insists that action is needed if we are to move forward with this issue.

Chapter 9 presents a framework by which to understand the ways that the cultural context influences a woman's experience of domestic violence. Marianne Yoshioka adopts a culture-general approach with three organizing factors: the individualist-collectivist continuum; the woman's relationship to the host society; and the unique social traditions. Drawing from first-hand research with Asian immigrant women living with domestic violence, this author provides a framework to help practitioners better understand how cultural differences manifest themselves when working in this field.

In Chapter 10 Senator Anne Cools offers an insightful account of her personal work with families affected by domestic violence over many years. She focuses on 'families' rather than individuals, as all those involved in this sad affair are affected by domestic violence, and she brings to the issue an understanding that pivots on the notion of social conflict. This draws into the frame the role of the police, the courts and professionals working together towards intervention.

Melanie Shepard, in Chapter 11, brings a great deal of clarity to the complex dynamic that exists within the IPV relationship. Focusing on battered women who then turn to violence themselves, Shepard makes the case for not calling these women 'batterers'. The reasons offered for this pivot on notions of self-defence, retaliation, initiation and control, among others, and these are central to the argument. This author goes on to argue that this has implications for practice which should be based on safety issues and that we should have specific programmes for battered women who turn to violence. Furthermore, we should not put women on male batterer programmes, as the issues are entirely different.

To what extent we, as health care professionals, can apply effective preventative interventions in IPV and what our roles may consist of is the focus of Chapter 12. Patricia O'Campo, Farah Ahmad and Ajitha Cyriac discuss these issues from the perspective of health care utilization for victims, disclosure, screening, physicians' barriers and chronicity. Clearly there is often major debate underpinning these thorny issues. These authors outline health care interventions that go beyond screening and identification and give pointers for future research. Although the general overall picture for IPV may appear bleak, this chapter offers some hope in moving forward.

If progress is to be made in intervening in domestic violence then multi-disciplinary working is of central importance. In Chapter 13 Karel Kurst-Swanger outlines structures, processes and outcomes of multi-disciplinary working and gives us clear indications of how to work together. Kurst-Swanger deconstructs the codes of professional groups to reveal how their boundaries, philosophies and language differ across traditions, and how this contributes to how they operate. This author offers a positive approach to overcoming the conflicts and tensions that can arise in multi-disciplinary work. Numerous operational processes are outlined to help professionals work effectively, learn from each other and tackle the difficult issues that confront them in this field.

The relationship between alcohol abuse and domestic violence has been well established and is considered a chronic condition with few reports of a one-off occasion. In Chapter 14 Julie Schumacher provides a comprehensive review of this relationship and reveals a disturbing picture of this apparently entrenched condition. However, this author suggests that those perpetrators who are referred to treatment programmes and who attend on a regular basis have better outcomes, and she argues for a more thorough approach both to referral and attendance on a number of training programmes, this being necessary if we are to reduce IPV.

Myths abound around domestic violence and in Chapter 15 Jay Peters argues that although these may serve a psychological purpose there may well be a social function regarding such myths. Such a function may be largely defensive for the perpetrator and revolve around trivializing the abuse and reducing the sense of guilt. Thus, it can be argued, that this can then marginalize the victim and indeed the social problem of domestic violence as a whole. This author argues strongly for the development of scales to measure the extent of the impact of myths and reports on just such a scale development.

Dana DeHart, in Chapter 16, gives us a rare glimpse into the offenders' experience of interventions for preventing violence. This chapter draws together the sparse research on this perspective and whets the appetite for further exploration into offenders' responses to treatment interventions. Without this research we are less likely to create effective programmes and, thus, remain ineffective at preventing this tragic condition. Without offenders' responses to domestic violence we will not be in a position to provide information for treatment approaches, which require sound evaluations as a matter of urgency.

The issue of treating IPV in conjoint settings is dealt with in Chapter 17. Danielle Mitnick and Richard Heyman make a convincing case for conjoint therapy when an assessment is made for appropriate couples. They argue that careful planning and clear treatment components need to be identified and general guidelines followed if interventions are to be effective. Although these authors are realistic in reporting outcomes they make an optimistic case for moving forwards with this difficult issue and state that although conjoint therapy appears to be a viable alternative for some, much work remains to be done.

In dealing with the family health perspective, in Chapter 18, Iona Heath blends together factual accounts and fictional narrative to highlight the complex relationships that exist between perpetrators and victims and other family members. This approach also reveals conflicts between families of domestic violence and health care professionals who have difficulty with the traditional medical model and its application to this form of crime. Focusing on the I-Thou relations that embrace notions of human compassion, the tensions become clear as the relations move to the I-It form.

In Chapter 19 Katherine van Wormer and Albert Roberts outline the severest cases of IPV in relation to homicide, including murder-suicide. In these extreme cases not only is there a death, either of the victim or the perpetrator as revenge, but also those remaining can often be incarcerated for many years. In this harrowing chapter we hear the accounts of three such females who each killed their abuser only to be sent to prison. Caught in a web of abuse, often with drugs and alcohol as contributing factors, these women give us a moving insight into their troubled lives.

Relationship conflict and abuse outcomes are the focus of Chapter 20 and are underpinned by an analysis of systems theory. Christopher Murphy and Christina Watlington deal with the substantial empirical support for the role of dyadic relationship conflict in understanding IPV. However, they also balance this with a clear delineation of the limitations of systems theory, which is only one perspective to understanding abuse. They conclude that the most important factors in understanding IPV are relationship conflict, mutual escalation of aggressive interchanges and poor communication.

In Chapter 21, Marybeth Mattingly and Laura Dugan discuss how female victims' responses to abuse affect the risk of future assaults by their male intimate partners. The major theme to emerge revolves around the popular response to victims of domestic violence to move to a shelter or seek help. However, these authors' research suggests that this may, in fact, make matters worse. They reveal that those victims who seek medical attention have a dramatically higher chance of being reassaulted. This alarming picture, again, shows the complexity of domestic violence and of our attempts to intervene.

Finally, in Chapter 22, we reflect on our attempts to view the problem of IPV in an interacive framework that comprises concerns regarding the reconition of the problem, society's fundamental reaction to it, the role of multi-professionals and their involvement, and the ultimate outcome for all concerned. Clearly IPV is far more complex than this but, simply stated, this framework gives us an anchorage from which we can explore the wider diverse issues.

Part one
Recognition

2   Abuse and the elderly

Georgia J. Anetzberger

Introduction: Willa and her family

Willa is 83 and widowed. She is a recovering alcoholic who is homebound, except for medical appointments, she is registered blind and suffers from multiple mental and physical impairments. These include bipolar disorder, chronic obstructive pulmonary disease, congestive heart failure, hypertension, diabetes and peptic ulcer. Although often depressed, Willa is alert and oriented, showing no significant cognitive decline. Willa's life has been characterized by hardship and violence. She was born into poverty, with an abusive mother. Her education ended in the fourth grade. She married five times, each marriage governed by alcoholism, deprivation, and both physical and verbal abuse. Willa has seven living children, two sons by her first husband and three daughters by her fourth husband. However, except for Edwina, who resides with Willa, none of her children live nearby.

Edwina is 60, has never married and is being treated by a psychiatrist for bipolar disorder. Frequently manic, she has not been employed outside of the home for more than two decades. Her time is spent caring for Willa, handling crises caused by her sister's daughter, Jennifer, and 'doing what I damn well please'.

Jennifer is 34, and was adopted by Willa as a teenager because of her mother's drug habit. As a result, she has lived with her grandmother intermittently for many years. Both Willa and Edwina describe her as headstrong, irresponsible, and out of control. She is also dependent on heroin. Recently she came to the house seeking money for drugs. When refused, Jennifer assaulted Edwina, broke furniture and dishes, and threw a lamp through the living room window. Willa fell attempting to intervene, which resulted in her hospitalization for bruises on the eye and knees.

Edwina struggles in her caregiving role. She always was at odds with her mother, but now the relationship is even more difficult because of Willa's many demands and complaints. Arguments between the two women are frequent, and occasionally have included threats and rough handling by Edwina. The visiting nurse and home care aide have expressed concern about Edwina's ability to manage Willa's 13 medications and dietary needs. They also worry about Willa's safety. Edwina frequently leaves her alone, locked in the house. During one such occasion, Willa fell while attempting to open the door for the aide. Edwina has also been known to refuse to seek the medical attention her mother requires. There are no family or friends willing to provide Willa and Edwina with support or assistance. Any that once existed are now estranged due to the constant conflict and chaos in the household. Still, Edwina feels some sense of responsibility for Willa, and Willa for Jennifer. At the same time, each one is fiercely independent, determined to pursue life on her own terms.

Problem recognition

There is nothing new about elder abuse. Throughout history older people have endured injury and suffering by family members or trusted others. More recent is recognition of elder abuse as a social problem, a public health concern, an important aspect of family violence, or as a crime. This recognition began barely more than a quarter of a century ago.

Family conflict and elder abuse are depicted in early legend and literature. Reinharz (1986) provides examples from Greek mythology and Shakespearean plays, framing them around the twin themes of loving and hating our elders. Stearns (1986) suggests that the tendency in some nineteenth-century European countries to construct small cottages for elderly kin to the rear of the main building was evidence of tensions common between older and younger relations. The mistreatment of older people was often associated with perceiving them as family or community burdens. Stenning (1958: 99) describes old age among the Fulani of West Africa as a time of giving away to the point of depletion all property to the children as they marry. In the end, the elderly parents reside as dependants, with old men in particular regarded as having little use, spending 'their last days on the periphery of the household'. Burch (1975) relates that various Eskimo societies abandoned elderly members when there was not enough food for everyone. Bever (1982) indicates that during the sixteenth and seventeenth centuries in Europe, many older women were accused of witchcraft and their lives threatened because of the strain they placed on family resources. Finally, Fischer (1978) recounts examples of adult children in colonial America turning away and despising their elderly impoverished mothers.

Early problem recognition

The earliest recognition of elder abuse as a problem emerged in the mid-1970s in both the UK and the USA. It was then that situations like that of Willa and her family began to capture public attention and the interest of practitioners, policy-makers and researchers. Professional acknowledgement initially came from the medical community, with physicians Baker (1975), Burston (1975), and Butler (1975) describing cases of elder physical abuse that they had encountered. Shortly afterwards, the phenomenon was placed into a family violence context, as Steinmetz (1978a: 7, 1978b) gave the first public testimony on the problem. Speaking before a Congressional committee exploring overlooked aspects of domestic violence, she discussed battered elderly parents, paralleling them to abused children and predicting that 'the '80s will be the decade of the battered parent'. Around the same time, the earliest studies into elder abuse were reported. All conducted in the USA, their purpose was to demonstrate the existence of elder abuse as well as to provide an early understanding of its nature and scope (e.g. Douglass *et al.* 1980). Although this research was only exploratory and used relatively unsophisticated investigatory techniques, it was important for establishing elder abuse as a problem affecting older adults. It also formed a profile of the victim, the perpetrator and the abuse that has changed little as a result of subsequent investigation.

Research into elder abuse in the UK and Canada began later than in the USA. Perhaps the earliest British contributor was Eastman (1984), who offered a case study qualitative analysis of the problem in domestic settings. Greater interest has surrounded elder abuse in institutional settings in the UK than in either of the other two countries (e.g. Clough 1999). Part of the reason has been ascribed to political ideology there, with left-wing concerns focused on breakdowns in *residential* care and right-wing concerns focused on breakdowns in *family* care (e.g. Kosberg *et al.* 2003). Turning to Canada, although elder abuse was recognized as a social problem among some provinces as early as the late 1970s (Beaulieu 1992) and research on the subject began shortly thereafter, scientific study of elder abuse was slow, halting and methodologically limited throughout the 1980s. Later, Podneiks (1992) played a critical role in portraying elder abuse as a national problem, sufficiently pervasive among elder Canadians to warrant broad public attention. Using methodology borrowed from American colleagues who had studied problem prevalence in the metropolitan Boston area (Pillemer and Finkelhor 1988), and considering four abuse forms, Podneiks uncovered a late life cumulative rate for elder abuse of 4 per cent and material abuse as the most common form at 2.6 per cent. Although Ogg (1993) tried to replicate the metropolitan Boston survey in London, there were methodological difficulties, and he was unable to determine problem occurrence in that city.

Problem recognition today

This first wave of problem recognition and research has been followed by steady growth and expansion in the attention given to elder abuse by researchers, practitioners and policy-makers. The attention is no longer concentrated in the USA, UK and Canada – it is now worldwide. Evidence of this comes from multiple sources. For example, growth is suggested by Stein (2006), who searched the database on 'abuse' of the Clearinghouse on Abuse and Neglect of the Elderly and found 558 published articles for the 32-year period 1959–99 and 1368 published articles for the 15-year period 1991–2006. Expansion is indicated by: (1) formation of the International Network for the Prevention of Elder Abuse (INPEA) in 1997, with current membership from both developed and developing countries; (2) publication of the World Health Organization (WHO) (2002) report on violence and health, which featured elder abuse; and (3) proclamation of World Elder Abuse Awareness Day on 15 June 2006, with recognition activities held in such countries as Japan, Uganda, Sweden and Albania.

Examining elder abuse

Definition and forms

Nearly everyone would categorize Willa and Edwina's situation as elder abuse. It falls under most elder abuse reporting, adult protective services or domestic violence laws found in the USA, Canada and the UK. It is consistent with elder abuse definitions proposed by various national and international groups, like the National Center on Elder Abuse (USA) and the WHO. Finally, it coincides with definitions derived through research by scholars like Margret Hudson and Tanya Johnson, who spent years attempting to standardize elder abuse definitions. Sample elder abuse definitions are found in Figure 2.1.

Johnson (1986: 180): elder mistreatment is a 'state of self-inflicted suffering unnecessary to the maintenance of the quality of life of the older person'.

Hudson (1991:14): elder mistreatment is 'destructive behavior that is directed toward an older adult, occurs within the context of a relationship connoting trust and is of sufficient intensity and/or frequency to produce harmful physical, psychological, social and/or financial effects of unnecessary suffering, injury, pain, loss and/or violation of human rights and poorer quality of life for the older adult'.

National Research Council (2003: 40): elder mistreatment is '(a) intentional actions that cause harm or create a serious risk of harm (whether or not harm is intended), to a vulnerable elder by a caregiver or other person who stands in a trust relationship to the elder, or (b) failure by a caregiver to satisfy the elder's basic needs or to protect the elder from harm'.

WHO (as cited in Lachs and Pillemer 2004): elder abuse is 'a single or repeated act, or lack of appropriate action, occurring within any relationship where there is an expectation of trust, which causes harm or distress to an older person' (Adapted by the British Action on Abuse of Older Persons and the Toronto Declaration on Elder Abuse.)

National Center on Elder Abuse (2006): elder abuse is 'any knowing, intentional, or negligent act by a caregiver or any other person that causes harm or a serious risk of harm to a vulnerable adult'.

Figure 2.1 Sample elder abuse definitions

However, widespread agreement on whether or not a specific situation qualifies as elder abuse is not the same as having universally accepted practical elder abuse definitions. These do not exist, although they have been recommended for over 20 years (e.g. National Research Council 2003). The difficulty in deriving definitions rests with disagreement about the place of several factors in definition construction, such as breadth of meaning, elder vulnerability, perpetrator intent and consideration of the frequency, duration, severity or effects of abuse. Of course, without universally accepted practical definitions, comparison of research findings and data collection results across public authorities is problematic. Moreover, practitioners and citizens are confused over what constitutes elder abuse and what does not (e.g. Wolf 1988).

Although nearly everyone might regard Willa and Edwina as elder abuse victims, they might not agree on the particular forms represented in their situation. The range of recognized elder abuse forms is considerable, from two to more than a dozen. Hudson (1991) illustrates the low end, with her two broad categories of elder mistreatment: elder abuse and elder neglect. The primary distinctions between the categories are: (1) nature of the act (i.e. aggressive or invasive behaviour for elder abuse, failure to act for elder neglect), and (2) role of the perpetrator (i.e. unacknowledged for elder abuse, a responsible party in providing assistance for elder neglect). The high end for recognized elder abuse forms is evident in the United Nations (UN) (2002) *Report to the Secretary-General* in preparation for the Second World Assembly on Ageing. Here five broad categories of elder abuse are identified: physical abuse; emotional abuse; financial exploitation; neglect; and self-neglect. These are followed by a list of 12 variations or additional categories mentioned in the scientific literature: sexual abuse; spousal abuse; medication abuse; abandonment or desertion; loss of respect; systematic abuse; economic violence; scapegoating; social or domestic violence; community violence; political violence and armed conflict; and HIV/AIDS-related violence. Somewhere in between these extremes are the National Center on Elder Abuse's (2006) six forms: physical abuse; emotional abuse; sexual abuse; exploitation; neglect; and abandonment. All six can be collapsed into Hudson's two broad classes, and some represent categories and others variations of categories in the UN's typology.

Applying the above recognized elder abuse forms to Willa and Edwina suggests that they have been subjected to multiple forms. This is typical for elder abuse victims. In fact, outside of self-neglecting elders, it is unusual for abuse victims to experience a single form. Using the National Center on Elder Abuse classifications, Willa has experienced physical abuse, emotional abuse and neglect; Edwina has experienced physical abuse, emotional abuse and exploitation. Using Hudson's dyad, Willa has been abused and neglected, while Edwina has been abused but not neglected. Finally, applying the major abuse categories identified by the UN finds the combination of Willa and Edwina victimized by four of the five abuse categories. Only self-neglect does not seem to be represented in their situation.

Prevalence and incidence

It is not known with certainty how often situations like Willa and Edwina's occur. National prevalence and incidence research has been conducted in only a handful of countries. Moreover, where it exists, investigations often are limited through use of flawed methods and incomparable definitions. Available studies suggest cross-national rates of 1–10 per cent. The best regarded prevalence study in the USA was localized to the metropolitan Boston area and examined three forms: physical abuse; chronic verbal aggression; and neglect. Through random sample telephone interviews, it was discovered that 3.2 per cent of respondents had suffered at least one abuse form since age 65, with physical abuse the most common (Pillemer and Finkelhor 1988). A decade later a national incidence study was conducted, revealing about 450,000 cases of elder abuse known to Adult Protective Services (the primary agency charged with handling elder abuse situations in the USA) or community agencies serving older people (National Center on Elder Abuse 1998).

Problem reporting to authorities like adult protective services tends to be low, even among professionals legally mandated to make referrals. Reasons include fear of litigation or eroding rapport established with a patient or client, lack of awareness about reporting procedures or confidence in the agency receiving reports, and a belief that reporting violates personal autonomy or makes no positive difference (e.g. Anetzberger 1993). Still, elder abuse reporting to Adult Protective Services has increased, from 117,000 in 1986 to 293,000 in 1996 (Tatara 1996). Most recent statistics suggest that almost 566,000 reports of elder and vulnerable adult abuse were received in 2004, with self-neglect and caregiver neglect most common (Teaster et al. 2005).

In the UK, Ogg (1993) found that 5 per cent of older respondents experienced verbal abuse, 2 per cent physical abuse and 2 per cent neglect. Prevalence rates elsewhere have varied widely, including 0.58 per cent for Australia (Boldy 2005), 5.7 per cent for Finland (Kivela et al. 1992), 8 per cent for Denmark and Sweden (Tornstam 1989) and 8.2 per cent for Korea (Cho et al. 2000). Similarly, elder abuse incidence has been established at 0.5 per cent for Israel (Iecovich et al. 2004) and five times that rate for Arabs in Israel (Sharon and Zoabi 1997).

Recognizing elder abuse

Theoretical explanations

Theoretical explanations for elder abuse abound, but none have been rigorously tested. Those that have the most support from empirical investigation include:

- *Psychopathological:* perpetrators of elder abuse exhibit abnormal behaviour, such as mental illness or substance abuse (e.g. Anetzberger et al. 1994).
- *Situational:* perpetrators inflict elder abuse under stressful circumstances where vulnerable elders are perceived to be associated with the stress (e.g. Lachs et al. 1994).
- *Symbolic interactional:* elder abuse results when perpetrators perceive disparities between the role that they ascribe to an elder and the actual behaviour exhibited by that person (Steinmetz 1988).

Returning to Willa and her family, each of the above explanations can apply. Edwina and Jennifer both exhibit psychopathology, mental illness and drug abuse. In addition, Edwina is stressed by life crises, including caregiving (situational) and Willa's difficult behaviours, which are contrary to her expectations (symbolic interaction). Perhaps because no single theory seems sufficient to explain elder abuse in all its complexities, recent efforts have been directed at combining theories into an over-arching perspective on the problem. For example, the National Research Council (2003) offers a transactional model, linking social embeddedness and individual-level factors of victim and perpetrator within a sociocultural context, considering relationship type, status inequity and power/exchange dynamics.

Detection

Elder abuse can be hard to identify, and may be confused with other problems. Manifestations can be subtle. Victims or perpetrators may deny the problem, or redefine it based on cultural, religious or family background. Detecting elder abuse requires problem awareness and suspicion (Abyad 1996), directed at presenting examples, signs and risk factors (Anetzberger 2001). 'Examples' are illustrations of elder abuse observed or reported by a reputable source. Jennifer assaulting Edwina is an example of the problem. 'Signs' are the result of elder abuse examples. They represent indicators that the problem may have occurred. Willa's bruises are signs of elder abuse; they are the consequences of her fall while intervening in Jennifer's assault on Edwina. However, signs are less definitive of the problem than examples, because they could be attributed to other causes as well. Finally, 'risk factors' are characteristics of the victim, perpetrator or situation thought to be associated with elder abuse as a result of research on the subject. Willa's difficult behaviours, Edwina's mental illness and Jennifer's drug abuse all are risk factors for abuse occurrences. Nonetheless, because, like signs, they can be ascribed to other phenomena, risk factors only suggest the *possibility* of elder abuse, not its certainty. Selected elder abuse examples, signs or risk factors are found in Figure 2.2.

Examples

- Slapping, shoving, or restraining
- Threatening with a knife, gun or other weapon
- Sexually assaulting or coercing
- Calling names or insulting
- Threatening placement in a nursing home
- Locking in a room
- Denying adequate care or supervision
- Failing to treat health problems
- Isolating from others
- Using money or property without consent
- Forging signature on legal documents
- Withdrawing money from bank accounts without knowledge

Signs

- Bruises, welts, or cuts
- Cigarette or rope burn marks

- Blood on person or clothing
- Sense of resignation or hopelessness
- Passive or withdrawn behaviour
- Fear or anxiety
- Unclean physical appearance
- Underweight, dehydration or weakness
- Unsafe environment, including insect or rodent infestation
- Missing money or cheques
- Unexplained changes in legal documents
- Unexplained decreases in bank accounts

Risk factors

- History of past abuse or neglect
- Evidence of current or past relationship problems
- Unrealistic expectations of the other person
- Anger, hostility or aggression
- Mental health or emotional problems
- Limitations in physical health or functional capacity
- Cognitive impairment
- Behaviour problems
- Financial dependence
- Social isolation
- Lack of social support
- Shared household

Figure 2.2 Examples, signs and risk factors of elder abuse

Screening or assessment instructions are helpful for detecting elder abuse and unravelling its dimensions. Several such tools have been developed, including the HALF (Ferguson and Beck 1983), Hwalek-Sengstock Elder Abuse Screening (Hwalek and Sengstock 1986), the Indicators of Abuse Screen (Reis and Nahmiash 1998), the Elder Assessment Instrument Revised (Fulmer *et al.* 2000) and STRP (Bass *et al.* 2001). They vary in format, focus and targeted profession or setting. The importance of screening or assessment instruments lies in their ability to ensure that clues are not missed and information is systematically collected and documented for clinical, legal or research purposes. Most tools have not been tested, and no tool has universal acceptance.

Multi-disciplinary teams can further enhance elder abuse detection and assessment by providing a more holistic perspective on the problem than could be offered by any single discipline or system (Anetzberger *et al.* 2005). Multi-disciplinary teams are groups of professionals or systems assembled by organizations or communities for case identification and recommendation (Teaster and Nerenberg 2004). Some have a limited function, such as financial abuse or fatality review. Some also are involved in programme planning, education and advocacy. Although the use of multi-disciplinary teams in elder abuse recognition has increased in recent years, they can be challenging to launch and sustain due to time demands, potential dominance by certain disciplines or systems, and territorial or interpersonal issues.

Conclusions

Responding to elder abuse requires a multi-faceted approach that includes: (1) research to understand the problem and how to effectively address it; (2) public and professional awareness to draw attention to the problem and its established interventions; (3) detection, prevention and treatment strategies to uncover the problem, address its consequences and avoid its reoccurrence; and (4) advocacy to promote policy and systemic change that effects better problem resolution.

Research on elder abuse has resulted in an increased understanding of the problem and how to address it. Still, as indicated previously, more and better study is needed across all elder abuse domains and in every country. This need was prioritized in the *Madrid International Plan of Action on Ageing*, which resulted from the Second World Assembly on Ageing (2002). The *Plan* also encouraged public awareness and professional education campaigns on elder abuse, using techniques like news stories, informational brochures, resource fairs and telephone hotlines. Such activities were highlighted during the 2006 World Elder Abuse Awareness Day when, for example, Ireland had balloon races where 500 purple balloons were launched and Cameroon conducted three days of radio talks and debates on elder abuse (Podneiks 2006).

Intervention strategies include elder abuse laws and services. Preliminary findings from the World Elder Abuse Environmental Scan conducted by the International Network for the Prevention of Elder Abuse (INPEA) suggest that elder abuse laws vary by country, and sometimes even within countries (Podneiks *et al.* 2006). For example, respondents from India, Lebanon and Nigeria – all developing countries – could identify no laws protecting older people from abuse. However, those from Canada, Sweden and the UK – developed countries – could identify national or local laws for that purpose. Elder abuse laws also are changing. In 2005 alone over a quarter of American states amended their existing adult protective services laws, typically to strengthen criminal penalties or to enhance staffing, training or practice (Steigel and Klem 2006).

Services to address elder abuse may include emergency shelters, discretionary funds, legal assistance, case management, counselling, respite and such supportive services as meals programmes and telephone reassurance. Services vary by locale, but gaps and barriers are most evident in developing countries, where diminished resources adversely affect the formation and maintenance of a service response to elder abuse. Most research on elder abuse-related services suggests that they tend to target victims, like Willa. Little assistance is offered to perpetrators, like Jennifer or Edwina, although they are more likely to accept and benefit from it. Victims most accept and benefit from concrete or empowerment services, like medical care or support groups. Perpetrators must accept and benefit from education, training and counselling (e.g. Nahmiash and Reis 2000).

Advocacy is evident in the elder abuse networks formed to improve problem recognition and response through public awareness activities as well as policy and system change. These formal coalitions of individuals and organizations are scattered globally and found at every level. They include the INPEA with representation in all six world regions and national networks in countries like Japan, Canada and Korea. Local illustrations include those in Ohio (USA), which has perhaps the oldest continually operating networks – the Consortium Against Adult Abuse founded for the Greater Cleveland area in 1980 and the Ohio Coalition for Adult Protective Service founded for statewide action in 1984. Advocacy has been critical worldwide for insuring that Willa and her family, along with other victims and perpetrators, receive the response required to treat elder abuse and prevent reoccurrence of this problem that diminishes the quality of their lives and even has the potential effect of extinguishing those lives altogether.

3 'Gender symmetry' in domestic violence: a falsely-framed issue

Michael S. Kimmel

Introduction

In recent years, debate has erupted among activists and scholars about the nature of domestic violence, and especially the gender of the perpetrators. Feminists now confront a growing chorus who claim that women and men are victimized by domestic violence in roughly equal numbers (e.g. Straton 1994). There are more than 100 empirical studies or reports that suggest that rates of domestic violence are equivalent (e.g. Archer 2000). In the USA, numerous studies have found that women and men are equally likely to report to researchers that they have hit their partner during the preceding 12 months. In the UK, 4.2 per cent of women *and* men said that they had been physically assaulted by a partner during the previous 12 months (Tendler 1999).

Thus, activists for 'men's rights' have suggested that policy-oriented efforts for women have been misplaced, because they focus entirely on women as the victims of domestic violence. Instead of the picture painted by feminist researchers and activists, these activists argue that, as one writer put it, 'men are the victims of domestic violence at least as often as women' (Brott 1994). Domestic violence, they argue, exhibits *gender symmetry* and an equal number of women and men are its victims.

While such activists draw our attention to the often-ignored problem of men as victims of domestic violence, their efforts are also often motivated by a desire to undermine or dismantle those initiatives that administer to women victims. To many, compassion seems to be a zero-sum game, and while we show any compassion for women who are the victims of domestic violence, we will never address the male victims.

These apparent discrepancies between claims of gender symmetry and claims of dramatic asymmetry have led to significant confusion among policy-makers and the general public. Is domestic violence a 'women's' issue, or do equivalent rates indicate that the 'problem' of domestic violence is one shared by women and men equally, or even not a problem at all? In this chapter, I examine the claims of gender symmetry in domestic violence. I review existing sources of data on domestic violence and suggest why the rates of such violence appear so varied. I offer some ways to understand and reconcile these discordant data, so that both scholars and policy-makers alike may acknowledge the male victims of domestic violence within the larger context of domestic violence. I argue that claims about gender symmetry exclude a thorough analysis of gender and how gender identity and ideology – the cultural definitions of masculinity and femininity – may help to clarify these seemingly discordant claims.

The idea of gender symmetry

Reports of gender symmetry run counter to existing stereotypes of male-female relationships, and thus often have the headline-grabbing value of a 'man bites dog' story. One review of the literature (Fiebert 1997) found 79 empirical studies and 16 reviews of literature that demonstrated gender symmetry among couples. In a more recent meta-analytic review of this literature, Archer (2000) looked at 82 studies that found gender symmetry.

These empirical studies raise troubling questions, but the questions they themselves *ask* are far from clear. For example, does gender symmetry mean that women hit women *as often* as men hit women? Or does it mean that an equal *number* of men and women hit each other? Does symmetry refer to men's and women's *motivations* for such violence, or does it mean that the *consequences* of it are symmetrical? These questions are often lumped together in reviews of literature and 'meta-analyses' which review existing data sets.

The two large-scale reviews of literature that demonstrate gender symmetry are useful indicators of the types of evidence offered and the arguments made by their proponents (Fiebert 1997; Archer 2000). Of the 79 empirical articles that Fiebert reviews, 55 used the same empirical measure of 'family conflict', the Conflict Tactics Scale (CTS), as the sole measure of domestic violence. This scale was also used in 76 out of the 82 studies that Archer examined. In addition, 28 of those studies noted by Fiebert discussed samples composed entirely of young people – college students, high-school students or dating couples under 30 – and not married couples. (These two groups overlap somewhat, as 13 of those studies of young, dating couples also used the CTS.) I discuss the CTS below, and also examine some of the reasons why studies of college-age and dating couples yield different rates of violence and aggression than studies of somewhat older married couples.

Of the nine studies in Fiebert's survey that used neither the CTS nor sampled only young, dating, unmarried couples, two were based on people's perceptions of violence, but offered no data about violence itself, while another was based on reports of witnessing violence that contained no useful data. One looked at spousal homicide that did not include homicides by ex-spouses (to which I shall also give some attention). Another, of young people, had no comparisons by gender (Mihalic and Elliot 1997). And one was based on violence in American comic strips in 1950 (Saenger 1963).

Of the three remaining studies, two were based on clinical samples undertaken by my colleagues (e.g. Tyree and Malone 1991). While these studies suggest that couples that seek clinical therapeutic help have high rates of mutual aggression, O'Leary has insisted that the age of the individuals dramatically changes the data (O'Leary 1999, 2000), and that clinical samples cannot necessarily be generalized to a national population. Even so, as Fiebert (1997) notes, the study by Tyree and Malone (1991) found that women's violence was a result of a 'desire to improve contact with partners', by which they meant that the women tended to slap or push their partner in order to get him to pay attention, but not to hurt him.

It would appear, therefore, that Gonzalez's unpublished masters thesis (1997), written apparently under Fiebert's supervision, is the only quantitative survey that purports to find gender symmetry without relying on the CTS. While it may be of interest that most of the women said their violence was a 'spontaneous reaction to frustration', Gonzalez did not survey males nor administer to a sample of males the same questionnaire, and thus one can make *no inferences whatever* about gender symmetry.

Fiebert's (1997) scholarly annotated bibliography thus turns out to be far more of an ideological polemic than a serious scholarly undertaking. But since it has become a touchstone for those who support a gender symmetry analysis, it is important to consider the studies on which it is based. Despite the vituperative ideological debates, there are serious and credible social science researchers who have used reliable social science and found gender symmetry. Below, I examine (1) the CTS, and especially what it measures and what it does not measure; and, (2) the effects of age and marital status on domestic violence.

Those who insist on gender symmetry must also account for two statistical anomalies. First, there is the dramatic disproportion of women in shelters and hospital emergency care facilities. Why is it that when we begin our analysis at the end point of the domestic violence experience – when we examine the serious injuries that often are its consequence – the rates are so dramatically asymmetrical? Second, claims of gender symmetry in marital violence must be squared with the empirical certainty that in every single other arena of social life, men are far more dispropor-tionately likely to use violence than women. Why are women so much more violent in the home that their rates approach, or even exceed, those of men, while in every other non-domestic arena men's rates of violence are about nine times those of women (on rates of violence generally, see Kimmel 2000).

How do we know what we know? Types of data

Our understanding of domestic violence has relied on a wide variety of evidence, from clinical observations to narrative accounts of victims and batterers, and the experiences of advocates, plus qualitative data gleaned from police and medical sources. Large-scale surveys have fallen into two distinct types (e.g. Bachman 2000; see also Walby 1999). These are 'crime victimization studies', which rely on large-scale aggregate data on crime victimization, and 'family conflict studies' which measure the prevalence of aggression between married or cohabiting couples. These two sources of data find very different rates of domestic violence – in part because they are measuring two different things.

Crime victimization studies

Data about crime victimization are gathered from a variety of sources. Some are obtained from household surveys, such as the National Violence Against Women in America Survey (NVAW), sponsored by the National Institute of Justice and the Centers for Disease Control and Prevention (e.g. Tjaden and Thoennes 1998, 2000a, 2000b) and the National Crime Victimization Study (NCVS) in which 60,000 households are surveyed annually. Police data typically relies on calls to domestic violence hotlines or calls to police departments.

Crime victimization studies have large sample sizes, in part because they are funded by national, state and local government agencies. They include a wide range of assaults, including sexual assault, in their samples. They ask not only about assaults by a current partner (spouse or cohabiting partner) but also by an ex-spouse or ex-partner. But they ask only about those events that the person experiences – or even reports to municipal authorities – as a crime, and therefore miss those events that are neither perceived as nor reported as crimes. They also find significantly lower rates of domestic violence than family conflict studies, ranging from less than 1 per cent to about 1.1 per cent of all couples. These lower rates of violence may be explained by the fact that crime victimization studies include all individuals in a household over age 12, even though rates of domestic assault are far lower for women over 65 and between 12 and 18. All family members are interviewed, which also may prevent some respondents from disclosing incidents of violence out of fear of retaliation (e.g. DeKeseredy 2000).

These studies uniformly find dramatic gender asymmetry in rates of domestic violence. The NCVS found females reported six times as many incidents of violence by an intimate as men did in 1992 and 1993 (Bachman and Saltzman 1995). The NVAW found that, in 1998, men physically assaulted their partners at three times the rate at which women assaulted theirs (Tjaden and Thoennes 2000b: 151).

Crime victimization studies further find that domestic violence increases in severity over time, so that earlier 'moderate' violence is likely to be followed by more severe violence later (Johnson and Ferraro 2000). This emerges also in discussions of spousal homicide, where significant numbers of women killed by their spouses or ex-spouses were also earlier victims of violence (e.g. Dugan *et al.* 1999). In sum, crime victimization studies typically find that domestic violence is rare, serious, escalates over time, and is primarily perpetrated by men.

Family conflict studies

By contrast, family conflict studies are based on smaller-scale nationally representative household surveys such as The National Family Violence Survey (Straus and Gelles 1990a) or the National Survey of Families and Households in the USA, and the British and Canadian national surveys. These surveys interview respondents once and ask only one partner of a cohabiting couple (over 18) about their experiences with various methods of expressing conflict in the family. Other survey evidence comes from smaller-scale surveys of college students or dating couples, and some draw from clinical samples of couples seeking marital therapy. Still other data are drawn from convenience samples of people who responded to advertisements for subjects placed in newspapers and magazines. According to Fiebert (1997), the total number of respondents for *all* studies that find gender symmetry is slightly more than 66,000; that is, slightly more than the single annual number of one of the crime victimization studies in any one year.

These surveys both expand and contract the types of questions asked to the respondents compared to crime victimization studies. On the one hand, they ask about all the possible experiences of physical violence, including those that are not especially serious or severe and that do not result in injury; that is, those that might not be reported, or even considered a crime. On the other hand, they ask questions only about cohabiting couples (and therefore exclude assaults by ex-spouses or ex-partners), and exclude sexual assault, embedding domestic violence within a context of 'family conflict'. So, for example, the CTS asks respondents about what happens 'when they disagree, get annoyed with the other person, or just have spats or fights because they're in a bad mood or tired or for some other reason' (Straus 1997: 217).

Family conflict studies tend to find much higher general rates of domestic violence than crime victimization studies – typically about 16 per cent of all couples report some form of domestic violence (Straus 1990a). One summary of 21 of the approximately 120 studies that have explored family conflict found that about a third of men and two-fifths of women indicated using violence in their marriages (Sugarman and Hotaling 1989). As surprising as it may be to see high levels of violence, the most surprising finding has been the gender symmetry in the use of violence to try to resolve family conflicts.

These studies also find much lower rates of injury from domestic violence, typically about 3 per cent (Stets and Straus 1990). When 'minor' forms of injury (such as slapping, pushing and grabbing) are excluded from the data, the yearly incidence falls significantly, from 16 per cent to around 6 per cent of all couples (Straus and Gelles 1986). They also find that violence is *unlikely* to escalate over time (e.g. Johnson and Ferraro 2000).

How are such different conclusions to be reconciled? A first step is to make the sources of data similar and make sure they are asking similar questions and comparing the same sorts of events. Crime victimization studies rely on two types of data – surveys of national probability samples that are representative of the population at large and 'clinical' samples (i.e. calls to police and shelters and visits to emergency rooms). Family conflict studies are based on three sources of data: nationally representative probability samples; clinical samples; and convenience samples based on responses to advertisements.

Nationally representative probability samples are the only sources of data that are consistently reliable and generalizable. While clinical samples may have important therapeutic utility, especially in treatment modalities, they are relatively easy to dismiss as adequate empirical surveys since they do not offer control groups from the non-clinical population and therefore offer no grounds whatever for generalizability.

Therefore, I shall omit from further discussion both types of clinical data – police, shelter and emergency room data, and data drawn from marital therapy cases.

Recruitment via advertisements in newspapers and magazines offers related problems of the representativeness of the sample and therefore undermines efforts at generalizability. Often people who respond to such advertisements do so because they have a 'stake' in the issue, and feel that they want to contribute to it somehow. The representativeness of such people to the general population is unclear at best.[1]

Virtually all the 'family conflict' surveys rely on CTS and CTS2, a survey measure developed by New Hampshire sociologist Murray Straus and his collaborators, so we must examine that scale a bit further. The CTS is enormously useful, especially for eliciting the quotidian, commonplace acceptance of violence as a means to 'communicate'. Let's begin our discussion where the CTS begins. Here is the opening paragraph to the survey as administered (Straus 1990a: 33):

> No matter how well a couple gets along, there are times when they disagree, get annoyed with the other person, or just have spats or fights because they're in a bad mood or tired or for some other reason. They also use many different ways of trying to settle their differences. I'm going to read some things that you and your (spouse/partner) might do when you have an argument. I would like you to tell me how many times ... in the past 12 months you ...

Such a framing assumes that domestic violence is the result of an argument, that it has more to do with being tired or in a bad mood than it does with an effort to control another person (for critiques of the CTS and CTS2 generally, see DeKeseredy and Schwartz 1998a, 1998b, 1998c).

The CTS asks about frequency, although only for one year. Asking how often in the past year either spouse or partner hit the other may capture some version of reality, but does not capture an ongoing systematic pattern of abuse and violence over many years. This is akin to the difference between watching a single frame of a movie and the movie itself.

Bringing gender into the equation

What is missing, oddly, from claims of gender symmetry is an analysis of gender. By this I mean more than simply a tallying up of which biological sex is more likely to be perpetrator or victim, and an analysis that explicitly underscores the ways in which gender identities and gender ideologies are embodied and enacted by women and men. Examining domestic violence through a gender lens helps clarify several issues.

For example, both women and men tend to see their use of violence as gender *non*-conforming, but the consequences of this non-conformity might lead women and men to estimate their use of violence and their victimization quite differently. Women are socialized *not* to use violence and, as a result, they would tend to remember every transgression. As Dobash *et al.* (1998: 405) write: 'women may be more likely to remember their own aggression because it is deemed less appropriate and less acceptable than for men and thus takes on the more memorable quality of a forbidden act or one that is out of character'.

Men however, might find it emasculating to reveal that their assumed control over 'their women' is so tenuous that they are forced to use violence to 'keep her in line'. They may find it difficult to admit that they cannot 'handle their wives'. *Thus, men might underestimate their violence and women might tend to overestimate theirs.*

What's more, in addition to overestimating their own violence, women may also tend to *underestimate* their partner's violence given the norms of domestic life, which frequently find women discounting, downplaying or normalizing their partner's violent behaviour, or even excusing it since they 'deserved' it. By the same token, in addition to underestimating their own violence, men may *overestimate* their partner's violence. American men, at least, believe violence is legitimate if used as retaliation for violence already committed (e.g. Kimmel 1996). Initiating violence is never legitimate according to the norms of traditional masculinity in America but retaliating against a perceived injustice with violence is always legitimate. *As a result, men will tend to overestimate their victimization and women will tend to underestimate theirs* (e.g. Bowker 1998).

Such a gendering of memory would have enormous consequences in a survey that asks only one partner to recall accurately how much they and their spouse used various 'conflict-resolution' techniques.

The causes and consequences of violence

A final substantive critique of the CTS is that it does not measure the consequences of physical assault (such as physical or emotional injury), or the causes of the assault (such as the desire to dominate). Straus (1997) responds that assessing causes and consequences may be interesting, but it is not a necessary part of the picture. He scolds his critics, saying that to fault his research on this question 'is akin to thinking that a spelling test is inadequate because it does not measure why a child spells badly, or does not measure possible consequences of poor spelling, such as low self-esteem or low evaluations by employers' (1997: 218).

Were Straus not a credible social scientist, one might suspect the reply to be disingenuous. As such, it is simply inadequate. It is more akin to a teacher who doesn't look at how far off the spelling mistakes are or whether there is a pattern in the mistakes that might point to a physiological problem like dyslexia or some other learning disability, as compared to academic laziness, and thus leaves the learning problem untouched and misdirects funds away from remediation towards punitive after-school programmes for lazy students. And even that analogy is imperfect because, unlike spelling, domestic violence is not about what happens to the perpetrator (the poor speller) but to someone else. Can one imagine any other issue in which causes and consequences are thought to be irrelevant?

The consequences of violence raise perhaps the most telling criticism of the CTS – a criticism not, incidentally, that Straus and his more thoughtful collaborators share, as I will discuss below. The CTS lumps together many different forms of violence, so that a single slap may be equated with a more intensive assault. In the

NVAW, for example, lifetime percentages of persons physically assaulted by an intimate partner found dramatic differences in some types of assault, but not others. For example, just under 1 per cent of men and women (0.9 per cent of women and 0.8 per cent of men) said their attacker used a knife in the attack, but 3.5 per cent of women and only 0.4 per cent of men said their partner threatened to use a gun; and 0.7 per cent of women and 0.1 per cent of men said their spouse actually did use a gun (Tjaden and Thoennes 1998: 7).

Even more telling are the gender disparities in serious physical injuries without weapons. For example, in a British study that found equal rates of reporting victimization violence, there were no injuries at all reported in the 59 per cent of incidents that involved pushing, shoving and grabbing (these are the behaviours more typically reported as being committed by women than by men). In the NVAW (a crime victimization-type study), half the number of men than women (4.4 per cent of men and 8.1 per cent of women) said their partner threw something at them, and three times as many women (18.1 per cent of women against 5.4 per cent of men) said their partner pushed, grabbed or shoved them, or that their partner slapped or hit them (16.0 per cent of women against 5.5 per cent of men). But over ten times as many women (8.5 per cent of women against 0.6 per cent of men) reported that their partner 'beat them up' (Tjaden and Thoennes 1998: 7).

The consequences of violence range from minor to fatal, and these are significant in understanding domestic violence in general and its gendered patterns. Far more men than women kill their spouses (and, of course, 'couples' in which one spouse killed the other could not participate in the CTS studies since both partners must be cohabiting at the time of the study). Rates of homicides of ex-spouses are even more gender asymmetrical. According to the FBI, female victims represented about 70 per cent of all intimate homicide victims in the USA during 1996 (see Bachman 2000). About a third of all female homicide victims in the USA were killed by an intimate compared with 4 per cent of male victims in 1990 (e.g. Bachman and Saltzman 1995).

Gender symmetry tends to be clustered entirely at the lower end of violence (Dobash *et al.* 1998: 382). According to some data, women are six times more likely to require medical care for injuries sustained by family violence (e.g. Stets and Straus 1990). Straus also reports that in family conflict studies the injury rate for assaults by men is about seven times greater than that for assaults by women (Stets and Straus 1990). This dramatic difference in rates of injury, found in both types of study, leads Straus (1997: 219), the researcher who is most often cited by those claiming gender symmetry, to write that:

> although women may assault their partners at approximately the same rate as men, because of the greater physical, financial, and emotional injury suffered by women, they are the predominant victims. Consequently, the first priority in services for victims and in prevention and control must continue to be directed toward assaults by husbands.

These different rates of injury are so pronounced that when injury data has been obtained in studies using the CTS, the rate of violence drops to that predicted by the crime victimization studies, and the gender asymmetry of such studies is also revealed (see Straus 1997). Both husbands and wives may be said to be 'aggressive' but many more husbands are 'violent' (Frude 1994: 153).

What the CTS leaves out

It is not only important to understand what the CTS measures, but to make explicit what it does *not* measure. First, the CTS does not include sexual assault. This is crucial, because a significant number of spousal assaults are sexual. The NVAW found that 7.7 per cent of all female respondents had been raped by an intimate partner at some point in their lifetime.

Second, the CTS only includes violence by a *current* spouse or cohabiting partner. It does not include violence by an ex-spouse or partner. Crime victimization studies do include such assaults. This is important because crimes by former spouses comprise a significant number of domestic assaults. It may be that when women exit a relationship, they have no 'need' for violence, while men tend to continue, or even escalate, their use of violence when women leave. The NCVS found that rates of intimate-perpetrated violence for separated women are over eight times higher than rates for married women (Bachman and Salzman 1995). It may be true that these types of assault are somewhat over-represented in crime victimization studies because people who are assaulted by a former spouse would be more likely to report it as a crime, since the former spouse clearly had no 'right' to aggress against the victim, and so it would clearly be seen as a crime and more likely to be reported. But to ignore these data would so skew any study and make it unreliable.

Failure to include sexual assault and assaults by ex-spouses or ex-partners compounds the problem that the CTS does not adequately measure rates of serious injury from domestic violence.[2] The NVAW found that 72.6 per cent of rape victims and 66.6 per cent of physical assault victims sustained injuries such as a scratch, bruise or welt, and that 14.1 per cent of rape victims and 12.2 per cent of physical assault victims sustained a broken bone or dislocated joint. Rape victims were far more likely to sustain an internal injury (5.8 per cent against 0.8 per cent), or a chipped or broken tooth (3.3 against 1.8 per cent). On the other hand, physical assault victims were more likely to sustain a laceration or knife wound (16.9 per cent against 6.2 per cent), a head or spinal cord injury (10.1 per cent against 6.6 per cent), and burns and bullet wounds (0.7 per cent against 1.8 per cent respectively; rape rates too low to estimate) (Tjaden and Thoennes 1998: 9).

Violence by ex-husbands also tends to be more serious. For example, the risk of spousal homicide goes up by about 50 per cent for women who leave abusive husbands. (This may also help explain the 'rationality' of the decision by women to stay in abusive relationships). Men may kill their ex-wives because their ex-wives left them; women may kill their ex-husbands because they believe that they will otherwise kill them for leaving. In both cases, then, the larger context for *both* women's and men's violence is men's violence. One study of spousal homicide (Barnard *et al.*1982) found that over half of all defendants were separated from their victims at the time they were accused of committing the murder.

Understanding aggression in domestic life

These two different types of study, crime victimization and family conflict, rely on two different theoretical perspectives and two different sources of data. They measure two different phenomena based on different conceptualizations of aggression in families. But they can be reconciled, conceptually and methodologically.

If one is interested in the level of aggression in family conflict, i.e. the likelihood of any type of aggression occurring when a couple has an argument, then the CTS may be somewhat useful. I say 'somewhat' because the utility of the CTS is limited, as previously noted, by the fact that it fails to take into account sexual assault and also assault by an ex-spouse. But it does enable us to see the overall amount of a particular kind of violence in families, what we might call *expressive* violence – the way a person might express anger, frustration or loss of control. If, however, one were interested in the ways in which one partner uses violence, not expressively but *instrumentally*, to achieve some end of control, injury or terror, then the CTS would be a poor measure. In this context crime victimization surveys will be more valuable because they measure serious injury, and include sexual assault and assaults by ex-spouses in their purview. These surveys may capture those family conflicts where the level of violence escalates beyond a mere 'conflict tactic' to something far more ominous and perhaps lethal.

Some violence by men against women is motivated not by the desire to express anger, frustration or some other immediate emotion during a family conflict, but by the desire to control. However, the use of violence may indicate not the experience of control but the experience of loss of control: 'Violence is a part of a system of domination ... but it is at the same time a measure of its imperfection' (Connell 1995: 84).

In that sense, we might say that many men who assault their partners or ex-partners indicate they are using violence when they fear that their control is breaking down, that their ability to control their partners by the implicit threat of violence is compromised, and they feel compelled to use explicit violence to 'restore' that control. Thus, men see their violence as restorative and retaliatory.[3] For example, in an earlier study, Dobash and Dobash (1979) found three antecedents of men's use of violence: sexual jealousy; perception that a woman has failed to perform a household task such as cleaning or preparing a hot meal; and a woman challenging the man's authority on financial matters. All of these are indicators of a breakdown of expected dominance and control.

This understanding of control-motivated, instrumental violence is particularly important in our understanding of claims of gender symmetry. For one thing, men's control over women has clearly broken down when their spouses have left them; thus, measures of physical assault that do not include assaults by ex-spouses will entirely miss these events. Second, breakdowns of men's control over women may be revealed not by physical assault, but by the woman's withholding or refusing of sexual intimacy. She may exert what limited power she may have by attempting to refuse sexual advances. Thus, measures that do not include sexual assaults among acts of aggression will be equally inadequate in assessing the problem.

Control-motivated instrumental violence is experienced by men not as an expression of their power but as an instance of its collapse. Men may feel entitled to experience that control over women, but at the moments when they become violent they do not feel that control. Masculinity, in that sense, has already been compromised: violence is a method to restore one's manhood and domestic inequality at the same time (Kimmel 1994, 1996, 2000). Such control-motivated, instrumental violence is more likely to escalate over time, less likely to be mutual and more likely to involve serious injury. This difference between expressive and instrumental violence is not simply a difference in purpose, but also in frequency, severity and initiation. It addresses whether the violence is part of a systematic pattern of control and fear, or an isolated expression of frustration or anger. These two types of violence are so different that Johnson (1995) and Johnson and Ferraro (2000) have come to call instrumental violence 'intimate terrorism' (IT) and the types of expressive violence measured by the CTS as 'common couple violence' (CCV).

Social control-motivated abuse can be illustrated in another form of domestic violence: stalking. Control-motivated abuse refers to intentionally inflicted physically or psychologically painful or hurtful acts (or threats) by one partner as a means of compelling or constraining the conduct, dress or demeanor of the other (Ellis and Stuckless 1996). Rates of stalking by an intimate, more prevalent than previously thought, can best be understood as an effort to restore control or dominance after the partner has left. Stalking exhibits dramatic gender asymmetry: nearly 5 per cent of American women and about half of one per cent (0.6 per cent) of men report being stalked by a current or former intimate partner at some time in their life (Tjaden and Thoennes 2000a).

Claims about the gender symmetry of 'conflict-motivated' expressive violence must be complemented with claims about the dramatic gender *asymmetry* in control-motivated instrumental violence. When these two are factored together, it is clear that women and men may express their anger or frustration during an argument more equally than we earlier thought. This, however, is by no means fully symmetrical because, as we know, the CTS leaves out two of the dominant forms of expressive conflict-motivated aggression – sexual assault and assault by an ex-spouse. And when control-motivated instrumental violence is added – the violence that more typically results in serious injury, is more systematic and is independent of specific 'conflict' situations – the gender asymmetry is clear (Johnson 2000).

Concerns about women's violence towards men

Despite the evidence that gender symmetry is largely a myth, we should nonetheless be concerned about women's violence for a variety of reasons. For one thing, compassion for victims of violence is not a zero-sum game; reasonable people would naturally want to extend compassion, support and interventions to all victims of violence. (It is an indication of the political intentions of those who argue for gender symmetry that they never question the levels of violence against women, and only assert that the level of violence against men is equivalent. Their solution, though, is not *more* funding for domestic violence research and intervention, but to *decrease* the amount of funding that women receive – even though they never challenge the levels of violence against women.)

Second, acknowledging women's capacity for intimate violence will illuminate the gender symmetry in intimate violence among gay male and lesbian couples. According to the NVAW, slightly more than 11 per cent of women living with a same-sex partner report being raped, physically assaulted or stalked by a female cohabitant (compared with 30.4 per cent of women with a live-in male partner). About 15 per cent of men living with a male live-in partner report having experienced violence (compared with 7.7 per cent of men with female live-in partners) (Tjaden and Thoennes 2000b).

Third, perhaps ironically, examining women's violence can better illuminate the dynamics of men's aggression against women. Since women's violence is often retaliatory or committed in self-defence, it may help to expose some of the ways men use violence to control women, and women's perceived lack of options except 'fighting back'.

Fourth, acknowledging assaults by women is important, Straus (1997: 210) writes, because they 'put women in danger of much more severe retaliation by men'. In an interview for the *Calgary Herald*, Straus elaborated that since women generally suffer greater fear and more injuries, 'when she slaps, she sets the stage for him to hit her. The safety of women alone demands we make a big deal of women hitting men' (Slobodian 2000).

Finally, men actually benefit from efforts to reduce their violence against women. It turns out that efforts to protect women in the USA have had the effect of reducing the homicide rate of men by their partners by almost 70 per cent over the past 24 years. According to James Alan Fox, Professor of Criminal Justice at Northeastern University, homicides by women of their spouses, ex-spouses or boyfriends have steadily declined from 1357 in 1976 to 424 in 1999 (Elsner 2001). Fox attributes this decline to the availability of alternatives for battered women: 'We have given women alternatives, including hotlines, shelters, counseling and restraining orders. Because more battered women have escape routes, fewer wife batterers are being killed', Fox told reporters (Elsner 2001). A 1999 study by the National Consortium on Violence Research found that the greater availability of hotlines and other resources for battered women, the greater the decline in homicide of their male partners (the study found that 80 per cent of these male domestic homicide victims had abused their partners and that nearly two-thirds of female murder victims had been abused before they were killed). It turns out that those very initiatives that have greatly benefited women (shelters, hotlines and the like) save *men's* lives as well.

Towards an inclusive explanation of domestic violence

It is certainly possible and politically necessary to acknowledge that some women use violence as a tactic in family conflict, while also understanding that men tend to use violence more instrumentally to control women's lives. Further, these two types of aggression must also be embedded within the larger framework of gender inequality. Women's violence towards male partners certainly does exist, but it tends to be very different from that of men towards their female partners: it is far less injurious and less likely to be motivated by attempts to dominate or terrorize the partner (Kaufman Kantor and Jasinski 1998).

Coupled with studies of parental violence towards children, which routinely find that more than 90 per cent of parents aggress against their children, family conflict studies are useful in pointing out the ubiquity and the casualness with which violence structures our daily lives. Coupled with data about intimate partner homicide, rape and other forms of sexual assault, crime victimization data are useful in pointing out the ways in which men's domination over women requires the implicit threat, and often the explicit instrumental use of violence, to maintain that power.

Claims of gender symmetry are often made by those who do not understand the data: what the various studies measure and what they omit. Others make claims of gender symmetry based on disingenuous political motives, attempting to discredit women's suffering by offering abstract statistical equivalences that turn out to be chimerical. Gelles and Straus (1999) themselves understand the political misuses to which their work has been put, and strongly disavow those political efforts. In a summary of their work, they write:

> Perhaps the most controversial finding from our 1975 National Family Violence Survey was the report that a substantial number of women hit and beat their husbands. Since 1975 at least ten additional investigations have confirmed the fact that women hit and beat their husbands. *Unfortunately the data on wife-to-husband violence has been misreported, misinterpreted, and misunderstood.* Research uniformly shows that about as many women hit men as men hit women. However, those who report that husband abuse is as common as wife abuse overlook two important facts. First, the greater average size and strength of men and their greater aggressiveness means that a man's punch will probably produce more pain, injury, and harm than a punch by a woman. Second, nearly three-fourths of the violence committed by women is done in self-defense. While violence by women should not be dismissed, neither should it be overlooked or hidden. On occasion, legislators and spokespersons ... have used the data on violence by wives to minimize the need for services for battered women. *Such arguments do a great injustice to the victimization of women.*
>
> (*Gelles and Straus 1999: 424, emphasis added*)

And Gelles (2000) underscores this disingenuous political use of their work with this clear and unequivocal statement: 'it is categorically false to imply that there are the same number of "battered" men as battered women' (note how he even puts the word 'battered' in quotation marks when describing men). It is not surprising that credible researchers disavow the political ends to which their work is often put.

Despite the dramatic differences in frequency, severity and purpose of the violence, we should be compassionate towards *all* victims of domestic violence. There are some men who are battered by their female partners, and these men are no less deserving of compassion, understanding and intervention than are women who are battered. And male domestic violence victims deserve access to services and funding, just as female domestic violence victims do. They do not need to be half of all victims in order to deserve either sympathy or services.

But just as surely, compassion and adequate intervention strategies must explore the full range of domestic violence – the different rates of injury, the different types of violence, including sexual assault, and the likelihood of violence by an ex-spouse. Such strategies must also understand the differences between violence that is an expression of family conflict and violence that is instrumental to the control of one partner by the other.

Conclusions

In conclusion, with all the caveats and modifications I have suggested to the family conflict model, and especially the CTS as the standard of measurement, I would argue that violence as an expression of family conflict is somewhat less than symmetrical, but does include a significant percentage of women. I would hypothesize that, including assaults and homicides by ex-spouses, spousal homicide and sexual assault, the gendered ratio of male-perpetrated violence to female-perpetrated violence is about 4:1.[4] On the other hand, violence that is instrumental in the maintenance of control – the more systematic, persistent and injurious type of violence – is overwhelmingly perpetuated by men, with rates captured best by crime victimization studies. Over 90 per cent of this violence is perpetuated by men.

When sexual violence and violence by an ex-spouse are considered, the evidence is overwhelming that gender *asymmetry* in domestic violence remains in full effect. Men *are* more violent than women, both inside the home and in the public sphere. The home is not a refuge from violence, nor is it a site where gender differences in the public sphere are somehow magically reversed. As citizens, we need to be concerned about all victims of violence. And we must also be aware that the perpetrators of that violence – both in public and in private, at home or on the street, and whether the victim is male or female – are overwhelmingly men.

Acknowledgements

An earlier version of this chapter was commissioned by the Irish Department of Education and Health and published in *Violence Against Women*. Subsequent debates in Ireland led to two pieces in *The Irish Times* (Kimmel 2001, 2002a). I am grateful to Harry Ferguson for comments and support. I am also grateful to two anonymous reviewers for their helpful feedback and to Sue Osthoff, Andrea Bible, Shamita Das Dasgupta, Aisha Baruni and Claire Renzetti for their careful readings and judicious editing.

Notes

1   In the best of these studies, O'Leary and his colleagues found that about 31 per cent of the men and 44 per cent of the women indicated that they had engaged in some aggression to their partners in the year before they were

married. A year after the marriage, rates had dropped for both groups and 27 per cent of the men and 36 per cent of the women indicated they had aggressed. Thirty months into the marriage the rates for the previous year were 25 per cent of the men and 32 per cent of the women (O'Leary *et al.* 1989: 264).

2 The CTS-2 does include a measure of sexual coercion, which seems to me a pretty cogent acknowledgement that it must be included in all understandings of gender symmetry.

3 It must be noted, of course, that the 'retaliation' is more often for a *perceived* injury or slight than any real injury (e.g. Beneke 1982).

4 As this is a conjecture based on estimates, it remains an empirical question to coordinate the synthesis of these two approaches.

4 Female victims of violence

*Marguerite L. Baty, Jeanne L. Alhusen,
Jacquelyn C. Campbell and Phyllis W. Sharps*

Introduction

Intimate partner violence (IPV) is a universal phenomenon existing in most countries, occurring across all demographic, ethnic, cultural and economic lines. Abused
women are more likely than their non-abused counterparts to experience negative
physical and psychological health symptoms, including stress-related and chronic
illnesses (Campbell *et al.* 2002a; Coker *et al.* 2002a). Therefore, health care professionals play an important role in identifying and caring for women with a current or past
history of abuse. However, recognition of IPV and its associated health outcomes is
challenging. The complex nature of such abuse requires understanding, and this
chapter provides a foundation for addressing IPV's impact. Specifically, an overview of
related epidemiology will be discussed, and IPV's bearing on women's health, both
physically and psychologically, will be addressed at length.

We use the term IPV, although other terms have been used interchangeably in the
literature, such as 'domestic violence', 'domestic abuse', 'spousal abuse' and 'battering'. We use a definition of IPV from the US National Center for Inquiry Prevention
and Control, a department within the Centers for Disease Control and Prevention
(CDC) (paraphrased): 'physical and/or sexual assault or threats of assault against a
married, cohabitating, or dating current or estranged intimate partner by the other
partner, including emotional abuse and controlling behaviors in a relationship where
there has been prior physical and/or sexual assault' (Saltzman *et al.*1999). Although
this definition applies to same-sex partners and women abusing male partners as well,
the primary focus of this chapter is women experiencing abuse from their intimate
male partners, since that is the largest relationship category of IPV and where most of
the research to date has concentrated, especially in terms of health outcomes.

Epidemiology

An estimated one in three women globally has experienced some kind of sexual,
physical or psychological assault, most often inflicted by an intimate partner (UNFPA

2000). In a recent, multi-country study, women in ten different countries shared their experiences of violence through a population-based survey. Lifetime prevalence of physical IPV ranged from 13 per cent in Japan to 61 per cent in rural Peru, with most women reporting between 23 and 49 per cent. Lifetime prevalence of sexual IPV ranged between 10 and 50 per cent (Garcia-Moreno *et al.* 2006). The United States' National Violence Against Women (NVAW) study indicated the following lifetime prevalence for assault by an intimate partner: 22.1 per cent for physical assault and 7.7 per cent for rape (Tjaden and Thoennes 2000a, 2000b), with past year prevalence of 1.5 per cent. A more recent population-based study of IPV among women in 12 major US cities found a prevalence of 9.8 per cent in the past two years (Walton-Moss *et al.* 2005). Women participating in a recent British crime survey reported 26 per cent lifetime prevalence and a 4.2 per cent past year prevalence of physical and non-physical IPV (Mirrlees-Black 1999). A New Zealand population-based study recorded a lifetime prevalence of IPV among women of 33 per cent in an urban setting and 39 per cent in a rural area (Fanslow and Robinson 2004). An Australian national survey reported 42 per cent lifetime prevalence among women, with 12 per cent reporting violence in their current relationship (Mulroney 2003). Abuse prevalence during pregnancy ranges from 3.4 to 11 per cent in industrialized countries (Mezey *et al.* 2001; Johnson *et al.* 2003) and from 3.8 to 31.7 per cent in developing countries (Garcia-Moreno *et al.* 2006).

Precise estimates of actual incidents of IPV are difficult. Even so, research estimates that nearly 5.3 million incidents of IPV occur per year in the USA, affecting 3 million women annually (Tjaden and Thoennes 2000a, 2000b; Chang *et al.* 2005). Both males and females can experience IPV, although 83 per cent of victims are female (United States Department of Justice 2005). Partners in same-sex relationships can also experience IPV, but men having sex with men are at greater risk than females in same-sex relationships (Tjaden and Thoennes 2000a, 2000b; Halpern *et al.* 2004).

Although both men and women can be victims of IPV, physical violence against females in heterosexual relationships tends to be most severe, placing them most at risk of being killed by their partners. In the UK between 1999 and 2000, 37 per cent of female murder victims were killed by an intimate partner, compared to 6 per cent of male murder victims (Home Office 2000; Aldridge and Browne 2003). In the USA, between 1976 and 2005, 30 per cent of femicides were committed by an intimate partner, but only 5 per cent of men who were murdered were IPV-related cases (Fox and Zawitz 2007).

A woman experiencing IPV will often present to a health care professional with a chief complaint other than abuse, although IPV may be underlying her symptoms and concerns. Recent research indicates high levels of both past year and lifetime prevalence for women presenting to health care settings. In hospital emergency departments, female clients report IPV lifetime prevalence of 37 to 50 per cent and past year prevalence of 15 to 18 per cent (Ernst and Weiss 2002; El-Bassel *et al.* 2003). Women attending primary care clinics have IPV lifetime prevalence of 37 to 50 per cent and past year prevalence of 8 to 29 per cent (Bauer *et al.* 2000a; Hegarty and Bush 2002). Women seeking obstetric and gynecologic services have a 6 to 21 per cent prevalence of IPV during pregnancy and 13 to 21 per cent prevalence post-partum (Campbell *et al.* 2000; Harrykisson *et al.* 2002). New Zealand women experiencing IPV were twice as likely to have visited a health care professional in recent weeks as non-abused women (Fanslow and Robinson 2004). Additionally, 41 per cent of women killed by an intimate partner in the USA utilized health care agencies for injury, physical or mental health problems in the year prior to femicide (Sharps *et al.* 2001a).

Women who are abused by their partners battle stigma and fear of reprisal if they report such abuse to justice authorities. According to the US Department of Justice, women suffering from IPV were six times less likely to report it to authorities than those victimized by strangers, because they feared reprisal by their partners (Catalano 2006). The willingness of women to disclose abuse may result in reported statistics substantially understating the true magnitude of the problem.

Risk factors

Although no single factor is most predictive of IPV, certain factors can increase a woman's risk. Women of all demographic backgrounds can experience IPV. In the USA, ethnic minority groups including African Americans, Native Americans and Hispanics are at increased risk, at least for past year IPV (Tjaden and Thoennes 2000a). However, any bivariate difference among ethnic/racial groups in the USA in IPV risk usually disappears (e.g. Walton-Moss *et al.* 2005) or decreases substantially (Schafer *et al.* 1998) when education, income and/or employment is entered into multivariate analyses. Any remaining differential risk for ethnic minority women in the USA for lifetime versus past year IPV can be attributed to discrimination and lack of resources, making it more difficult for these women to escape violent relationships, rather than an inherent or cultural increase in the risk of IPV occurring in the first place. In Australia, Aboriginal women experience IPV at a rate ten times higher than non-Aboriginal women, and they are at a higher risk of femicide by their intimate partners, indicating they are at higher risk for severe abuse (Mulroney 2003). Native American women in the USA are also at higher risk for both IPV and intimate partner femicide. How much of the difference in risk can be attributed to differences in social, demographic and environmental factors and the women's willingness to disclose is not entirely clear. The historical and current trauma of colonization and oppression are undoubtedly factors (Atkinson 2002).

Socioeconomic status plays a role in IPV risk. Women living below the poverty line are at increased risk of IPV in the USA (Tjaden and Thoennes 2000a). In both industrialized and developing countries, economic dependence on the male partner, poverty, low levels of formal education and traditional gender norms suggesting submissiveness of women were identified as risk factors for IPV (Tjaden and Thoennes 2000a; Garcia-Moreno *et al.* 2006). Cohabitation instead of formal marriage increases IPV risk as does ex-partner status, although the cross-sectional nature of most studies makes it impossible to tell if the dissolution precedes or follows the IPV (Walton-Moss *et al.* 2005).

Younger women are at higher risk of IPV, although it can occur at any point during a woman's life. Pregnancy and new motherhood can increase the risk of abuse in both industrialized and developing countries, as IPV can begin or worsen during the prenatal and post-partum periods (Garcia-Moreno *et al.* 2006). However, the most common pattern of IPV in the childbearing year in the USA is IPV before, during and after the pregnancy, or physical and/or sexual violence before and after pregnancy, but not during, although emotional abuse may even worsen during pregnancy. Young age, low education and income, minority race/ethnicity and unmarried status compound IPV risk both before and during pregnancy. Unwanted or unplanned pregnancies pose a threefold increase in risk of physical abuse over a planned pregnancy (Goodwin *et al.* 2000; Pallitto and O'Campo 2005).

A past history of physical and sexual child abuse is closely linked to IPV and unhealthy, unbalanced relationships as an adult. Women who experienced child abuse or witnessed IPV in their family of origin have been found to be two to three times as likely to be involved in current abusive relationships (Coker *et al.* 2000b, 2000c). Similarly, a woman with a history of violent relationships may be caught in a cycle of violence, re-engaging in that violent relationship or new relationships with violent partners.

Substance abuse, especially in the primary perpetrator, has been consistently linked to the occurrence, reoccurrence and severity of IPV as well as intimate partner homicide (Sharps *et al.* 2001b; Lipsky *et al.* 2005a). IPV risk increases tenfold for a woman with a substance-abusing male partner, and if both partners are substance abusers, IPV risk is 13 times that of a non-using couple (Coker *et al.* 2000a).

Femicide risk for an abused woman increases if she is leaving an abusive relationship, if the abuser is unemployed, if the abuser has access to a gun and/or has made previous threats with a gun, or if a child resides in the house who was not fathered by the abuser (Campbell *et al.* 2003). In addition, pregnancy is not protective against IPV-related femicides. McFarlane *et al.* (2002) found femicide to be a significant cause of maternal mortality. Among 437 cases of attempted/completed femicide, 5 per cent of victims were murdered during pregnancy. Those abused during pregnancy were at three times higher risk of femicide than those who were abused but not during pregnancy. Chang *et al.* (2005) found that 31 per cent of maternal injury deaths from 1991–9 were femicides with African American women most at risk.

Impact on health

The relationship between IPV and health is complex. Long-term negative health consequences of IPV for survivors, even after the abuse has ended, result in lower health status and lower quality of life as well as higher utilization of health care services (Tjaden and Thoennes 2000a). Health care professionals' awareness of the physical and mental health manifestations of IPV and willingness to screen for IPV in clients can contribute to early identification, possible intervention and potential prevention of more severe health consequences.

Physical health consequences of IPV

IPV has been linked to a host of immediate and long-term health outcomes including physical, sexual, reproductive, psychological and behavioural health consequences.

Many women experiencing IPV are injured by the abuser, and over a third seek medical treatment for their injuries (Bachman and Saltzman 1995; Sharps and Campbell 1999). Injuries to the head, face, neck, upper torso, breast or abdomen are common physical signs. Soft tissue injuries, including bruises and cuts, are the most common non-fatal injuries followed by strains/sprains, fractures/dislocations, head injuries, eye injuries, stab wounds and sexual assault (Mullerman *et al.* 1996; Bhandari *et al.* 2006). Abused women can also present with burns, dental injuries, gunshot wounds, spinal cord injuries and poisoning (Varvarro and Lasko 1993). Pain and decreased function related to the trauma are immediate health consequences.

The physical health effects of IPV may also manifest as less apparent, long-term health complications. Abused women are more likely to rate their physical and mental health as fair to poor (Campbell 2002b; Campbell et al. 2002; Coker et al. 2002a), as IPV can affect nearly every body system. Many abused women (10–44 per cent) experience choking, or incomplete strangulation, as well as blows to the head (Sharps et al. 2001a). This can result in loss of consciousness and potentially serious medical problems including neurological sequelae such as seizures, visual disturbances, headaches, fainting spells and chronic pain (McCauley et al. 1995). The exact mechanism of these conditions has not been established but could include repeated injury or stress, alterations in neurophysiology or a combination of the two (Campbell et al. 2002).

Self-reported gastrointestinal symptoms such as decreased or loss of appetite, eating disorders and diagnosed functional gastrointestinal disorders such as chronic irritable bowel syndrome, dyspepsia and chronic abdominal pain occur at rates higher than average among battered women (Campbell et al. 2002; Coker et al. 2000a). These disorders may begin during an acutely violent, stressful relationship, may be related to a history of childhood sexual abuse, or both (Leserman et al.1998).

Cardiovascular conditions, such as hypertension, angina and palpitations are highly correlated with sympathetic nervous system reactivity and are common complaints of IPV survivors (Coker et al. 2005). Stress hormones elevate blood pressure, increasing the blood flow to mount the 'fight or flight' reaction. Exposure to the chronic stress of IPV can increase alpha-adrenergic tone, thereby increasing peripheral vascular resistance and sustained hypertension.

Additional research has shown that the stress-related effects of IPV may lower the immune response in women. Battered women exhibit more signs, symptoms and illnesses associated with viral infections, such as colds and flu, as a result of long-term exposure to psychological stress (Leserman et al. 1998). Woods et al. (2005) found that abused women had higher circulating total leukocyte and lymphocyte counts than non-abused women. These findings suggest that a compromised immune system may place abused women at greater risk of increased morbidity.

Sexually transmitted infections

Generally, sexually transmitted infections (STIs) are associated with, but not limited to, poor birth outcomes, ectopic pregnancy, infertility and cervical cancer. STIs also represent an integral component of morbidity among women at highest risk of IPV (poor, minority women of childbearing age). As such, they warrant a comprehensive overview.

IPV is associated with up to a fourfold increased risk for STIs including human immunodeficiency virus (HIV), and several mechanisms may explain how exposure to IPV increases a woman's risk of STIs. At baseline, women are more biologically vulnerable than men to protracting STIs, including HIV. Additionally, STI risk may be mediated through the sexually coercive behaviours (discussed in great length in Chapter 6) of the abusive partner within the relationship (Wu, *et al.* 2003; Raj *et al.* 2004). Forced sex occurs in approximately 40 to 45 per cent of physically violent intimate relationships and is associated with a two- to tenfold increased risk of STIs as compared to physical abuse alone (Campbell and Soeken 1999b; Wingood *et al.* 2000). Forced sex may cause genital injuries which facilitate disease transmission (Liebschutz *et al.* 2000).

Indirectly, STI risk may also be exacerbated by the victim's psychological trauma of violence and abuse leading to impaired decision-making, substance abuse and greater risk-taking (Campbell and Lewandowski 1997). IPV also impairs open communication between partners regarding safe sex practices including condom negotiation, monogamy or HIV status disclosure. Kalichman *et al.* (1998) found that women with abusive partners were more likely to fear negotiating condom use, believing that insistence may be seen as implying unfaithfulness or untrustworthiness of either partner. Additionally, women feared being threatened or assaulted when requesting condom use. Conversely, a history or diagnosis of an STI may be an initiating factor for partner violence (Medley *et al.* 2004).

The increased risk for abused women of pre-invasive cervical neoplasia and invasive cervical cancer illustrates the direct and indirect mechanisms of transmission (Coker *et al.* 2000a). Repeated sexual assaults may cause cervical trauma that, when combined with the introduction of human papillomavirus (HPV), can initiate cervical carcinogenic process. Additionally, physical or sexual IPV may indirectly affect cervical cancer risk by increasing chronic stress, suppressing immune function and reducing the body's ability to mount an effective immune response to HPV infection (Hildesheim *et al.* 1997)

Reproductive health

IPV affects reproductive health outcomes as well. It affects a woman's reproductive life through her partner's use of forced sex and manipulation of contraception. Lack of contraception control can result in unintended pregnancy. Perhaps the most comprehensive research investigating the relationship between IPV and unintended pregnancy was based on Colombian data. The adjusted odds of an unintended pregnancy for a woman in the past five years were 41 per cent higher if she had ever been physically or sexually abused by her partner (Pallitto and O'Campo 2005).

IPV is also associated with considerable health issues during pregnancy. Low weight gain, anemia, infections, bleeding in the first and second trimesters and pre-term labour are positively correlated with IPV (Cokkinides *et al.*1999). Premature birth, uterine rupture, haemorrhage and maternal or foetal death are also associated with exposure to IPV (El Kady *et al.* 2005). Some studies have demonstrated a significant relationship between IPV and lower birth weights, while others have found no association. A recent meta-analysis of eight studies, across the USA and Canada, used a fixed-effects model to determine that women who reported IPV during pregnancy were 40 per cent more likely to give birth to a low birth-weight baby (Murphy *et al.* 2001). McFarlane and Soeken (1999) found that among an ethnically stratified cohort of 121 women who experienced abuse during pregnancy, infant weight gain from 6 to 12 months was significantly greater for infants of mothers reporting an end to the abuse.

Chronic pelvic pain, premenstrual syndrome, dysmenorrhea, pelvic inflammatory disease and sexual dysfunction are noted more frequently among sexually abused women than non-abused women (Leserman *et al.* 1998; Coker *et al.* 2002a). Research has found women reporting only physical abuse are equally likely to report a gynecological problem as those who report sexual abuse; however, women with a history of sexual abuse have more gynecological health complaints (Campbell *et al.* 2002). In a large, highly representative, US population-based study, the odds of victims of spouse abuse having a gynecological problem were three times greater than average (McCauley *et al.* 1995). The increased findings of pelvic pain, dyspareunia, fibroids and urinary tract infections in abused women are consistent with the descriptive accounts provided by abused women of forced anal, vaginal and other abusive sexual practices (Campbell *et al.* 2000).

Mental health consequences

The mental health consequences of living in an abusive relationship are also substantial, in part due to the repeated exposure to trauma that many women experience. Nearly 66 per cent of the women surveyed for the NVAW study reported two or more incidences of physical violence by the same partner, with an average of seven. Over two-thirds were victimized by the same partner for more than a year (mean: 4.5 years) (Tjaden and Theonnes 2000a). More than 25 per cent of women in abusive relationships are beaten cyclically, many on a weekly basis (Plichta 1992).

Physical abuse is often mixed with emotional and sexual abuse as a mechanism of coercive control. Between 40 and 45 per cent of physically abused women are forced into sex or sexually degrading acts in the relationship (Plichta 1992). Subsequently, a battered woman lives in realistic fear of further beatings, rape, injury and possible death, and the repeated abuses may cause her to battle feelings of trauma-related guilt (Street *et al.* 2005). The level to which IPV and subsequent fear and guilt impact mental health sequelae may be mediated by several structural factors within the abusive relationship including social isolation, lack of social support systems, restricted educational opportunities, job instability and financial insecurity. These are all significantly associated with poorer mental health symptoms (Coker *et al.* 2003; Nurius *et al.* 2003; Zink and Sill 2004).

The myriad mental health sequelae among abused women include depression, post-traumatic stress disorder (PTSD), phobias, anxiety, panic disorders and substance abuse disorders (Carbone-Lopez *et al.* 2006; Pico-Alfonso *et al.* 2006). A comprehensive meta-analysis by Golding (1999a) showed that abused women were three to five times more likely to experience depression, suicidality, PTSD, alcohol abuse and drug abuse than the general population. Results from the NVAW study support the links between IPV and depression, heavy alcohol use and drug use (Tjaden and Theonnes 2000a). This study did not measure suicidality or PTSD, but smaller studies have shown positive correlations between abuse and depression, PTSD and suicidality in women (Nixon *et al.* 2004; Houry *et al.* 2006). Power and control as forms of abuse were most highly associated with these health outcomes, although all forms of abuse were significantly related to increased risk (Coker *et al.* 2002a).

Depression and PTSD are complex issues with many mediating influences. Depression in abused women has been associated with daily stressors, childhood abuse, forced sex in the relationship, marital separations, change in residence, increased number of children, and child behaviour problems (Campbell and Lewandowski 1997; Cascardi *et al.* 1999). Factors influencing PTSD in abused women include dominant partners, social isolation, severity and number of violent episodes, presence of forced sex, a past history of child sexual abuse, trauma-related guilt and avoidant coping strategies (Astin *et al.* 1995; Street *et al.* 2005; Vitanza *et al.* 1995). Over time, an abused woman's level of depression lessens with lessened IPV, but PTSD persists long after the abuse has stopped. Woods (2000) found that 66 per cent of abused women continued to have PTSD symptoms despite being out of the abusive relationship for an average of nine years (range 2–23 years). This hallmark characteristic of PTSD appears in the general population as well.

Abused women experience depression and PTSD as co-morbidities at a much higher rate than non-abused women. Two studies specifically examining the co-morbidity of major depressive disorder and PTSD in abused women found that in 49 to 75 per cent of cases, major depression occurred in the context of PTSD (Stein and Kennedy 2001; Nixon *et al.* 2004). Another large case-control study of racially balanced, highly educated, middle-class working women confirmed these results: 19.7 per cent of abused women suffered from both PTSD and depression versus 4.5 per cent of their non-abused counterparts (O'Campo *et al.* 2006).

While partner substance abuse is a risk factor for IPV, abused women often battle co-morbidities of alcohol, tobacco and recreational and prescription drug abuse, with a mean prevalence of 18.5 per cent for alcohol abuse or dependence and 8.9 per cent for drug abuse or dependence (Golding 1999a). A community-based survey in California showed that women reporting abuse were eight times as likely to experience alcohol abuse or dependence as their non-abused counterparts. Even when controlling for family history of alcohol use, age and income, these women were still at a fivefold risk of alcohol abuse (Lown and Vega 2001). This co-morbidity can seriously impact physical health outcomes, social functioning and quality of life (Ballenger *et al.* 2004). The few studies that found no association between substance use and IPV had key limitations. One study utilized a chart review which did not indicate how substance use had been assessed (Letourneau *et al.* 1999) and another did not have a non-abused control group (Wingood *et al.* 2000). Despite these conflicting findings, the majority of research supports an increased prevalence of substance use among women experiencing IPV. The temporal relationship between IPV and substance abuse among abused women has yet to be proven, but indications are that trauma precedes substance use, rather than – or at least more often than – the converse (e.g. Schuck and Widom 2001).

Conclusions

IPV is globally increasing and is of paramount concern. Health care professionals are well positioned to identify women experiencing IPV because they frequently access the health care systems. Because the consequences of abuse are extensive, and both current and long-term health effects gravely impact these women both physically and psychologically, health care professionals can have a substantial impact on the well-being of these individuals. Early recognition and subsequent care of those affected can facilitate more positive short- and long-term health outcomes.

5 A child psychiatry perspective: children as victims of adult-adult violence

Adrian Sutton

Introduction

The argument for protecting children from mistreatment is both moral and clinical. Children's vulnerability and dependence places an obligation on adults to manage their own behaviour and curtail certain aspects of this in deference to the needs of children. Failure to do so can produce symptoms and signs of distress and disorder with the potential for both short- and long-term effects (e.g. Kolbo *et al.* 1996).

There is an increased risk of child mistreatment when violence, whether physical, verbal or both, exists in the relationship between parents or adult domestic partners (Hester *et al.* 2000; 30). There may be physical, sexual and emotional abuse directly comparable to that observable in the adult relationship, but that only tells part of the story. The Royal College of Psychiatrists' document *Domestic Violence* (2002: 15) states that 'Domestic violence or serious conflict between adults in the home is especially harmful to children and, when persistent, should be considered as a form of emotional abuse and a child protection issue'. The UK Court of Appeal also emphatically underlined this: 'It may not necessarily be widely appreciated that violence to a partner involves a significant failure in parenting – failure to protect the child's carer and failure to protect the child emotionally' (Court of Appeal UK 2000: 623).

The combined effect of witnessing violence and the fact of that violence being from one person upon whom the child is dependent, can be profound. Although the impact may not be as obvious to a potential observer as the violation caused by physical or sexual abuse, nor the humiliation in emotional abuse, the assault on the senses and the confusion of emotions can be profoundly damaging.

A child psychiatric perspective

Child psychiatry is involved with understanding concerns which arise about a child's emotions, behaviour, relationships and learning and, when a disturbance is identified, advising on the child's particular needs. The aim is to promote care which will be more closely attuned to that child and to offer specific interventions if available. It is a comprehensive approach which takes full account of the child in his or her own unfolding development, within the particular context of the home, community and educational environment.

Assessment: getting the full picture

Appreciating the significance of *continuities* and *discontinuities* in the way a child presents is essential. Development is a complex interweaving and unfolding of underlying physical potential with life experiences. Chromosomal, genetic, antenatal or later health problems may all affect both physical and psychological development, sometimes giving rise to specific disorders. Life experiences may build a greater or lesser degree of resilience or vulnerability in a child, and consequently equip or handicap that person in relation to the degree to which they will be able to contend with or, alternatively, be traumatized by, adverse events. Resilience can be enhanced by ensuring that the challenges children face are ones that they are equipped to respond to, either through their own resources or the strength in their relationships. When properly supported through adverse events, children may also come to realize more of their own capabilities and potential. Similarly, there are qualities of experience that may leave them more vulnerable: this will lead to avoidable suffering and, potentially, ill health or an inability to use relationships to good purpose.

It is not possible to proceed from a single description of any specific behavioural or emotional concern about a child to a conclusion about its cause, its significance or what response may be required. A child behaving in a particular way may represent something positive in one situation but in another it may indicate significant or serious problems. The absence of upset at the loss of an important person may be as concerning as a persisting inability to function because of upset at such a loss. Information is required about the immediate concerns (presenting problems and their history), what is happening in the current situation of the child and their family (social history), the child's previous experiences and development (personal, developmental and medical history), his or her progress educationally and, if possible, similar details of key facts in the parents' and siblings' lives and wider community. This information is formalized in the 'multi-axial system of classification' (World Health Organization 1996). This is synthesized into a 'diagnostic formulation' which summarizes an understanding of the child, his or her present situation and overall development (including how these interact), what may need to be done to maintain or alter the process of that development and what the outcome is likely to be with or without intervention. It is of the greatest importance that a part of the picture is not mistaken for the whole.

Sometimes children make direct statements about domestic violence, deliberately or consciously wishing to communicate upset or outrage. However, comments may arise 'in passing', without the child appearing to be driven by the need or wish to communicate to a trusted adult nor with the expectation that such comments will be perceived as an issue of concern. In all these situations, the general principles about safety and welfare should be followed. The statements should be taken seriously and a considered response formulated in conjunction with those responsible for the child. The primary issue is to ensure the child's safety while making a comprehensive assessment.

Describing the behavioural features a child may manifest, Hester *et al.* (2000: 4–5) list 27. In fact, the same list could be given for children who have experienced physical abuse, sexual abuse or no abuse. Such lists give non-specific indicators of the need for exploration of the child's mental health requirements. There is no uniquely identifiable constellation of symptoms and signs caused by domestic violence: an event is not a person. Rather, we must understand the child and his or her individual needs, including the need for the cessation of violence.

Loud and silent casualties

Staff at his school were concerned about 9-year-old Peter: for four months he had stopped focusing on his work and seemed worried about writing anything down. During a classroom session where 'families' was the topic, his younger sister, Jane (6), mentioned that their parents had recently separated. Peter's teacher spoke to his mother who said she had been worried about Peter: sometimes he was weepy, quiet and withdrawn but at other times aggressive. There were also outbursts when he said he wished he wasn't alive and he had said, 'What would really make me happy would be if my dad was dead.' His mother told the teacher that since she had been pregnant with Jane there had been times when her husband drank a lot and became violent towards her. Peter had seen this but his father had never attacked him. She had recently taken legal action to prevent her husband being in the family home or having direct contact with her: contact arrangements with the children had also been determined by the court. It was arranged that they stay at paternal grandparents' house alternate weekends and see their father there. However, Peter was now saying that he would not meet his father. When his mother attempted to force him, he ran away saying he would rather be dead than see his father again.

Such changes at home and school are clear indicators of psychological disturbance. On first consideration, it might be reasonable to link the onset of Peter's problems with what sounds like a further period of alcohol-associated violence. However, might one not then have expected that the father leaving the family home would have had a positive effect on Peter? Peter has very strongly expressed his fury with his father and that to be forced to see him would feel like a 'fate worse than death', and even suicidal wishes. However, there is sufficient information for a full formulation and examples of some further considerations include:

- Might Peter's behaviour indicate continuing violence or the threat of this?
- Peter might feel relieved that his father is no longer living with them but the contact with his father may contain disturbing experiences (e.g. his father saying he is 'going to get his mother back' for taking legal action. The grandparents might be critical of Peter's mother and denigrate her to him.

- Peter may have been feeling this bad for a long time but only now feels safe to express it.
- Perhaps there is relief about the father's departure but worry about how the mother is coping.
- Some different process, which is not dependent upon anything outside Peter, may have taken place *inside* Peter. He could have become depressed with this process taking on a 'life of its own' rather than the misery he experiences being only a reaction to the outside events.

The above examples are neither exhaustive nor mutually exclusive but they indicate how symptoms and signs can be 'reactive' or 'internally generated'. More information will indicate what may be maintaining, amplifying or perpetuating Peter's presentation. The immediate issue is to keep Peter safe from the very real threat of violence to his mother by his father and from the threat that he may be *to himself* because of his feelings of hopelessness.

Child psychiatry referrals are perhaps more likely to be made on the basis of behaviour that is impinging adversely on others. Winnicott (1956) emphasized that viewing behaviour in only moral terms can cause serious misunderstanding of the child's clinical state. The behaviour is an indicator that the environmental demands upon the child are beyond what they are able to manage. However, a significant number of children do not show distress or disturbance in such readily identifiable ways. Children who, despite adversity, are not so vocal, literally or metaphorically, may need just as much consideration.

The assessing child psychiatric staff enquired about Peter's sister, Jane, although nobody had raised any concerns about her. She was described as having always been a shy girl, behind in her reading and writing but not showing any recent signs of upset or behaviour changes. She went to contact with her father without any complaints and always behaved herself. Overall she was described as 'no trouble'.

The practice in military combat is that the casualties who should be attended to first are the silent ones: they may not be crying out because their airway is blocked; they cannot breathe. A comparable warning needs to be heeded for children such as Jane. Her shyness could all too easily be attributed to 'temperament' when there could be many other causes. In conjunction with her reading and writing difficulties, and the absence of signs of reactions in her emotions or behaviour despite major changes and events in her life, there are powerful indicators that she may well be suffering from major, chronic inhibitions in her emotional life. The question to be asked is: 'Is her emotional airway blocked?' Assessment would need to establish the extent of this and the balance of influences maintaining and perpetuating it.

Being held in trust

Having ensured that the clinical response is on the basis of understanding the child and not on the basis of a pre-formed idea of the impact of domestic violence, the task is to help avoid avoidable suffering, ensure general and therapeutic support through inevitable suffering, and minimize the effects of any developmental distortions consequent upon adverse experiences.

Ensuring the child's welfare involves understanding the need for both real safety and a sense of safety. Some children may be able to assimilate the experiences of domestic violence without fundamentally pathological processes ensuing. However, there has to be a sufficient experience of being 'safe-enough' in having thoughts and memories about, or talking about, what has happened. This requires a form of care that is closely enough attuned and adapted to the needs of the particular child and which provides the external safety of what could be called an 'ordinarily predictable nurturing environment'. The foundation is demonstrably living in *real* safety: talking comes next. Child mental health *specialists* can only be effective child mental health *therapists* if the child is being cared for reasonably, which is the ultimate achievement of the combined effects of well-adapted care (which itself may be therapeutic) and, when required, specific treatments (e.g. psychotherapy).

Contact in physical and psychological space

As illustrated in the case of Peter and Jane, children may continue to be adversely affected in the absence of actual violence, even in the context of legally defined contact arrangements. In relation to the dynamics of mental life, 'having contact with' can continue within a person even without the violent person being actively present. If there is no certainty of safety from the perpetrator, living with fear means that inside the child (in the *inner world*) the attacks continue simply because they remain a possibility. Post-traumatic stress disorder (PTSD), in which symptoms occur over an extended period of time after the traumatic event or events, is one manifestation of this. In this condition, associations, which may or may not be apparent to the person or to those around them, set off re-experiencing, in the present moment, of elements of the original events or the whole of them (i.e. 'flashbacks' or intrusive thoughts or memories).

Pamela and Leanne were in care after their father killed their mother. They had seen the murder and witnessed many more attacks. In one particular consultation, Pamela described persistent trouble falling asleep. When the bedroom light was turned off, she kept seeing flashing lights. She shared a room with Leanne who told her that she could not see anything. The psychiatrist enquired more closely about these experiences. The lights were blue and Pamela felt frightened when she saw them.

The psychiatrist asked the girls if it reminded them of anything or made them think about anything else. They said it did not. It reminded him very powerfully of the events of the murder. These had been reported to him by the girls' social worker but neither girl had been able to talk with him about what they had witnessed. In fact, both girls had been vehement in their reaction to enquiry about it, telling him that it was all written down (the statements they had given to the police) and he could read it but they would not talk about it. The flashing blue lights sounded like they could be a flashback relating to the lights of the police cars and the ambulance that had come to the house on the night of the attack. The psychiatrist felt this link needed to be tested, both to show the girls that he could cope with thinking and talking about the murder and because, if his idea was correct, it was likely to assist

Pamela in 'moving on' emotionally. At the same time, it was important to approach this with full respect for the girls' fear – to even think about the attack was to experience it all over again as if in the present. He told them that they were not going to like him mentioning it, but he thought the lights were about the night of the attack and that they were to do with the police cars and ambulance. Although startled, the girls were able to cope with this link and did begin to give their account. Subsequently Pamela's sleep settled.

A familiar scenario in the consulting room is the child who, in the underlying emotional life of the mother with whom they are still living, has a resemblance to the abusive parent in appearance or manner. The care of the child brings that parent 'in contact' with the abuser day in, day out. This can profoundly affect the way the parent behaves towards the child and lead to serious difficulties. The resemblance may simply be an issue of gender, or more specific (e.g. 'He looks just like his father'). Since the primary perpetrators of the physical violence in domestic violence are male, this leaves boys more commonly vulnerable to the impact of these processes.

A child's past experience of the abusive parent may contain very different aspects. The parent who was violent may at other times have been the parent who was consistently able to meet certain of their needs, perhaps in ways the other parent could not. The child will need to be able to 'join these up' inside themselves if they are to make proper judgements of people in ongoing and future relationships: the child will need to learn that opposite aspects may coexist within the same person. If not, there may be unmanageable inner turmoil. In psychodynamic terms, this needs to be understood as involving both conscious and unconscious processes. The process of 'splitting and denial' may lead not only to an inability to maintain personal safety through proper recognition of the violent potential in a partner, but may also perpetuate an idealized image of that person or cause self-denigration.

Being a fit parent

Being a parent means accepting a different form of personal rights, freedoms and limitations. Certain liberties are lost because of the responsibilities that parenthood brings. This may seem a rather negative description of parenthood when, for most people, the good experiences far outweigh the bad. However, it does also convey how a person's freedom to act upon his or her impulses, wishes or desires should be governed by ' ... rejection of injury, of coercion, of slavery, of indifference' (O'Neill 2002: 95), particularly in fulfilling parental obligations.

When we are assessing parenting, we look to find that quality of person that the child needs the parent to be. The fit must be a close enough one – this is what is meant by 'fitness to parent'. Assessment seeks to identify the presence, absence or relative balance of different abilities. If aspects are absent or insufficient then we seek to find out whether this can be altered within a time frame that is adequate for the needs of the developing child. The potential for a minimum sufficient change to occur may depend upon many different factors. The availability of sufficient economic resources or formal and informal social support may be crucial. The parents' own internal resources, including their potential to develop new abilities, may be the fundamentally important elements.

The clinical significance of authority

The ability to take charge of intense emotions and thoughts relating to violent and aggressive impulses is a component of ordinary development and can be understood as the establishment of an appropriate *healthy internal authority*. A failure in this respect is at the heart of violence in intimate relationships. Such internal authority is less likely to develop if it is not experienced in the key caring relationships. Where domestic violence has occurred, there is a need to establish for the child an experience of healthy external authority that will take charge and lead to the cessation of that violence.

Balancing responsibilities and preventing 'false engagement'

In the practitioner-parent relationship, the professional seeks to enter into a cooperative venture with the parent or parents, with all parties putting themselves 'in the service' of the child (for detailed discussion of psychodynamic issues in work with parents see Sutton and Hughes 2005). However, this may not always be achievable. The professional has a particular responsibility to examine whether the approach taken may be contributing to or even causing difficulties. However, a dangerous perversion of the relationship may occur if the responsibilities or obligations of all parties are not appreciated (e.g. if a failure to reach agreement is assumed to be a failure in professional practice since there may be specific difficulties in one or both parents that result in them not having the ability or perhaps the will to cooperate). The professional may become engaged in trying to make himself or herself acceptable to the parent in a way which inadvertently loses sight of the child as the subject of concern, and distorts the professional's actions. Rather than speaking with professional authority on the child's needs and engaging respectfully with the parent as a parent, a sub-plot may develop. In this, the parent inadvertently becomes defined as the patient/client. Unconsciously, the parent's needs become paramount, creating the illusion of a truly 'cooperative' venture. A 'false engagement' in which the paramount needs of the child are lost is established.

Another complication may arise when a parent who has been the victim of attack is unable to remove herself and the child from the violent relationship, or she may have fundamental problems in providing for the basic care of the child. To say that this person is not capable of protecting her child may seem very harsh or may unconsciously feel like a further attack on that person. The description of parental ability must not be confused with a moral judgement, nor must the concerns or fears for the adult take precedence. For those working in children's services it is perhaps easier to do this, since we can hold to the idea that we are only meeting the particular adult(s) because there are children involved, and this may avoid some of the pressure to develop the 'false engagement' described above. However, those working in services for adults have no less an obligation to hold the child in mind.

Creating a healthier order

In current practice, the aim is to work with parents without the involvement of the courts *wherever possible*. This is obviously desirable providing that in those cases where it is not possible the authority of the court is always sought. Unfortunately there can be a level of expectation put upon professionals to achieve a solution without recourse to the court that subtly acts to promote a belief that to do so is a failure. Interventions of an inappropriate or lesser degree may be attempted but these may simply waste everybody's time and, more importantly, fail the child. If the nature of concerns exceeds a certain threshold then the professional(s) must seek *alternative authorisation* (i.e. the authorization of the court) if they are to proceed, as this provides an explicit definition in law of the power to act on professional opinion. This process of seeking authorization can be essential in delineating the extent of individual autonomy and authority for parents and professionals alike. Asking the court to decide what should or should not be done, or who should be making decisions about any actions, is consistent with the earlier description of the need for a *healthy authority* to be present at all levels of the system involved with the child's life.

The mechanisms and methods involved in defining authority in this way are actually part of a *clinical* process, not simply a legal exercise. The unfolding process of making explicit that one must act to the limits of one's proper powers *and not beyond* can clarify the real nature of the relationship between all the parties and challenge underlying, perhaps unconscious, confusions. Of particular importance are those that may arise from the experiences of the parent(s) in their own childhood (this general process is termed 'transference'). Experiences in childhood in which those who had power acted in ways that were authoritarian or abusive may result in any relationship where there is a perceived discrepancy of power being unconsciously experienced in the same way as that earlier relationship. The reality of that earlier relationship may be confused with the current relationship with the professional: the latter is then perceived as having powers and motivations that they do not have and they will be behaved towards as if they do. The professional must manage the impact of these perceptions upon them (the 'countertransference') in such a way as to avoid acting beyond his or her actual powers and authority, creating a self-fulfilling prophecy. In extreme situations this can only be demonstrated by seeking the decision of the court as to whether or not they should be authorized to act upon professional (clinical) opinion. This may be the only route to challenging the underlying beliefs.

Managing interprofessional relationships

Child care and protection can evoke complicated responses in professionals. Kraemer (1988: 256) has described this in relation to sexual abuse: 'Under the influence of the deceptive confusions ... there is often a strong temptation to bend the rules in some way, as if the case in question were not really like the others; but it is a dangerous course to take ... it is better to stick to cumbersome regulations, even if it seems at the time to be unnecessary or even positively unhelpful ... ' Comparable factors can occur in domestic violence where powerlessness, violence and sexuality are interlinked. There is an obligation upon professionals to be aware of these, to manage them in themselves and to seek to work within structures that properly support good practice.

Confusion in relation to authority and responsibility may arise in the relationships between the various professionals involved. Disagreements and disputes usually reflect the seriousness with which each person approaches the situation. However, in contact with the vulnerability of the child, this can lead to an individual over-valuing his or her position in the total picture of the child's life. The net result is that proper appreciation of the usefulness to the child is lost. A professional must appreciate that the benefit to the child arises solely from fulfilling his or her defined role well, and with full acceptance of its limits and boundaries. The frustrations that may arise in the course of this process must be tolerated and the organization within which the professional is working must provide proper support for the stresses that result.

Rivalries can often be seen in a concentrated form during care proceedings. The application of the 'full force of the law' can bring forward complex dynamics relating to the experience of authority by the various parties (whether lay or professional). An argument presented earlier was that an essential element for progress in domestic violence is the establishment of a 'healthy authority': this is in contrast to the abuse of power which operates when authoritarian activity takes place, or the failures which result from irresponsibly unauthoritative behaviour. While there cannot be an indiscriminate trust in the correctness of the outcome of the legal process, there is a danger that areas of insufficient trust may become magnified because of the very nature of the events which have brought about the problems for the parents and children (i.e. untrustworthy 'authority figures'). A consequence of reliance on, or being at the mercy of, such figures can be a profound sense of humiliation: these experiences are central to the understanding of violence (Gilligan 2000). There is danger that the legal process, which at its best is healthily humbling, becomes destructively humiliating if the underlying unconscious dynamic of the abuse of power or the failure of the application of healthy authority become enacted. Professionals' training and practice must therefore include reflecting on perceptions and beliefs about power and authority.

An additional component of managing the dynamic can be through full appreciation of the *legal process* as part of the *clinical service* to the child. This may require a change in the perception of these as somehow separate processes in a hierarchical rather than complementary relationship to each other. This was central to the earlier discussion of clinicians' and practitioners' understanding of the ways in which they are or are not given authority to act (or are prevented from acting without proper authority) acting as a tool in managing relationships with both children and adults.

Conclusions

The importance of the physical evidence of bruises, broken bones or other physical impingements or intrusions, and the emotional sequelae of these, are well established. Domestic violence is a different type of impingement: the child is intruded upon through the eyes and ears by seeing and hearing violence inflicted upon a key person in their lives by another key person. This can create a state in the child's 'inner world' which has profound effects on their ability to live a reasonable life and to make healthy developmental progress. Our understanding of the concept of 'the paramountcy of the child's needs' must take full account of this in practice and in planning for children's services. The impact will vary from child to child, so assumptions about the needs consequent upon such experiences must not be made.

When considering parents' wishes and desires, their abilities and inabilities in managing impulses in relationships, and their ability to protect a child from another person's inabilities must be looked at through the lens of their children's emotional and developmental needs. The fundamental test is whether the parties can or cannot achieve a situation in which the child is protected from adults' difficulties in managing their aggressive and violent impulses. The range of considerations and responses in relation to domestic violence, including in relation to children's mental health, are as extensive as those that apply when other child protection issues arise.

6 Sexual coercion and domestic violence

Poco Kernsmith

Introduction

Sexual aggression, particularly in the context of existing relationships, can take many forms, ranging from subtle emotional pressure to physical force (e.g. Basile 1999). Although some forms are less severe and violent, each ultimately results in an unwanted sexual experience (Basile 1999). In a physically abusive relationship, the dynamics of sexual consent, coercion and marital rape are confounded by the threat of physical violence.

Rape of one's spouse first began to be recognized as a result of the feminist movement in the 1970s (Brownmiller 1975). Feminist theory identifies that in a patriarchal society, women are dominated and oppressed emotionally, socially, financially and sexually (Ward 1995). In this system, male violence against women, particularly in relationships, is condoned by society through rape culture (Herman 1984). Research by Finkelhor and Yllo (1985) and Russell (1990) documented the extent to which sexual violence in marriage occurs. Since that time, laws in many western countries have begun to change to forbid rape of a spouse (e.g. Regan and Kelly 2003). However, laws in the USA commonly include exceptions that make prosecuting spouses for sexual assault more difficult than other assaults (Monson and Langhinrichsen-Rohling 1998).

Sexual coercion and marital rape

Sexual coercion is the act of pressuring an unwilling partner to engage in sexual activity (Basile 1999). This can include such categories of behaviour as persistence, deception, threats of violence or emotional consequences, assault while sleeping, use of alcohol and drugs, physical restraint and physical force (e.g. Stermac *et al.* 2001). It may be as subtle as social expectations of a woman's responsibility to engage in sex in marriage (Basile 1999).

Sexual coercion is not synonymous with rape. Finkelhor and Yllo (1985) express concern that recognition of the more subtle forms of coercion may minimize the definition of, and the understanding of the impact of, forcible rape. In actuality, the impacts of each form vary substantially (e.g. Basile 1999). However, in the context of an abusive relationship, even the most subtle forms of coercion can have a profound impact on the victim. Yet, most of these cases do not meet the legal definition of rape. This is particularly problematic in marital relationships because laws commonly include exceptions for all but the most physically violent incidents (Monson and Langhinrichsen-Rohling 1998).

Prevalence

Estimates of rape in marriage indicate that between 7 and 14 per cent of married women have been raped by a partner (e.g. Tjaden and Thoennes 1998). Women raped by a spouse are ten times more likely to experience repeated assaults than those raped by a stranger or acquaintance (Mahoney 1999). Of those who report being raped by a spouse, between 70 and 85 per cent report experiencing more than one rape, and 30 to 55 per cent report being raped more than 20 times (e.g. Mahoney 1999). Therefore, it is estimated that 38 per cent of all rapes are perpetrated by a current or former husband (Russell 1990).

It is difficult to estimate the extent to which women in abusive relationships are coerced into having unwanted sex. Basile (1999) identifies that the victim's ability to freely choose when to have sex is obstructed by the ever-present threat of violence. Therefore, women who have agreed to unwanted sex to avoid violence may not identify that experience as rape. Instead, it is a method of self-protection.

Males are far more likely than females to commit forcible rape (Spitzberg 1999). However, research has indicated that females perpetrate sexual coercion at nearly the same rate as males (e.g. Hogben *et al.* 1995), though the reactions to and the interpretations of these behaviours are quite different (Struckman-Johnson and Struckman-Johnson 1994). Additionally, some research indicates that females perpetrate physical domestic violence at rates similar to males (e.g. Archer 2002). Other research suggests that the context in which the violence occurs, often being self-defence or retaliation for ongoing abuse, demonstrates that females are not typically the primary aggressors in violent relationships (e.g. Kernsmith 2005a). Therefore, they would be unlikely to commit acts of sexual violence. Although violence does occur by females against males and in same-gender relationships, the complexities of the differences in dynamics are beyond the scope of this chapter.

Domestic and sexual violence

Sexual abuse in marriage most commonly occurs in relationships characterized by severe and frequent physical violence. Campbell and Soeken (1999b) identified marital rape as associated with a greater number of risk factors for domestic homicide than other abusive relationships that did not include sexual violence. Between a third and a half of all abused women report sexual violence (e.g. Mahoney 1999). Even more may have been coerced but not identified that experience as sexual abuse.

Because the dynamics and motivations are often similar, various forms of intimate partner violence, including physical violence, sexual assault and stalking, commonly coexist. Nearly half of battered women in one sample reported also being raped by the abusive partner (Campbell and Soeken 1999b). The National Violence against Women (NVAW) study (Tjaden and Thoennes 1997) revealed that nearly a third of women who had been stalked by a partner were also sexually assaulted by the same partner. Therefore, a woman who is sexually abused by a partner is likely to have experienced other forms of violence or stalking by that same partner.

Sexually coercive individuals, much like domestically abusive individuals, tend to accept stereotyped gender norms about sex roles and sexual relationships, view relationships as adversarial, and have a willingness to use force or violence to manage conflict (Craig 1990). These males accept the traditional sexual script in which males are viewed as having an insatiable sexual appetite and valuing sexual access with little regard for the means of obtaining it or the choice of sexual partner (Check and Malamuth 1985).

Although some sexual coercion is characterized as a result of social incompetence on the part of the perpetrator, it is at least as likely that the perpetrator is quite skilled and adept at obtaining sex from an unwilling partner (Muehlenhard and Falcon 1990). This is particularly likely in domestically violent relationships, in which the abusive partner attempts to control all aspects of the relationship (Pence and Paymar 1986). Sexual violence may serve as one more tactic with which to terrorize the victim. Alternatively, unobstructed sexual access to the partner may be a goal or 'reward' of the emotional and physical violence for the perpetrator.

Consenting to unwanted sex, either verbally or without discussion, is a means of keeping the peace in both non-violent and violent relationships. Basile (1999) reports that acquiescence occurred in non-violent relationships to avoid consequences such as pouting, withholding other affection, guilt and being angry or unkind. In violent relationships, the threat of verbal or physical abuse as a punishment for refusing sex may be used to coerce unwanted sexual behaviour.

The level of control abusive partners exhibit, and the threat of violence or harm should a woman not comply with the demands, makes it virtually impossible to view sexual relationships in a severely abusive relationship as truly consensual (MacKinnon 1983 cited in Basile 1999). Basile identifies 'rape by acquiescence' as a woman consenting to unwanted sexual activities in order to avoid the negative consequences of refusing. One example that illustrates this dynamic is 'Robin' (Basile 1999: 1052): 'There were a lot of times, I did say no, and there was a few that I didn't say anything because he was gonna do whatever he wanted to anyway whether I said no or whether I didn't. There was a lot of times, instead of raising an issue, I wouldn't say anything'.

Consenting to sex may be a coping mechanism in which women attempt to decrease the chances of being beaten or raped by an abusive partner. Over time, the woman may lose the ability to feel sexual desire or experience sexual satisfaction (e.g. Howard *et al.* 2003). Then, as in the case of 'Robin', over time all sexual acts may be characterized as unwanted. The violence decreases the likelihood that a woman will have sexual interest while simultaneously demanding that it continue to occur.

Impact

Rape by a spouse is generally perceived by the public to be less serious than other forms of rape. However, victims of spousal rape generally endure more physical violence and greater injury than victims of acquaintance rape (Stermac *et al.* 2001). This may be due to the correlation between physical and sexual abuse in relationships, or women's reluctance to seek assistance in all but the most violent cases.

In addition, psychological trauma is greater than in other forms of rape (Culbertson and Dehle 2001). Psychological impacts include hypervigilance and intrusion symptoms which are part of post-traumatic stress disorder (PTSD). The increased psychological impact of the assault may be due in part to the continued contact with the rapist if they remain in the relationship (Finkelhor and Yllo 1985). The nature of the continued relationship increases hypervigilance and intrusive symptoms (Culbertson and Dehle 2001). Victims also experience self-blame and a decreased sense of self-efficacy (Culbertson and Dehle 2001; Howard *et al.* 2003). Because the victim chose the abuser as her partner and is unable to stop the often repeated abuse, these impacts are magnified for victims of marital rape. Marital rape erodes one's sense of dignity and self-worth, leading to depression and anxiety (Finkelhor and Yllo 1985).

In addition, women may be less likely to seek social support due to isolation, economic dependence or fear of retaliation (Mahoney 1999). Domestic violence frequently includes attempts to isolate the victim from potential support systems (Pence and Paymar 1986). Women reporting both physical and sexual violence are even less able to identify and use social supports than those experiencing physical violence alone (Howard *et al.* 2003). In addition, they may experience shame or guilt, because of feeling responsible for the assault or for having 'consented' (e.g. Howard, *et al.* 2003)

Most women who have survived a physically violent sexual assault by a spouse recognize that experience as rape. However, they may not define it as rape until much later, often after the relationship has ended (e.g. Basile 1999). Women who are pressured to have sex or consent due to the implicit *threat* of violence do not commonly identify this as rape (Basile 1999). For these reasons, and the cultural stigma against rape victims, women who have experienced multiple forms of violence have the most difficulty labelling and discussing rape (e.g. Mahoney 1999).

Research has indicated that maritally raped women make significant improvements in emotional and psychological well-being following counselling interventions, although the level of well-being is still lower post-counselling than that of physically abused women who have not experienced sexual violence (Howard *et al.* 2003). Perhaps due to the difficulty of discussing these forms of abuse, survivors may benefit from group counselling with others who have experienced similar abuse. This may serve to decrease the sense of shame and isolation by sharing and hearing the experiences of others. Advocacy services may also be beneficial as women can be assisted with pressing charges against their husband, filing for divorce, and obtaining a job and housing.

Health consequences

Physical traumas associated with sexual violence include vaginal and anal tearing and bleeding, urinary tract infections and urine leakage (Campbell and Soeken 1999b). Victims of marital rape who sought services in the hospital emergency room sustained greater injuries than those assaulted by a non-partner, despite being less likely to have resisted the assault (Stermac *et al.* 2001). These injuries included bruises, lacerations, fractures and internal injuries.

During pregnancy, physical and sexual violence have been shown to increase (e.g. Browne 1997). Those women who had experienced both sexual and physical violence were found to be at the greatest risk of being abused during pregnancy (Campbell 1989). This abuse is related to a variety of negative health outcomes, including miscarriage, stillbirth and infertility (e.g. Campbell and Soeken 1999b).

In addition, domestic violence has been found to be associated with repeated unwanted pregnancies and abortion (Jacoby *et al.* 1999). Eby and Campbell (1995) identified that victims of spousal rape are also at greater risk of contracting sexually transmitted diseases. Both unwanted pregnancy and disease transmission are associated not only with forcible rape, but also with the partner's use or threats of violence if the victim requests safer sex practices, such as wearing a condom during consensual sex (e.g. Campbell and Soeken 1999b). The control exerted by the abusive partner extends to control of the woman's body and physical well-being.

Women who have been raped by a partner are less likely to report the incident or seek medical or psychological services as compared to others who have been assaulted by someone they know (Mahoney 1999). Those who seek assistance have typically been assaulted many times. When a woman does report to the police, she is more likely to complete a physical examination and a forensic evidence kit at the hospital than other rape survivors (Stermac *et al.* 2001). This is likely to be due to the repeated and escalating nature of domestic violence. Therefore, it is likely that women who choose to report after a history of assaults are perhaps at the point of being ready to terminate the relationship.

Conclusions

Women in abusive relationships are at high risk of sexual coercion and assault. The constant threat of violence makes it difficult to determine which sexual acts are consensual or coerced. The physical and psychological trauma experienced by the victim is magnified by her continued relationship with the perpetrator and the chronic nature of the abuse. Health care providers play a critical role in the detection of physical and sexual relationship violence.

7 Evolutionary psychological perspectives on men's violence against intimate partners

Aaron T. Goetz and Todd K. Shackelford

Introduction

Modern evolutionary psychological perspectives have been used to predict and understand a wide array of human behaviours, from cooperation and competition to mating and morality. Evolution is the centerpiece of biology, and in the last few decades many psychologists have recognized the value of using an evolutionary perspective to guide their research. With a focus on evolved mechanisms and associated information-processing features, evolutionary psychology has risen as a fruitful approach to the study of human psychology and behaviour. In this chapter, we use an evolutionary psychological perspective to address violence between intimate partners.

Paternal uncertainty and the function of male sexual jealousy

Jealousy is an emotion that is experienced when a valued relationship is threatened by a real or imagined rival, and generates responses aimed at stifling the threat. Jealousy functions to maintain relationships by motivating behaviours that deter rivals from mate-poaching and deter intimate partners from infidelity or outright departure from the relationship (e.g. Buss *et al.*1992). Because ancestral men and women recurrently faced the adaptive problems of retaining partners and maintaining relationships over human evolutionary history, men and women today do not differ in the frequency or intensity of experienced jealousy (e.g. White 1981). However, a sex difference is evident when considering two basic types of jealousy – emotional and sexual – and this sex difference coincides with sex differences in the adaptive problems that ancestral men and women recurrently had to solve over human evolutionary history in the context of their relationships (Buss 2000). Ancestral women's adaptive problem of securing the paternal investment needed to raise offspring exerted a selection pressure for women to be more sensitive to, and more distressed by, cues associated with a partner's *emotional* infidelity. However, ancestral men's adaptive problem of paternal uncertainty exerted a selection pressure for them to be more sensitive to, and more distressed by, cues associated with a partner's *sexual* infidelity. Because emotional infidelity and sexual infidelity have been highly correlated throughout evolutionary history (i.e. if an individual were engaging in one type of infidelity, he or she was often engaging in the other type), researchers studying sex differences in jealousy have used forced-choice methods in which participants are asked to select which partner infidelity type upsets them more, although some researchers, such as Sagarin *et al.* (2003) and Wiederman and Allgeier (1993) have also found a sex difference in jealousy using continuous measures. At least two dozen studies have provided evidence of this sex difference in jealousy, documenting that men experience greater jealousy in response to the sexual aspects of an intimate partner's infidelity, whereas women experience greater jealousy in response to the emotional aspects of an intimate partner's infidelity. These results are corroborated by experimental data (e.g. Schützwohl and Koch 2004), physiological data (Buss *et al.* 1992), patterns of divorce (Betzig 1989) and the behavioural output of jealousy, such as mate retention behaviours (e.g. Buss and Shackelford 1997).

Men's sensitivity to, and distress as a result of, a partner's sexual infidelity are not surprising given the severe reproductive costs to men of cuckoldry – the unwitting investment of resources into genetically unrelated offspring. Some of the costs of cuckoldry include the potential misdirection of a man's resources to a rival's genetic offspring, his partner's investment in a rival's genetic offspring, and reputational damage if the cuckoldry becomes known to others (e.g. Platek and Shackelford 2006). Perhaps with the exception of death, cuckoldry is associated with the most severe reproductive costs for an individual man, and it is therefore likely that selection will have resulted in the evolution of male strategies and tactics aimed at avoiding cuckoldry and decreasing paternal uncertainty.

Intimate partner violence and sexual jealousy

Male sexual jealousy is one of the most frequently cited causes of intimate partner violence (e.g. Russell 1982; Frieze 1983; Daly and Wilson 1988; Buss 2000; Gage and Hutchinson 2006). Intimate partner violence is a tactic used by men to restrict a partner's sexual behaviour (Daly and Wilson 1988; Wilson and Daly 1996) and may be best understood as a behavioural output of male sexual jealousy. A man may afford his partner many freedoms, but these freedoms only rarely include sexual activity with other men (Buss 1996, 2000). Men are hypothesized to have evolved mechanisms dedicated to generating risk assessments of a partner's sexual infidelity. These mechanisms include, for example, assessments of the time spent apart from his partner (i.e. time during which she might have been sexually unfaithful), the presence of potential mate-poachers, his partner's reproductive value (i.e. expected future reproduction) and fertility (i.e. current likelihood of conceiving), and his partner's likelihood of committing infidelity (e.g. Shackelford and Buss 1997; Schmitt and Buss 2001; Shackelford *et al.* 2002; Goetz and Shackelford 2006). Moreover, the male mind may be designed to be hypersensitive to cues of his partner's sexual infidelity, motivating more false positives than false negatives because the benefits of the former outweigh the costs of the latter (Haselton and Nettle 2006). Together with assessments of the likelihood of a partner's sexual infidelity, contextual factors – such as social and reputational costs, proximity of the partner's adult male kin (who might be motivated to retaliate for a man's violence against his partner), and economic dependency (Figueredo and McClosky 1993; Wilson and Daly 1996) – are processed by mechanisms of the male mind to inhibit or motivate men to inflict violence on their partners.

Occasionally, men's use of violence against their partners is lethal. As with non-lethal partner violence, male sexual jealousy is a frequently cited cause of intimate partner homicide across cultures (Daly and Wilson 1988). Killing an intimate partner is costly, but under specific circumstances might the benefits have out-weighed the costs enough for selection to produce a psychology that motivates partner killing? According to Daly and Wilson (Daly and Wilson 1988; Wilson *et al.* 1995a), killing an intimate partner is not the designed product of evolved mecha-nisms, but instead is a byproduct of mechanisms selected for their non-lethal outcomes. This byproduct or 'slip-up' hypothesis states that men who kill their partners have 'slipped up' in that their violence – which was intended to control an intimate partner's sexual behaviour – inadvertently results in the partner's death.

The byproduct hypothesis is attractive in that it would seem too costly to kill an intimate partner. Why kill a partner and risk the enormous costs that often flow from such actions, when a man could simply end the relationship with the woman he suspects of sexual infidelity? But consider this. If killing an intimate partner is a slip-up or accident, as argued by Daly and Wilson, why are so many partner homicides apparently premeditated? Hiring someone to kill a partner, aiming at and shooting a partner with a firearm and slitting a partner's throat appear to be intentional killings, not accidental killings. Although some partner homicides may be accidental, too many seem premeditated and intended. This is one observation that led Buss and Duntley (1998, 2003) to propose that many intimate partner homicides are motivated by evolved mechanisms designed to motivate killing under certain conditions. Discovering a partner's sexual infidelity, Buss and Duntley argue, may be a special circumstance that motivates partner homicide. This 'homicide adaptation theory' does not argue that discovering a partner's infidelity inevitably leads to homicide, but that this circumstance would activate mechanisms associated with weighing the costs and benefits of homicide, and that under certain circumstances partner killing might be the designed outcome (for a fuller treatment see Buss 2005).

Daly and Wilson's (1988; Wilson *et al.* 1995a) and Buss and Duntley's (1998, 2003; Buss 2005) competing hypotheses have not yet been examined concurrently so that a single hypothesis remains that best accounts for the data (but see Shackelford *et al.* 2003), and our intention is not to critically evaluate these competing hypotheses. We intend to argue that intimate partner homicide, by design or as a byproduct, is often the behavioural output of male sexual jealousy stemming from paternal uncertainty.

Men's 'mate retention' or 'mate-guarding' behaviour is another example of the behavioural output of jealousy. Buss (1988) identified specific mate-guarding behaviours, such as vigilance (e.g. dropping by unexpectedly to check up on a partner) and concealment of mate (e.g. taking a partner away from a social gathering where other men are present). These mate-guarding behaviours vary in ways that suggest that they are produced by mechanisms that evolved as paternity guards. For example, a man guards his partner more intensely when she is of greater reproductive value (as indexed by her youth and attractiveness) and when the perceived probability of her sexual infidelity is greater (Buss and Shackelford 1997). In addition, men who are partnered to women who have characteristics that make them more likely to commit sexual infidelity guard their partners more intensely (Goetz et al. 2005), and men guard their partners more intensely when they are near ovulation – a time when an extra-pair copulation or sexual infidelity would be most costly for the in-pair man (Gangestad et al. 2002).

Recognizing that men's mate retention behaviours are manifestations of jealousy, Shackelford et al. (2005) investigated the relationships between men's mate retention behaviours and intimate partner violence, specifically whether some mate retention behaviours and seemingly innocuous romantic gestures may be harbingers of violence. Securing self-reports from men, partner reports from women and cross-spouse reports from married couples, Shackelford and his colleagues found that men's use of particular mate retention behaviours was related to partner violence in predictable ways. For example, men who dropped by unexpectedly to see what their partner was doing or who told their partner that they would 'die' if the woman ever left them were most likely to use serious violence against their partners, whereas men who attempted to retain their partners by expressing affection and displaying resources were least likely to use violence. These findings corroborated the results of research conducted by Wilson et al. (1995b), who found that women who affirmed statements such as, 'He insists on knowing who you are with and where you are at all times' and 'He tries to limit your contact with family or friends', were twice as likely to have experienced serious violence by their partners.

Sexual violence in intimate relationships and sexual jealousy

Between 10 and 26 per cent of women experience rape in marriage (e.g. Russell 1982; Finkelhor and Yllo 1985; Watts et al. 1998; Hadi 2000; Dunkle et al. 2004). Rape also occurs in non-marital intimate relationships. Goetz and Shackelford (2006) secured prevalence estimates of rape in intimate relationships from a sample of young men and from an independent sample of young women in a committed relationship for at least one year, but not necessarily married. Goetz and Shackelford documented that 7.3 per cent of men admitted to raping their current partner at least once, and 9.1 per cent of women admitted that they had experienced at least one rape by their current partner. Questions concerning sexual coercion and rape in relationships are emotionally loaded and may be subject to social desirability concerns. These percentages therefore may be underestimates of the prevalence of rape in intimate relationships among young men and women who are not married.

Many hypotheses have been generated to explain why, across cultures, women are sexually coerced by their partners. Some researchers have hypothesized that sexual coercion in intimate relationships is motivated by men's attempts to dominate and control their partners (e.g. Frieze 1983; Bergen 1995, 1996; Watts *et al.* 1998; Gage and Hutchinson 2006) and that this expression of power is the product of men's social roles (e.g. Yllo and Straus 1990). Results relevant to this hypothesis are mixed. Several studies have found that physically abusive men are more likely than non-abusive men to sexually coerce their partners (e.g. Finkelhor and Yllo 1985; Donnelly 1993), a result that is consistent with the domination and control hypothesis. Gage and Hutchinson (2006), however, found that women's risk of sexual coercion by their partners is not related to measures assessing the relative dimensions of power in a relationship, such as who has more control over decision-making. That is, women partnered to men who hold the dominant position in the relationship are not more likely to experience sexual coercion by their partners than women partnered to men who do not maintain the dominant position in the relationship, a result that does not support the domination and control hypothesis. Although many researchers agree that *individual men* may sexually coerce their partners to gain or maintain dominance and control in the relationship, proponents of the domination and control hypothesis often argue that men are motivated *as a group* to exercise 'patriarchal power' or 'patriarchal terrorism' over women (e.g. Yllo and Straus 1990).

An alternative hypothesis has been advanced by researchers studying sexual coercion from an evolutionary perspective: sexual coercion in intimate relationships may be related to paternal uncertainty, with the occurrence of sexual coercion related to a man's suspicions of his partner's sexual infidelity (Thornhill and Thornhill 1992; Wilson and Daly 1992; Camilleri 2004; Lalumière *et al.* 2005; Goetz and Shackelford 2006). Sexual coercion in response to cues of his partner's sexual infidelity might function to introduce a male's sperm into his partner's reproductive tract at a time when there is a high risk of cuckoldry (i.e. when his partner has recently been inseminated by a rival male). This sperm competition hypothesis was proposed following recognition that forced in-pair copulation (i.e. partner rape) in non-human species followed female extra-pair copulations (sexual infidelities; e.g. Cheng *et al.* 1983; Lalumière *et al.* 2005) and that sexual coercion and rape in human intimate relationships often followed men's accusations of their partners' sexual infidelity (e.g. Russell 1982; Finkelhor and Yllo 1985). Before considering the case of partner rape in humans, we review briefly the animal literature on forced in-pair copulation. Examining the adaptive problems and evolved solutions to these problems in non-human animals may provide insight into the adaptive problems and evolved solutions in humans (and vice versa). Shackelford and Goetz (2006), for example, argued that because humans share with some avian species a similar mating system (social monogamy) and similar adaptive problems (e.g. paternal uncertainty, paternal investment in offspring, cuckoldry), humans and some birds may have evolved similar solutions to these adaptive problems.

Forced in-pair copulation in non-human animals

Instances of forced in-pair copulation are relatively rare in the animal kingdom, primarily because males and females of most species (over 95 per cent) do not form long-term pair bonds (Andersson 1994). Without the formation of a pair bond, forced in-pair copulation, by definition, cannot occur. Many avian species form long-term pair bonds, and researchers have documented forced in-pair copulation in several of these species (Goodwin 1955; Cheng *et al.* 1983; Birkhead *et al.*1989). Forced in-pair copulation reliably occurs immediately after female extra-pair copulations, intrusions by rival males and female absence in many species of waterfowl (e.g. Cheng *et al.* 1983; McKinney *et al.* 1983) and other avian species (e.g. Goodwin 1955; Birkhead *et al.* 1989; Valera *et al.* 2003). Forced in-pair copulation following observed or suspected extra-pair copulation in these avian species is often interpreted as a sperm competition tactic (Cheng *et al.* 1983; Lalumière *et al.* 2005).

Sperm competition is a form of male-male post-copulatory competition. Sperm competition occurs when the sperm of two or more males concurrently occupy the reproductive tract of a female and compete to fertilize her egg(s) (Parker 1970). Males can compete for mates, but if two or more males have copulated with a female within a sufficiently short period of time, males must compete for fertilization. Thus, the observation that in many avian species forced in-pair copulation immediately follows female extra-pair copulations has been interpreted as a sperm competition tactic because the in-pair male's forced in-pair copulation functions to place his sperm in competition with sperm from an extra-pair male (Cheng et al. 1983; Birkhead et al. 1989). Reports of forced in-pair copulation in non-human species make it difficult to claim that males rape their partners to humiliate, punish or control them – as is often argued by some social scientists who study rape in humans (e.g. Pagelow 1988).

Mounting evidence suggests that sperm competition has been a recurrent and important feature of human evolutionary history. Psychological, behavioural, physiological, anatomical and genetic evidence indicates that ancestral women sometimes mated with multiple men within sufficiently short time periods so that sperm from two or more males concurrently occupied the reproductive tract of the woman (e.g. Smith 1984; Baker and Bellis 1993; Wyckoff et al. 2000; Pound 2002; Shackelford et al. 2002; Gallup et al. 2003; Goetz et al. 2005; Kilgallon and Simmons 2005; Shackelford and Goetz 2007). This adaptive problem led to the evolution of adaptive solutions to sperm competition. For example, men display copulatory urgency, perform semen-displacing behaviours, and adjust their ejaculates to include more sperm when the likelihood of female infidelity is higher (Baker and Bellis 1993; Shackelford et al. 2002; Goetz et al. 2005).

The selective importance of sperm competition in humans, however, is an issue of scholarly debate. Those questioning the application of sperm competition to humans (e.g. Dixson 1998; Birkhead 2000) do not contend that sperm competition in humans is not possible or unlikely, but that it may not be as intense as in other species with adaptations to sperm competition. When considering all the evidence of adaptations to sperm competition in men and current non-paternity rates (e.g. Bellis *et al.* 2005; Anderson 2006), it is reasonable to conclude that sperm competition may have been a recurrent and selectively important feature of human evolutionary history. Below, we discuss theory and research related to forced in-pair copulation in humans. In keeping with the established animal literature and a comparative evolutionary perspective, we often refer to partner rape in humans as forced in-pair copulation – the forceful act of sexual intercourse by a man against his partner's will.

Forced in-pair copulation in humans

Noting that instances of forced in-pair copulation follow extra-pair copulations in waterfowl and documentation that forced in-pair copulation in humans often follows accusations of female infidelity (e.g. Russell 1982; Finkelhor and Yllo 1985), Wilson and Daly (1992) suggested in a footnote that 'sexual insistence' in the context of a relationship might act as a sperm competition tactic in humans as well. Sexual coercion in response to cues of his partner's sexual infidelity might function to introduce a male's sperm into his partner's reproductive tract at a time when there is a high risk of cuckoldry.

Thornhill and Thornhill (1992) also hypothesized that forced in-pair copulation may function as an anti-cuckoldry tactic designed over human evolutionary history as a result of selective pressures associated with sperm competition. Thornhill and Thornhill argued that a woman who resists or avoids copulating with her partner might thereby be signalling to him that she has been sexually unfaithful and that the forced in-pair copulation functions to decrease his paternal uncertainty. Thornhill and Thornhill argued that the fact that the rape of a woman by her partner is more likely to occur during or after a break-up — times in which men express greatest concern about female sexual infidelity – provides preliminary support for the hypothesis. Thornhill and Thornhill, for example, cited research by Frieze (1983) indicating that women who were physically abused and raped by their husbands rated them to be more sexually jealous than did women who were abused but not raped. Similar arguments were presented by Thornhill and Palmer (2000) and Lalumière et al. (2005) suggesting that antisocial men who suspect that their female partner has been sexually unfaithful may be motivated to engage in forced in-pair copulation.

Both indirect and direct empirical evidence supporting this hypothesis has been documented. Frieze (1983) and Gage and Hutchinson (2006), for example, found that husbands who raped their wives were more sexually jealous than husbands who did not. Shields and Hanneke (1983) documented that victims of forced in-pair copulation were more likely to have reported engaging in extramarital sex than women who were not raped by their in-pair partner. Studying men's partner-directed insults, Starratt et al. (2007) found in two studies that a reliable predictor of a man's sexual coercion is his accusations of his partner's sexual infidelity. Specifically, men who accuse their partners of being unfaithful (endorsing items such as 'I accused my partner of having sex with many other men' and 'I called my partner a "whore" or a "slut" ') were more likely to sexually coerce them.

Direct empirical evidence supporting this hypothesis is accumulating. Camilleri (2004), for example, found that the risk of a partner's infidelity predicted sexual coercion among male participants but not female participants. It is biologically impossible for women to be cuckolded, so one would not expect women to have a sperm competition psychology that would generate sexually coercive behaviour in response to a partner's sexual infidelity. Goetz and Shackelford (2006) documented in two studies that a man's sexual coercion in the context of an intimate relationship is related positively to his partner's infidelities. According to men's self-reports and women's partner reports, men who used more sexual coercion in their relationship were partnered to women who had been, or were likely to be, unfaithful, and these men were also likely to use more mate-retention behaviours.

Because cuckoldry is associated with substantial reproductive costs for males of paternally investing species, men are expected to have evolved adaptations to address the adaptive problem of paternal uncertainty. One such adaptation may be a sperm competition tactic whereby sexual coercion and forced in-pair copulation function to increase the likelihood that the in-pair male, and not a rival male, sires the offspring that his partner might produce. It may be that a proportion of sexually coercive behaviours (in the context of an intimate relationship) are performed by antisocial men who aim to punish, humiliate or control their partners independent of their perception of cuckoldry risk. We are not arguing that all sexual coercion and forced in-pair copulations are the output of evolved mechanisms designed to reduce the risk of being cuckolded. Instead, we are suggesting that sexual coercion might sometimes be the result of male-evolved psychology associated with male sexual jealousy.

Conclusions

It is possible to study intimate partner violence with little or no knowledge of evolution. Most do. Those who study intimate partner violence from an evolutionary perspective often ask questions that are different from those asked by most clinical and forensic psychologists. Evolutionary psychologists are interested in ultimate (or distal) explanations, referring to the evolved function of a trait, behaviour or mechanism. This is in contrast to proximate explanations, which refer to the immediate causes of a trait, behaviour or mechanism. Although the explanations are different, they are compatible and equally important (Sherman and Alcock 1994). A fuller understanding of intimate partner violence will be reached when both ultimate and proximate explanations are provided.

8 Effective educational strategies

June Keeling

Introduction

The aim of this chapter is to explore some of the issues incumbent on educators when developing educational programmes for health care providers on the subject of intimate partner violence (IPV). The chapter does not advocate any specific educational programme but instead identifies some of the key concepts that should be considered when developing such a programme.

At national policy level, IPV and training in health services often remain segregated, despite the framing of both issues as essential components of health and the growing evidence connecting them to psychological and physical morbidity factors associated with survivors of the abuse. Despite all the rhetoric about evidence-based policy, the Department of Health in the UK states that 'all trusts should be moving towards routine enquiry' (DoH 2000, 2005), and the inclusion of IPV training being advocated by professional bodies, including the Royal College of Nursing (RCN 2004) and the Nursing and Midwifery Council (NMC 2004), educational programmes that explicitly address intimate partner abuse are seldom integrated into a pre-registration nursing programme or medical schools (Keeling and Birch 2002). In the USA, health professional organizations state that violence against women is a public health epidemic (Bryant and Spencer 2002). An endorsement by the American Medical Association and the American College of Obstetricians and Gynecologists (1995) that physicians should routinely enquire about domestic abuse with all female patients is equally rhetorical as research has demonstrated that on average only 10 per cent of physicians screen female patients for IPV (Rodriguez *et al.* 1999; Elliott *et al.* 2002).

It is generally accepted that the implementation of an educational programme specific to the dynamics of domestic abuse would be beneficial to health professionals and it is suggested that such a change would have a positive influence on rates of disclosure (Mezey and Bewley 1997; McGuigan *et al.* 2000; Keeling 2002). Indeed a recent research study by Lo Fo Wong in the Netherlands tested whether, following a 1.5-day training course for general practitioners (GPs), disclosure of partner violence increased (Wong *et al.* 2006). The resultant increased disclosure rates are an interesting phenomenon. The debate about routine enquiry into IPA is ongoing and detracts somewhat from the issues surrounding the development of effective and relevant educational programmes. Of course, educational programmes and protocol and policy for those disclosing are inextricably linked, but the development of an educational programme may be planned somewhat individually. Thus for the purpose of this chapter, the emphasis lies with the educational learning needs of the student and the key skills of the educationalist required to design and facilitate a relevant learning programme.

Curriculum development

Educators need to plan thoroughly, systematically and creatively to facilitate educational programmes which will inform and energize health professionals to empower and effectively support survivors of abuse. The programme needs to acknowledge the complexities of teaching an emotive subject such as IPV, the overlying issues of which may negate student learning, including personal experiences of domestic violence (victim/perpetrator), and misconceptions and misnomers which may have a direct effect on the student's learning experiences (Davison 1997). In the USA, it has been reported that annually there are 5.3 million incidents affecting women aged 18 and over, and 3.2 million incidents affecting men (Tjaden and Thoennes 2000a). Similar statistics in the UK demonstrate that 26 per cent of women have experienced IPV at some stage in their life. Globally, one in three women experiences some form of abuse (Garcia-Moreno *et al.* 2006). This therefore implies that the learning experience for many students may be encumbered by previous life experiences. The term 'student' refers to any individual undertaking formal study of an educational programme, pre- or post-registration, undergraduate or postgraduate.

A systematic construction to the educational programme is required to ensure that a logical and coherent evidenced-based approach to IPV is achieved (Aggleton and Chalmers 2000). An awareness of curriculum theory and how various programme designs are developed to assist adult learners is essential to maximize the adult learners' experiences and knowledge acquisition and prevent re-traumatization for those students who have experiences of abuse. Four simple components to designing a learning experience for students have been described as: determining the training needs; designing the programme; providing the teaching; and then evaluating the programme (Long 1983). A lengthy approach using nine stages has also been recognized (Houle 1972). However, a five-stage programme has been outlined by Boone (1985) incorporating: an understanding of the organization where the educational programme will be taught; linking with people and places; designing the programme; implementing the programme; and evaluating the programme. This appears to embrace a more holistic approach to IPV and the delivery of an educational programme in higher education institutions and clinical arenas. A unique aspect of the learning experience is the 'linking of people and places' to IPV, which can be translated into students' past experiences as survivors or perpetrators. Caution is required to prevent re-traumatization. However, a skilled facilitator can support the student who chooses to share his or her experiences in order to process some of these events and constructively utilize those experiences in the learning process. This can relate to experiences of statutory and voluntary agencies within the community that play a vital role in providing support. Some survivors of abuse access an educational programme as a cathartic process. Therefore, the presence of, and rapid access to, support networks is fundamental when delivering any IPV programme.

There appears to be a disparity between professional bodies' recommendations and practice in the educational arena. Most educational programmes involving IPV are taught as a 'stand alone' lecture, in isolation from the rest of a curriculum. This may leave students with inadequate skills and knowledge that are removed from the learner's clinical practice, thereby losing any impact in terms of progressive learning (Alpert *et al.* 1998). The student may be prevented from achieving higher cognitive and affective taxonomies (Reece and Walker 2003). Ideally, IPV should be a *recurrent theme* throughout any training programme for health providers, a constant thread, woven into all the theoretical and practical components of the curriculum.

Having a symbiotic relationship, the theoretical component of any educational programme will have a direct impact on the associated skill acquisition involved in the practical element. A philosophical approach to IPV is crucial to bring about this symbiosis. A further benefit of this approach is the anticipated strengthening and higher achievement in the cognitive and affective taxonomies reached by the students on completion of the module (Reece and Walker 2003). The philosophical approach may lie between experimentalism and reconstructionism. Reconstruction-ism issues are central to the tenet of domestic violence which revolves around inequality and dominance, and control of one person over another. Although the purpose of these two approaches differs, an inclusion of parts of both may be appropriate. In terms of experimentalism, the educative qualities need to be planned to enable the students to understand their own life experiences of abuse and then relate them to the theoretical underpinning of IPV (Uys and Gwele 2005).

Groups

Having had the privilege of working alongside key facilitators in New Zealand on behalf of the New Zealand College of Midwives, I was able to co-facilitate their excellent approach to group work utilizing role play. Using given scenarios, health providers (in this instance midwives) worked in groups of three, one taking the role of the health provider, one being the client who embraces the role of a survivor of abuse, and one being an observer to the interaction between the 'nurse' and the 'client'. Each member of the group rotates through each role. I have found this approach promotes a deeper understanding of the challenges faced by health providers in the provision of support, and by survivors in their struggle to voice their experiences.

Group interaction, discussion and debate need to be carefully facilitated, and when utilized in conjunction with reflective practice can be an effective strategy to turn the students' experiences into learning (Boud *et al.* 1985). The ideological advantage of group work is that skills required for supporting a survivor of abuse can be developed in the classroom and replicated in the clinical environment by utilizing role play. Effective group work has been described as work comprising of two or more individuals who interact with each other, and are aware of the other members as they all strive towards a common goal (Johnson and Johnson 2003). Reece and Walker (2003) further endorse this approach by stating that it may enable learners to reach higher cognitive and affective taxonomies. The utilization of life events may indeed result in a greater depth of learning for the students. A fundamental element of learning involves behaviour change which can be achieved through reflective practice and analysis of past events (Mackintosh and Colman 1995). This approach is mirrored by the humanistic approach as described by Rogers, who believed that education should facilitate the process of change in an individual so that she or he may function fully (Rogers 1983). Indeed, learning has also been defined as 'the transformation of experience into knowledge, skills, attitudes, emotions, values, beliefs, senses etc.' (Jarvis 1995: 58).

Behaviour changes can be challenging to the student, in particular to those health providers whose behaviour may have remained unchallenged for many years. I remember vividly that having worked as a midwife for 15 years, I heard an older colleague state that the women she cared for in her locality were 'not the type of women to experience IPV'. This dreadful stereotyping can only do harm and resonates the inadequate service offered by all too many health providers.

The facilitation of group work is essential to prevent one student dominating or intimidating the other students and to encourage an equal participation and contribution from all (Brookfield 1990). It can become problematical if a student chooses to utilize the group work as a cathartic process for their past experiences of IPV and dominates the group. Rogers identifies that the principle role of the educationalist is to allow a student to learn in order to satisfy their appetite for knowledge (Rogers 1983), and to enhance the depth of learning students should be encouraged to utilize their own experiences and, through the process of reflection, identify positive changes to their clinical practice (Alexander *et al.* 1994). It is the responsibility of the educator/facilitator to ensure all students have an equal opportunity to learn and contribute. The services of a student support department or occupational health department should offer support to students who feel they require individual assistance or counselling. Adult learning is complex and by utilizing a humanistic approach the facilitator can work alongside the students in an atmosphere of mutual respect, with a resultant unity of working towards a shared goal (Rogers 1983). Reflective listening and the synthesis of information are crucial in the response to survivors of abuse (Bolstad *et al.* 1992). Therefore students need to be taught these skills and knowledge in order to begin to synthesize and reflect on information, and to understand the insidious effect that IPV has on a family.

Health professionals in contemporary society are expected to be able to demonstrate evidence-based clinical excellence while simultaneously demonstrating empathy, exercising professional judgement and working within a professional code of conduct (NMC 2004). When studying IPV, students should be expected to demonstrate an ability to support survivors of abuse in complex situations when there may be conflicts of interest (e.g. child protection concerns versus a mother's wishes to return to an abusive partner). Unlike many educational programmes in nursing curricula or medicine, where the student learns to 'perfect' a skill (e.g. phlebotomy or hand-washing), or demonstrate their knowledge of a subject (e.g. health promotion), when supporting a survivor of domestic abuse it may be necessary to initially offer support but in actuality do nothing if the survivor of abuse so chooses, after a risk assessment and assessment of child protection issues. This often creates a paradox with the health professional who is so used to 'doing'. Empirically this appears to be a challenge for many students undertaking formal educational programmes on IPV. Piaget and Dewey both state that people develop philosophically and psychologically (Piaget and Inhelder 1969; Dewey 1997), with Kohlberg (1969) adding that moral reasoning also progresses. Thus the student will develop and gradually accept that it may only be appropriate to listen to a survivor, depending on their request and circumstances.

A plethora of reasons why health providers fail to enquire about IPV, even when there is compelling evidence to suggest the client is being abused, have been cited. They include fear of offending the client, lack of self-confidence, inadequate training and lack of time in clinical situations (Hathaway *et al.* 2002; Keeling 2002; Bacchus *et al.* 2003). Public health nurses consider that asking about domestic abuse is within their professional remit, but in a study by Shepard *et al.* (1999) only 24 per cent of nurses felt able to discuss this subject and concerns were identified that more training was required. Perhaps the most significant deterrent for disclosing domestic abuse is a deficiency in the interpersonal skills of the health care professional due to a lack of knowledge and understanding of the issues surrounding IPV, which may result in them appearing insincere, ineffectual and even a danger (i.e. they may take inappropriate action and unwittingly place the survivor of abuse in more danger than if they had not disclosed) (Chambliss *et al.* 1995; Hathaway *et al.* 2002).

Assessment strategies

The assessment criteria must be designed to meet the academic rigour demanded by the relevant professional body in the country where the programme is being delivered. Assessment of learning has been described as 'the means used to measure what students have learned' (Eaton 2001). The assessment criteria may be formative or summative. It is useful to develop the assessment criteria to ascertain how acquired knowledge from the module can be applied to the student's individual working environment. The student should be able to demonstrate appropriate application of their knowledge, analysis of current literature, and the ability to synthesize a preset topic that is pertinent to their individual workplace at the appropriate level of study (Quinn 2000). However, a theoretical assessment criterion disregards the necessary assessment of the skill acquisition which is vital to effectively support a survivor of domestic abuse in the clinical arena.

A written assignment would demonstrate the acquisition of theoretical knowledge in relation to practice, however in order to assess students' approach in responding to a survivor of domestic abuse with the newly-acquired/developed practical skills, a skills-based assessment via an objective structured clinical examination (OSCE) should be considered. It has been identified that this method of assessing is one of the fairest for the students as it is an objective assessment against preset criteria, thus increasing the validity of the assessment (Maden 1997). The true value of this form of assessment is that all learners who reach the required standard can demonstrate that they have at least achieved a minimum standard which it is anticipated will enhance their confidence in clinical practice (Eaton 2001). Furthermore, the assessment enables early detection of difficulties being experienced by a student, following which remedial action can be taken (Nicklin and Kenworthy 1996). This is particularly relevant to a module involving domestic abuse where 1 in 4 women and 1 in 12 men have experienced family violence at some stage in their life (Lovendski and Randall 1993) and where the personal experiences of abuse may have a direct effect on students' learning (Davison 1997). These difficulties would be apparent during an OSCE but not necessarily in a written assessment.

A multi-professional approach

It is widely acknowledged that survivors of IPV benefit from effective multi-professional collaboration (Bacchus *et al.* 2003; Sully *et al.* 2005). This approach has also been advocated by both researchers and government departments alike (e.g. Home Office 1998; Bacchus *et al.* 2003) and has been further endorsed by survivors of abuse (Sully 2002). Co-facilitation of an educational programme of IPV should be representative of both statutory and voluntary organizations, including members of the police service, women's refuge services, alcohol and drug services, maternity providers, social workers, public health nurses and the judiciary. Although this list is far from exhaustive, it does identify some of the key personnel required in the provision of a holistic educational programme. Each representative should identify their role in the support of survivors of abuse and how they collaborate with the other agencies. This approach is central to the efficacy of any intervention programme which lies adjacent to an educational programme. The benefits of multi professional working cannot be overstated.

Conclusions

The health service is unique as it is often perceived to be a 'safe place' for survivors of abuse, even though this has been disproven many times. The author has witnessed curtains being drawn around a client and the partner claiming 'she likes her privacy'. This was not the case but rather to enable the abuse to continue. Similarly, a patient who had been critically ill in intensive care then improved and was moved to a high dependency unit. There, she was forced to sign for her state benefit by her threatening and abusive partner.

As educationalists we understand how adult learners learn and it is our responsibility to work with caregivers to promote the most effective educational programme that addresses the learning needs of the students in respect of the complexities of IPV.

It is our responsibility to develop an appropriate educational programme to meet the needs of both the adult learners in a clinical arena and subsequently the needs of abuse survivors.

Debate continues on the appropriateness of routine enquiry concerning IPV. While we await a definitive answer it must be acknowledged that the lack of education and training for health care providers is having a detrimental effect on survivors who choose to disclose. The role of the health provider in the provision of appropriate support for and the empowerment of survivors is paramount and in its absence leaves this vulnerable group of people with possible adverse outcomes through negligence and inappropriate advice.

Part two
Reaction

9 The impact of the cultural context on the experience of domestic violence

Marianne R. Yoshioka

Introduction

Over the past decade, increasing attention has been given to cultural variations in the experience of domestic violence. For example, Rabin *et al.* (1999) studied the differences in domestic violence experiences of Jewish and Arab women, reporting that the difference in cultures shaped differences in experience. Tran and DesJardins (2000) focused attention on Vietnamese and Korean American battered women, identifying similarities and differences in their experiences. McClusky (1999) has documented cultural variations in the partner abuse experiences of indigenous women in Belize, acknowledging the powerful influence of the cultural, economic and political context. Finally, Finkler (1997) detailed the culturally unique experiences of women in Mexico living with partner abuse, identifying cultural and systemic barriers to addressing the abuse. This literature has been invaluable in articulating the needs and perspective of particular groups. However, what is missing is a more holistic understanding of the ways in which the cultural context of individual ethnic groups may be understood. Extrapolating from the existing research, along what dimensions does the experience of domestic violence vary? Because many cultural groups have not been targeted in this ethno-specific approach, we have been left with gaps in the knowledge base. Increasingly, as scholars, researchers and practitioners, we have had to answer for ourselves what meaningful cultural differences in the experience of domestic violence look like.

The goal of this chapter is to describe a model to explain the ways in which the cultural context impacts on the experience of domestic violence. By adopting a culture-general approach, a framework will be described that identifies and organizes aspects of the cultural context across groups. This work stems from existing research that suggests that the cultural context status will influence the type of violence a woman experiences, a woman's perception of the options that are available to her to address the violence, and to whom she reaches out for help. This framework is based on years of research with battered Asian immigrant women. Based upon qualitative and quantitative research, three contextual factors have been identified that can help practitioners and researchers to understand how domestic violence experiences vary by cultural group. These factors are: (a) individual versus collectivist orientation; (b) relationship with host society; and (c) social traditions. While this framework was developed based on research with Asian immigrant women, it is highly informed by the practice and research literature addressing multiple cultural communities. As such, it may be applicable to all women living with domestic violence. This framework is useful for identifying questions about how the cultural context influences the behavioural and mental health outcomes of women living with violence. It can help to guide the development of effective assessment and intervention strategies to address cultural differences. By developing an understanding of how the cultural context impacts a woman's experience of domestic violence, practitioners and researchers will be better prepared to understand their clients' situations.

Why is the cultural context important?

This work begins with the assumption that understanding the sociocultural context is critical when working with culturally different women, because it is the lens through which abuse is defined and options for change are weighed (Kawamoto 2001). Based on focus groups with adults from four ethnic groups – African American, Anglo American, Mexican American and Korean American – Sorenson (1996) documented the ways by which sociocultural factors converged to shape women's experience of violence and their perceived options to address it. The multiple contexts of social and economic inequity, immigration and culture were identified as powerful backdrops to understanding interpersonal relationships. For example, within these contexts, the study participants struggled to understand American conceptions of abuse. They discussed their hesitancy to involve the police in private matters, their lack of resources, and the unwelcoming or discriminatory treatment they received from formal service providers. Religious institutions and belief systems may both provide solace *and* constrain women from acting independently. Sorenson concludes that ethnicity, immigration and beliefs about gender and marriage are key variables to understanding women's experience of partner abuse.

Drawing on work such as Sorenson's, we can begin to distil the elements of culture and the critical related variables of acculturation and immigration that are important to a woman's experience of partner abuse. Culture has been defined most broadly as a way of life determined by prescribed norms of behaviour, beliefs, values and skills (Gordon 1978). It is comprised of a myriad of rules governing social protocol and the maintenance of important traditions and rituals. Knowledge of these rules is critical to performing in culturally appropriate ways. A disregard of them can result in insult and/or humiliation.

A framework to understand the impact of culture

Understanding the ways by which culture shapes a woman's experience of domestic violence requires us to adopt an ecological perspective. This perspective focuses the woman's situation within the multiple environments that influence her perception, her resources and her cultural belief systems. A woman living with violence is embedded in complex cultural systems that impact her emotional and problem-solving processes, family, peer, community and institutional responses, and community beliefs of gender and power.

Guided by Bronfenbrenner's (1977) ecological model, there are three primary systems within which a woman defines what is abusive and what will be helpful. The 'micro-system' represents those elements of the woman's environment that directly influence, or are influenced by, her. This includes her immediate and extended family and her informal support network. The 'exo-system' represents elements of a woman's environment that have indirect influences on her functioning and resources. This system includes characteristics of cultural community (e.g. how large it is, how well established it is, whether there are culturally specific resources available to her), and her relationship with the host country in terms of citizenship status. The 'macro-system' represents those cultural beliefs and values that influence women's perceptions and choices through their impact on elements of the other systems. This system may include culturally informed beliefs and attitudes about gender, marital roles and partner violence. It also includes culturally informed social protocols through which respect and structure are communicated. Within these three systems, a woman ascribes meaning to her experiences and her choices. She brings into this system her own sense of identity and value of the roles of wife and mother, her culturally influenced coping style and her attitudes toward help-seeking. By adopting an ecological perspective, we are able to examine the multiple and simultaneous influences of the culture context.

Understanding the impact of the cultural context

Primacy of the individual or the group

Extensive research has identified the constructs of individualism and collectivism as the single most powerful dimensions by which to understand cultural differences in social behaviour (Triandis 1995). Collectivist cultures are characterized by a deep value placed on interdependent relationships within social groups. The goals of the group are given priority over individual goals and individual behaviour is shaped primarily by group norms. As such, social behaviour is regulated by duty and obligation.

Individualist cultures place an emphasis on independence. Accordingly, a person's behaviour is deeply shaped by individual-level attitudes and preferences (Triandis and Suh 2002). Ting-Toomey (1988) has argued that when members of an individualist culture like the USA are engaged in an interpersonal conflict, they will behave in ways that will save their own sense of face. In contrast, members of collectivist cultures will behave in ways to save the face of others. As a result, individuals from collectivist cultures tend to prefer passive and collaborative conflict resolution strategies that will maintain relationships even when there are personal costs (Ohbuchi *et al.* 1999). In individualist cultures, high personal costs justify the breaking of the relationship (Kim 1994). Members of an individualist culture prefer more assertive, confrontational and possibly adversarial approaches to achieve equity, because justice is given priority over relationship.

Interwoven with these concepts of collectivism and individualism is the 'tightness' or 'looseness' of the culture – that is, the level of tolerance of diverse behaviour. In tight collectivist cultures there are specific norms and rules that regulate social interaction and there are strong negative consequences for individuals who deviate from role-prescribed behaviour. These consequences typically take the form of shame and loss of face for oneself and one's family. In looser cultures, there is much greater tolerance for behavioural variation (Triandis and Suh 2002), as definitions of normative behaviour become more broad. In loose individualist cultures there is greater acceptance of women taking on a wider variety of roles (e.g. living independently outside of a marriage), and behaving in ways that address their own needs and desires.

If these concepts are coupled with the research into stigma disclosure, much can be learned about how the individualist-collectivist orientation of a culture and its tightness or looseness impacts a woman's experience of domestic violence. Research on stigma disclosure has found that decisions to share personal information are based on the topic of the disclosure and the social acceptability of being perceived outside of normative bounds (e.g. Serovich 2001). It is for these reasons, for example, that disclosure of sexual abuse among Puerto Rican females is particularly stigmatized by strong cultural values of virginity (Fontes 1993). In a culture where female virginity at the time of marriage is highly valued, there is a social penalty for deviating from this expectation for any reason.

In tight collectivist cultures, a disclosure of domestic violence is particularly stigmatizing because it requires the woman to place herself, the abusive partner and, by association, their families, outside normative roles and behaviour. In most cultures, marriage and motherhood occupy a central location in the role of a woman and are important vehicles for women to accrue status (e.g. Gillespie 2000). In tight collectivist cultures a disclosure that threatens these roles is weighed carefully against living with violence. This point is well illustrated by my findings (Yoshioka 2001a) based on a community sample of Korean American adults living in the metropolitan area of Boston, Massachusetts. Almost 29 per cent of this immigrant sample of 103 men and women recommended keeping the violence a secret as the best option for a battered woman and her family. What is implied is that the social cost to the woman and her family is high enough to warrant secrecy.

In an examination of the experience of violence in the lives of South Asian women, Yoshioka *et al.* (2003) found that in many cases the abusive partner and/or his family members threatened the woman with divorce. In the tight, collectivist culture from which these women come, the threat of divorce is part of the abusive process because a divorce brings a powerful loss of face for the woman, her parents, and very possibly her sisters, whose marriage potential may be diminished. There is little acceptance for a woman whose husband is alive to live independently with children outside of a marriage. Similar findings have been reported for Jewish and

Arab women (e.g. Adelman 2000). Women coming from tight collectivist cultures may not readily perceive independence as a possible or desirable outcome. Rather it may be viewed as an extraordinary cost.

These experiences lie in contrast to those for women coming from looser collectivist cultures where there is greater variation in religious influences and women's roles and rights. For example, within Jamaican immigrant communities, a woman living with children independent of a husband or father is one of the many accepted family configurations for a woman (Francis 2001). Because the norms for women's behaviour are broader, the meaning and implications of a threat of divorce for a Jamaican woman are different than for an Arab woman.

Developing a keen understanding of a woman's cultural orientation will help to evaluate the real costs and benefits they must face when making decisions about addressing domestic violence in their lives. There may be real differences in the options available to women, depending on whether they come from a loose, individualistic culture or a tight, collectivist one.

Relationship to the host society

A second key way that the cultural context shapes a woman's experience of domestic violence is her immigration, colonization and/or acculturation status. These all impact on the relationship between a woman and the host society in terms of her legal standing (i.e. eligibility for assistance programmes and employment opportunities), the size of the cultural community with which she identifies, her familiarity with social, political and cultural systems, and the real and perceived receptiveness of these systems to the woman.

'Immigration' is a powerful, long-term process that is often complicated by the stress of financial strain, the loss of a stable and geographically accessible social support network, lack of language fluency and lack of social familiarity (e.g. Mehta 1998). It is through these mechanisms that immigration status may not only exacerbate a woman's risk of partner abuse (e.g. Erez 2000) but may also be a *source* of abusive behaviour. 'Colonization' refers to a process whereby individuals from one society force those from another to live within their own cultural context. It is applicable in circumstances of forced migration (i.e. slavery) and uninvited national expansion (e.g. Europeans in North America). The literature documenting the legacy of colonization on indigenous people has shown that community trauma, loss, and forced social disorganization impact on the individual experience of partner abuse (e.g. Kawamoto 2001). The legacy of oppression and racism continues to alter family and community dynamics (e.g. Brownridge 2003) for generations post-independence (Kebede 2001). Finally, 'acculturation' is a complex social process that is initiated when members of one cultural group are exposed over an extended period of time to members of another (Laroche *et al.* 1998). It refers to the adoption of the values, preferences and behaviours of the host society (e.g. Williams and Berry 1991). Although, over time, individuals within the colonized community may experience a shift in values to those of the dominant society (i.e. acculturation), this process occurs within a racist context (Weaver 2001). Similar to immigration, the colonization experience defines the individual's relationship to the host society in terms of legal standing, state eligibility, and social and language fluency. However, it carries with it a significant psychological process of self-devaluation as messages of the racist environment are internalized.

How a woman came to be in a country is an important dimension to understanding the impact of the cultural context on the domestic violence experience. The experience of partner violence and the options available to a battered woman are different if she is a highly acculturated citizen from a non-colonized group, if she is an immigrant of 20 years in a large cultural community, if she is a recent refugee who has relocated into a small cultural community, or if she is a member of a community that has been subjugated across generations. There is a range of individual- and community-level factors that vary across these dimensions. The individual factors involve her fluency with social services, her perceptions of mobility within the environment, and her ability to speak the language of the majority. They include her experiences of the receptivity of formal support systems to her concerns, and the number of family members available to her locally and nationally. The community factors include the availability of social services in her first language, the level of privacy within the community that she can expect when seeking assistance, the types of services that she can receive, and the historical relationship between her community and the helping professions, including law enforcement and faith-based organizations.

Beyond shaping alternatives to domestic violence, immigration status itself may pose risks of certain kinds of abusive acts. There is growing documentation of the direct link between immigration status and the types of violence to which a woman is exposed. This is most commonly found in situations where the woman has a more tenuous immigration status than the abusive partner. In many cases, because the partner has more secure legal status, has a greater familiarity with the host nation's social systems, and/or is more fluent in the national language, an immigrant woman must rely upon him and others to navigate her environment. Immigration-related abusive behaviours include: taking a woman's passport and refusing to return it to her; threatening to report the woman for deportation; refusing to file applications for residency or threatening to withdraw applications; threatening to take the children out of the country; and lying to her about her immigration status (e.g. Yoshioka 2001b).

Social traditions

The third and final way to understand the impact that the culture context may have on a woman's experience of domestic violence is to examine specific cultural social protocols and traditions and their involvement in the violence experience. Social traditions refer to culturally specific obligations, duties and rituals associated with social situations. For example, traditions of gift-giving, dowry or bride price (e.g. Olatubosun 2001) at the time of marriage, culturally-based rules or norms of sexual intimacy within marriage (Cwik 1995), use of honorific titles (e.g. Wang 1990), and treating others in keeping with their social role. All follow social protocols. An understanding of culturally informed social traditions and obligations can facilitate the identification of culturally specific forms of abuse and/or the ways that sociocultural tradition may facilitate the violence.

For example, in Asian cultures, mothers-in-law occupy a unique position of power and authority over the brides of their sons (e.g. Nakazawa 1996). Traditionally, the role of the mother-in-law was to train the 'junior wife' in how to care for her husband and the household (Masuda 1975). Yoshioka (2001a, 2001b) found in interviews with 110 South Asian battered women that 25 per cent reported severe forms of psychological assault by their in-law parents including having their possessions destroyed. Additionally, 25 per cent reported having been punched, beaten up, or having had their arms or hair twisted or pulled by their mothers-in-law.

The power relationship between mothers- and daughters-in-law is found in other cultural communities in addition to those of Asia. Mitchell (1994) reports that in some cultural segments of Peru, older female relatives occupy positions of unmitigated authority over younger ones. Similarly, this culturally sanctioned arrangement can lead to abuse (Mitchell 1994). Simic (1983) discusses the same power relationship in Slav families. Nested with dual systems of patriarchy and familism, a woman's status and power increases as her son ages and gains the power attributed to a man. The mother-in-law is able to wield her power over the other younger woman.

Hassouneh-Phillips (2001, 2003) describes the ways in which the religious beliefs of Muslim women can be used to facilitate domestic violence and create forms of abuse unique to these women. Women's powerful beliefs in accruement of spiritual rewards for the acceptance of suffering and an unblemished performance of one's family roles in the face of domestic violence leads them to strive to be uncomplaining, patient and accepting. Hassouneh-Phillips documents the men's manipulation of sociocultural protocols to create culturally unique forms of abuse. In some cases, the abusive partners were found to misrepresent portions of the Koranic text to exert control over their wives. In other cases, they engaged in the practice of polygamy in discordance with Islamic dictates and in ways to humiliate the first wife (Hassouneh-Phillips 2001). This included marrying the wife's sister, unequal treatment of the wives, and forcing a wife to participate in the marriage ceremony to a co-wife. In some instances, the co-wife was also a perpetrator of abuse.

A deep understanding of the culturally informed social rules, protocols and expectations for personal conduct by which women live their lives can help practitioners to view domestic violence from a multi-cultural perspective. If mainstream definitions of abuse are the only lens through which behaviour is understood, much of the complex and culturally unique dynamics of domestic violence will be missed.

Conclusions

The experience of domestic violence is a complicated one, made more so by culturally based differences in beliefs, preferences and behaviours. In this chapter, a model has been presented to understand the three primary ways by which cultural differences may manifest themselves. Practitioners working with culturally diverse populations may use this model to better understand the ways in which cultural influences impact not only the type of violence and abuse a woman has experienced but how she understands who can help her and her choices. Its value is as an organizing framework, bringing together both the micro and macro manifestations of culture and requiring the practitioner to place his or her focus as much on the larger systems of family and community within which a battered woman resides as on the woman herself.

Practitioners should begin by understanding where the immigrant community is situated on the individualist-collectivist continuum and its relative tightness or looseness. To do this will require the social worker to seek out cultural consultants and other experts, spend time in the community, and listen carefully to the priorities and values embedded in his or her clients' stories. This information will shed light on the pressures to which a client is responding, the kind of responses she will feel are most appropriate, and to whom she feels accountable.

Practitioners must accept that there are powerful dynamics that are set in motion by one's relationship to the host society, as this defines opportunity, familiarity and receptivity. We should develop an understanding of the migration and/or colonization history of a client's cultural community. Determining the size and longevity of the community will help the practitioner to understand client concerns of privacy and the availability of within-culture services. Conceptualizing a client's experience of domestic violence within the context of colonization is an important step toward understanding the reality of her situation.

Finally, practitioners must be attentive to the myriad of ways that violence and abuse may manifest themselves. Mainstream measures of domestic violence are important tools, yet they will not identify behaviours and threats that have meaning only within the cultural context. Practitioners working with specific cultural communities must document these culturally unique forms of abuse for the education of others.

One of the inherent dilemmas of an examination of cultural differences pertains to the decision of what to do about them. Do we seek to understand so that we may help our clients to fit into our system better? Clearly, with support and information, women from many different cultural communities have used the law enforcement options available to them, learning to live independently and free from violence. Or do we change our systems to meet our clients' needs better? In the USA, the system of services offered to women living with abuse is oriented toward living independently of the abusive partner. This is a critical service that has undoubtedly saved the lives of thousands of women. In many areas of Asia, models of community mediation are used to address family disputes, including cases of domestic violence and in some cases the result of the mediation is divorce (Madaripur Legal Aid Association 1996). This is not to suggest that all situations of domestic violence should be handled in this manner, but to illustrate that from a collectivist perspective there are ways to address domestic violence that involve both sides of the family and individuals influential in the community.

The ultimate answer is that we must do both. At present, most of our efforts are spent helping our clients to fit into our system better. Questions for the helping professions are whether we can conceive of other responses that equally ensure a woman's safety. If we embrace collectivist values to what extent would such an approach better serve our many and diverse client populations?

10 The political, societal and personal interface of abuse

Senator Anne Cools

Introduction

As a Canadian senator born in the British West Indies, I am pleased to contribute to this book in the sincere hope that some will use it to advance their knowledge of, and their responses to, those difficult human problems which attend intimate relationships. I am indebted to the international leaders on domestic violence, in whose work the treatment and study of family violence originated. In particular, I thank Erin Pizzey, who in England in the early 1970s founded the world's first women's shelter, and Dr Murray Straus, an American who in the USA initiated the research into and scholarship on domestic violence. Their contributions are truly remarkable. About her initial experiences at her shelter, on 5 July 1998, Erin Pizzey wrote in *The Observer*: 'Of the first 100 women coming into the refuge, 62 were as violent as the partners they had left. Not only did they admit their violence in the mutual abuse that took place in their homes, but the women were abusive to their children' (Pizzey 1998: 24).

Dr Straus, in his article 'Physical assaults by wives: a major social problem' in the 1993 book, *Current Controversies on Family Violence*, wrote about his and his colleagues' work on the National Family Violence Survey: 'Of the 495 couples in the 1985 National Family Violence Survey for whom one or more assaultive incidents were reported by a woman respondent, the husband was the only violent partner in 25.9% of the cases, the wife was the only one to be violent in 25.5% of the cases, and both were violent in 48.6% of the cases' (Straus 1993: 74).

The foremost American scholars, Dr Murray Straus, Dr Richard Gelles, Dr Susan Steinmetz and Dr Jan Stets have found symmetry and reciprocity in rates of violence between men and women. In Canada, their findings have been confirmed by Canadian scholars Dr Donald Dutton, Dr Kim Bartholomew, Dr Marilyn Kwong, Dr Eugen Lupri, Dr Merlin Brinkerhoff and others. Canada's pre-eminent scholar Dr Donald Dutton wrote about these data in an article entitled 'Transforming a flawed policy: a call to revive psychology and science in domestic violence research and practice'. Critical of the prevailing American Duluth model, he said: 'Most professionals are still unaware of these data patterns. In fact, in many states a court mandated "intervention programme" that specifically eschews psychological treatment is in place, based on the notion that interpersonal partner violence is a form of gender oppression akin to slavery ... ' (Dutton and Corvo 2006: 460).

In writing, I offer my experience working with families in the 1970s and 1980s as the Canadian pioneer in social services, assisting families afflicted by domestic violence. I say 'families' because my helping work has always included men. Simultaneously, from 1980 to 1984, I also served on the National Parole Board and denied, granted and revoked paroles to many inmates, some in certain domestic homicides then called 'passion crimes'. I also offer my work as a senator, especially on the divorce law, which, like the criminal law, has been ravaged by ideological, mean-spirited and misandrous practices. My perspective is that of balance, fairness and equilibrium, grounded in the notion that human beings and human relationships are extremely complex, and that intimate family relationships involve personal vulnerabilities, elusive dynamics and multiple emotions. Managing human relations and human dynamics is challenging even for the well-equipped personality. For the not so well-equipped, managing human relations is daunting and sometimes nearly impossible. Life and human intimacy is a difficult road for many. Human emotions such as love, anger, expectations and disappointments are driving forces. Human needs and human emotions are compelling. Human complexity is further complicated by the fact that human beings frequently have little or no understanding of what and why they feel, and little or no insight into the effects of their own behaviour on those with whom they live. Jesuit priest Father Thomas Green, in his 1984 book, *Weeds Among the Wheat*, employs Jacques Guillet's work on personal discernment (Guillet 1970). Father Green quotes Guillet: ' ... there is the darkness in man himself who is incapable of seeing his own heart clearly, incapable of grasping completely the seriousness of his actions and the results deriving from them ... ' (Green 1984: 29).

On observing human behaviour, the inescapable conclusion is that human beings, both men and women, are afflicted by their own imperfections, frailities and woundedness. This condition governs most human behaviour. Interestingly, the more imperfect and wounded a person is, the less tolerant that person is of imperfection and woundedness in others. Human capacity for misunderstanding is great. Men and women are equally capable of vice and virtue. Vice and virtue are human characteristics not gendered ones. I have politically repudiated the too-prevalent notion introduced into the public discourse by radical gender feminist ideology that women are morally superior to men, that men are morally inferior to women and that somehow men are naturally morally defective. The false proposition of women's inherent virtue and men's inherent vice has dominated and deformed family and criminal law policy for the past three decades. Much public policy on domestic violence, particularly arrest, charging and prosecuting policy, has been founded on this deformity, wreaking havoc in the lives of people, most of whom are ill-prepared and ill-equipped to handle such havoc. These policies have bequeathed incalculable pain and suffering and unspeakable tragedy. The empirical evidence on violence within intimate partner relationships and within families confirms that domestic violence has been falsely framed as violence against women and as a gender issue, a women's question. Men and women are equally capable of violence and aggression, and have perpetrated them on each other for centuries. Violence and aggression are a pathology of intimate relations, not a pathology of the male of the species.

In the 1970s, Erin Pizzey broke new ground. She introduced to the world the notion that domestic violence was a social problem needing the attention of policy-makers, government, helping professionals and academics. Having started the world's first shelter for women and children fleeing violent homes, she soon thereafter wrote the first popular book on domestic violence, *Scream Quietly or the Neighbours Will Hear* (Pizzey and Forbes 1974). Pizzey had great influence in Canada and the USA. During the 1970s in Canada, I created the first of my two shelters in Toronto. I also assisted in the creation of many other shelters in Ontario, working successfully with municipal and provincial governments on funding formulas and operating standards for them. In 1977, with the Ontario Institute for Studies in Education, I organized Canada's first conference on domestic violence, 'Couples in Conflict'. Its featured speaker was Dr Richard Gelles, who had studied with Dr Murray Straus. I endeavoured to advance the public consciousness of the undesirability of family violence, and, simultaneously, lobby for public support for the amelioration of those who suffered. This work led me to enter federal electoral politics as a candidate in the 1979 federal general election with Pierre Elliott Trudeau, then prime minister of Canada. In 1984, when inviting me to join the Senate of Canada, Mr Trudeau asked for and received my promise that I would maintain my work with families in conflict. This was an easy pledge for me to make.

By the late 1980s, the 1970s' humanistic concerns about close relationships had succumbed to radical gender feminist ideology. Family relationships and man-woman intimate relations became battle grounds, subject to the ideological notions known as 'the patriarchy' and 'men's power and control over women'. Public policy and the administration of justice took a terrible turn away from helping and healing families and towards persecuting and punishing men – in a word, coercion. 'Battered women's syndrome', 'recovered memory syndrome', 'Svengali influence' and other empirically questionable, even dubious phenomena, dominated the legal consciousness. Some, with whom I disagree, called it 'feminist theory'. Mere accusations of physical or sexual assault were treated as *findings*. Some ideologues even argued that, based on women's credibility, mere accusations of violence were sufficient to obtain convictions. This atmosphere fostered the growth of much unscrupulous behaviour, often rewarded by awards of spousal support, child support and exclusive possession of the family residence. False accusations abounded. Wrongful convictions were plentiful. It was a dark era in human relations, particularly male-to-female relations. Radical feminist ideological orthodoxy prevailed. It was all very simple: women were angels and men were devils. Any person – social worker, academic, lawyer or judge – who questioned the orthodoxy faced derision and career ruination in very nasty and mean-spirited public circumstances.

Patriarchy, heterosexism and the feminist lens: the menace of ideology for families and its wreckage

Around 1990, the government of Canada sponsored a multi-million dollar project called the 'Canadian Panel on Violence Against Women'. Its 1993 report was named *Changing the Landscape: Ending Violence – Achieving Equality*. Its titles and subtitles were steeped in radical feminist nomenclature. Part 1 was called 'The context' and Chapter 1 was entitled 'The feminist lens'. Chapter 1 also contained a section called 'Looking through a feminist lens'. Another section was called 'Patriarchy and violence' while another was entitled 'Heterosexism'. The report informed that the concept of patriarchy was essential to the Panel's analysis of the nature of gender inequality and violence against women (Canadian Panel on Violence Against Women 1993: 14). The report explained patriarchy thus: 'Patriarchy is not just a central concept in feminist analysis. For many women it is also a daily reality – the most violent and profound expression of patriarchal power sits at their dinner tables every evening and sleeps in their beds at night' (p. 17).

The report described heterosexism: 'Heterosexism is the assumption that a woman's life will be organized around and defined in relation to a man' (Canadian Panel on Violence Against Women 1993: 16). The report also told us that 'Canadian society is organized around compulsory heterosexuality', and that 'Heterosexism is imbedded in all state institutions that women are likely to call upon – the police, the justice system and religious institutions' (p. 16). These concepts had more to do with constructing an ideological framework and little to do with assisting families in crisis. This was a sorry example of money wasted on ideologically-driven initiatives to the neglect of families.

By the time of this report, I had been distancing myself from the radical gender feminists' attempts to subject troubled human relations to dubious ideology, by which all human behaviour was adjudged by an artificial, even fictitious construct, termed the 'patriarchy' and 'men's power and control over women'. This contrived construct was a subversion of justice itself. By quoting two women, I would like to illustrate by their words why I had taken a different road away from this rapacious and devouring ideology. The first is Sally Miller Gearhart, an American who described herself as a radical lesbian feminist. Her article 'The future, if there is one, is female', was published in her 1982 book, *Reweaving The Web of Life: Feminism and Nonviolence*. Gearhart wrote: 'To secure a world of female values and female freedom we must, I believe, add one more element to the structure of the future: the ratio of men to women must be radically reduced so that men approximate only ten percent of the total population' (p. 280).

The second is Justice Bertha Wilson, a Supreme Court of Canada judge from 1982 to 1991. In her 1990 speech entitled 'Will women judges really make a difference?', she asked: 'Will this growing number of women judges by itself make a difference? The expectation is that it will; that the mere presence of women on the bench will make a difference' (1990: 16). Justice Wilson cites the work of Carol Gilligan, a US feminist professor and the author of the 1982 book, *In a Different Voice: Psychological Theory and Women's Development*. Justice Wilson said:

Gilligan's work on conceptions of morality among adults suggests that women's ethical sense is significantly different from men's. Men see moral problems as arising from competing rights; the adversarial process comes easily to them. Women see moral problems as arising from competing obligations, the one to the other, because the important thing is to preserve relationships, to develop an ethic of caring. The goal, according to women's ethical sense, is not seen in terms of winning or losing but rather in terms of achieving an optimum outcome for all individuals involved in the moral dilemma. It is not difficult to see how this contrast in thinking might form the basis of different perceptions of justice.

(Wilson 1990: 20)

I repudiate the unsupportable claim that women are more ethical, caring or moral than men. This was symptomatic of the moral and intellectual bankruptcy of radical feminist ideology and its stranglehold over the public discourse.

Challenging orthodoxy, ideology and shibboleths: breaking the stranglehold

On International Women's Day, 8 March 1995, while speaking to a large meeting of government employees to warm applause, I said a few unplanned words that challenged the orthodoxy of radical feminist ideology. In mentioning domestic violence, and in my words the 'other side of the equation', I said that ' ... behind every abusive husband is an abusive mother'. My remarks were like a thunderbolt. They immediately became the dominant media story of print, television and radio from coast to coast. I gave media interviews by the dozen. My remarks dominated the media for days, especially the talk shows. Supportive letters and phone calls deluged my office. Unknowingly, I had performed a much needed national service. The country was relieved that someone finally – a woman – had said that women were capable of violence too. This public expression went on for several days. My remarks and I were sustained. For example, on 8 March 1995, Toronto's CFRB radio station held a survey during its all-day talk show about my remarks. CFRB put the question to its listeners: 'When you were growing up, which parent was more abusive – your mother or your father?' Of 200 respondents, 62 per cent said mothers, and 38 per cent said fathers. In Ottawa, CFRA radio's *The Lowell Green Show* found that 70 to 80 per cent of the callers agreed with me. On 9 March 1995, *Maclean Hunter Broadcast News* placed my remarks before its viewers asking: 'Do you agree?' Of the 273 respondents, 57 per cent agreed and 43 per cent disagreed. Though not scientific, these three public dialogues – a few among many – revealed the extent, the magnitude, of the public discussion, and the public's interest in this subject.

The abuse of abuse: false allegations of violence, vexatious and malicious prosecutions: a heart of darkness in the body politic

One example of false allegations of domestic violence is the 1998 case, *R.* v. *Ghanem*, in the Provincial Court of Alberta, Canada. On 31 October 2000, I testified before the Standing Committee on Justice and Social Policy of Ontario's Legislative Assembly, about Bill 117, the Domestic Violence Protection Act 2000 (Official Report of Debates 2000). In asking the government of Ontario to rethink this bad bill, I cited this judgement. Mr Ghanem, the defendant, had been charged with assaulting his wife. He was tried and acquitted of this charge. Mr Ghanem's wife, supported by her mother, had him charged in an effort to imperil him in their divorce proceeding. Mr Ghanem was elsewhere when the assault was alleged to have taken place. He had an alibi. About this alibi, Judge Fraser stated, at paragraph 2: 'I am advised the alibi was formally disclosed to the Crown. It was also disclosed to the police officer immediately upon being told of the allegations. The officer chose not to investigate the alibi and instead just laid the charge. Apparently he didn't feel he had any responsibility to do so'.

Judge Fraser, at paragraph 19, in stating his reasons for acquitting Mr Ghanem, said about the wife, 'I find the evidence of the complainant and her mother to be contradictory, confusing, contrary, conflicting, irreconcilable and quite frankly, false' (Fraser 1998). Judge Fraser spoke of the dangers of the zero tolerance policy in domestic cases and said, at paragraph, 21:

> I want to make two further comments because one is curious as to how a man could be falsely accused in these circumstances right up to and including a trial. The reasons are quite clear to me and disturbing. First, the police apparently have a policy of zero tolerance in domestic assault cases. Any zero tolerance policy is dangerous. It is especially dangerous when it is not properly applied.
>
> (*Fraser 1998*)

There are many cases like this. I chose Ghanem because it was a criminal proceeding seeking to damage a husband in a civil divorce case. Interestingly, despite an acquittal, under Bill 117, someone like Ghanem, though acquitted, would find himself back in court. Bill 117 was passed, but it has not been proclaimed. Happily to date it is not in force.

I shall cite another divorce-related case of false accusations of abuse, within a civil proceeding of child custody in the Ontario Court of Justice (Provincial Division) in Milton, Ontario. In the 1995 judgement, *A.L.J.R.* v. *H.C.G.R.*, Judge Fisher stated at paragraph 17: 'I find that the father committed no physical or sexual abuse and the mother programmed her child to give fictitious complaints' (Fisher 1995). Continuing at paragraph 23, Judge Fisher confessed, 'When, in the past, I have read evidence of alleged abuse, I have decided to err on the side of caution and order supervised access. Judges often do this. I confess to have been taken in by the mother's evidence.

However, it appears in making such an order that I simply erred. It is to be hoped that this order corrects that error' (Fisher 1995).

The precondition of false accusations of abuse is the reliable expectation that women must always be believed, that men must always be disbelieved and doubted, because women are virtuous truth-tellers and men are liars of dubious moral character who are naturally inclined to hurt, rape or maim their wives and children. This has caused enormous injustice and unspeakable pain and suffering. It has destroyed families. It has undermined the basis of the helping professions. It has undermined the administration of justice. This plethora of false accusations of physical or sexual abuse by mothers against fathers is a heart of darkness. It is soul destroying.

Police and prosecutorial responses to intimate partner violence: the need for study and reform

I shall cite Grant A. Brown, a PhD from Oxford University and a lawyer in Edmonton, Alberta. He wrote an article entitled 'Gender as a factor in the response of the law-enforcement system to violence against partners', about prosecutorial and judicial responses to intimate partner violence. This was published in the 2004 journal *Sexuality and Culture*'s special issue on gender and partner violence. Not surprisingly, there is little data in Canada on the role of prosecutors in determining outcomes in cases of partner violence. Yet all know that men are disproportionately prosecuted, and that practice is most uneven. Dr Brown wrote:

> Canadian judges sometimes comment from the bench on the differences in treatment they perceive to exist between men and women who are accused of partner violence. In finding Darryl Arsenault not guilty of assaulting his common-law partner Susan Himmer, B.C. Provincial Court Judge Brian Saunderson said, 'There are far too many prosecutors declining to make the hard decisions, lest they offend some interest group or incur the displeasure of their superiors who themselves are subjected to pressure from the same groups ... The result can be made to work hardship in individual cases.' The judge ruled that Arsenault was defending himself when he slapped Himmer after she verbally abused and assaulted him. Himmer testified that she was drunk and in an 'out of control ' rampage after Arsenault's ex-wife insulted her. Judge Saunderson criticized the Crown for not charging Himmer for her assaults, saying it created a double standard. 'The mere fact of this prosecution sends a very clear message: a woman in a relationship with a man can provoke him, degrade him, strike him and throw objects at him with impunity, but if he offers the least physical response, he will be charged with assault ...',
>
> (*Brown 2004: 37–8*)

Conclusions

Governments in Canada, the USA and elsewhere must reconsider their misguided and foolish policies on domestic violence. They must turn away from ideology towards a more humane and balanced approach. My Senate office files are bursting with correspondence, judgements, affidavits, press clippings and scholarly research that describe heartbreak, pain, fathers' suicides, children's suicides, psychic injury and terrible injustice. Thousands of distressed people appeal to me for help. The patriarchal notion, a contrived and artificial construct introduced at the instance of radical gender feminist ideologues, drove out common sense, reason, law and humanity from the treatment of family violence. Governments, in adopting policies based on feminist ideology to treat complex, intimate human relations, chose policies which were not only deeply flawed, but were doomed to failure because they misunderstood and underestimated human needs and human actions as ideology usually does. This public policy, by severing male-female relations from our sense of humanity and justice, drove out all other human considerations such as weakness, psycopathy, emotional immaturity, character disorders, couple dynamics, identity disturbances, jealousy, mental problems and deviances such as drugs and crime. It also drove out all other human and personal factors like psychic injury and the tendencies described by Erin Pizzey as 'violence-prone'. This artificial construct in public policy was superimposed upon all male-female relationships, denying all the empirical data, and even proper treatment itself. This ideological construct ran amok and was akin to a mental disease, a disorder in the mind of the body politic, raging to criminalize manhood and to drive many men into the criminal classes and the underclass.

That our governments, despite the compelling and conclusive evidence to the contrary, would adopt this construct as public policy and thereby put its full coercive power behind it, pitting itself against its own citizens, testifies to the paucity of politics. It testifies to the paucity of the human condition, and proves the notion that evil frequently masquerades as good. These artificial constructs have menaced human relations and family relationships while offering no healing to families in need. The challenge of the future is to recast these policies, to take up the cause of families afflicted by domestic violence and to continue its treatment by assisting families in need. We must assist research by probing deeply into the hearts and minds of human beings who use violence. We must endeavour to understand the recesses of the mind, the pathologies that surface and act out in intimate family relationships, and to discern and correct the dynamics, thereby offering hope and renewal.

11 Battered women who use violence: implications for practice

Melanie Shepard

Introduction

Women's use of violence in heterosexual relationships has been a source of controversy since researchers began to study domestic violence three decades ago. Researchers' early claims that women were as violent as men did not fit the experience of battered women's advocates, criminal justice practitioners and health professionals, who saw the fear in women's faces and the injuries to their bodies. Counterarguments that suggested women were rarely violent or, mostly, passive victims of violence also did not ring true. In recent years, there has been a trend toward criminalizing women's use of violence toward their abusive partners and conceptualizing their use of violence as being a similar phenomenon as that used by men. This effort to be 'gender neutral', as if 'gender equality' truly existed, does not fit with the reality of women's daily lives. It has serious ramifications for the safety and well-being of battered women and their children.

The line between victim and assailant is becoming murky for practitioners on the front lines, although most recognize that the violence used by men and women is not the same. Increasingly, women are being arrested for domestic violence in the USA (Hirschel and Buzawa 2002). Criminal justice reforms, such as mandatory or preferred arrest policies, that were designed to protect battered women, have unintentionally resulted in women being arrested for their use of violence and court-ordered to attend batterer treatment programmes. Most women who are court-ordered to attend groups for domestic assault are battered women themselves (Miller 2005). In a study comparing domestic violence victims with women enrolled in a batterer intervention programme both groups were found to report high levels of victimization (Abel 2001). This chapter will explore some of the differences between the use of violence by men and women in heterosexual relationships and provide guidelines for intervention.

Gender differences in battering behaviour

A critical distinction exists between 'using violence' and 'battering' in intimate partner relationships. Battering involves the use of a range of controlling tactics,

TOURO COLLEGE LIBRARY

including physical, psychological and sexual abuse, to achieve and maintain dominance in intimate relationships (Pence and Paymar 1993). It is purposeful behaviour that seeks to maintain a climate of intimidation and fear so that the 'batterer' controls the life of the 'victim'. Physical and psychological abuse can take place in response to 'battering' in the form of retaliation or self-defence. Most women are not in a position to be 'batterers', simply because they lack the physical strength, resources and/or motivation to do so.

There is evidence of gender differences in terms of the type of *abusive behaviours*, *motivations* and the *consequences* for using violence in intimate partner relationships. Researchers disagree about whether women commit violent acts as frequently as men, although there is more agreement on the greater severity of men's violence. One only needs to open a daily newspaper to find evidence that this is the case. While Straus (2005: 56–7) argues that women 'initiate and carry out' physical assaults on their partners as often as men and 'despite the lower probability of injury resulting from attacks by women, women produce a substantial percentage of all injures and fatalities from partner violence', Kimmel (2002b: 1355–6) points out that women's violence 'is far less injurious and less likely to be motivated by attempts to dominate or terrorize their partners'.

A closer look indicates that men use a wider range of physically and sexually *abusive behaviours* when compared to women (Dobash and Dobash 2004). Women are much more likely to report that they are afraid of their partners (e.g. Swan and Snow 2003), most probably because they are at greater risk of serious injury (e.g. Swan and Snow 2003). The reality is that many of the women seen in hospitals, shelters and community agencies are in danger for their lives because of the severity of violence committed toward them by their abusive partners. Sexual violence remains the hidden and under-prosecuted form of intimate partner violence (IPV), perpetrated significantly more often by men (Tjaden and Thoennes 2000a, 2000b). It is estimated that between a third to a half of battered women have been victims of sexual violence by their partners (Bergen 1998), while being rarely charged or prosecuted in the criminal justice system (Hasday 2000).

The fear that women face speaks to one of the prime *motivations* for using violence. Women more often report that self-defence was the motivation for their use of violence (Swan and Snow 2003). The definition of what constitutes self-defence becomes murkier when perceptions of self-defence are compared with legal definitions or research categories developed for measurement purposes. Women may believe they are acting in self-defence to prevent imminent harm, but their actions may not be construed that way by authorities relying on narrow definitions of what constitutes self-defence. The interpretation of 'self-defence', 'retaliation' or 'initiation' depends upon the perspective of those viewing the behaviour and for what purpose. In a series of in-depth interviews with women, Dasgupta (1999: 217) reaches the conclusion that 'the most pervasive and persistent motivation for using violence was to end abuse in their own lives'.

Central to our understanding of battering is the idea that abusive behaviour is used in a systematic way to maintain ongoing control over one's partner. A number of studies have provided evidence that men are more likely to use violence to control their partner (e.g. Barnett *et al.* 1997). Dasgupta (2002: 1378) finds that 'women try to secure short-term command over immediate situations, whereas men tend to establish widespread authority over a much longer period'. While the intention may be to control what is happening in a given situation, the abusive behaviours do not generate the level of fear and intimidation that is typical of battering. Strategies to address women's violence must differ from those addressing men's because the underlying motivations for using violence are typically not the same.

Women face serious *consequences* for their use of violence in intimate relationships. As noted earlier, women are at greater risk than men of being injured in domestic violence incidents (e.g. Swan and Snow 2003). Since the adoption of mandatory arrest or preferred arrests in the USA and elsewhere there has been a dramatic increase in domestic violence – including the arrest of women by themselves or in dual arrests where both parties are arrested. The arrest rates for women vary widely across the USA (Hirschel and Buzawa 2002). In a study of over 6000 arrests, 'female arrestees were significantly less likely than males to have histories that warrant concern regarding the potential for future violence' (Henning and Feder 2004: 69).

Anecdotal accounts suggest that battered women who are arrested are reluctant to turn to the criminal justice system in the future for protection, which is likely to place them at greater risk of harm. The label of 'batterer' may limit women's access to essential victim services, which are needed for the safety and protection of themselves and their children. Women who are arrested may lose all rights and privileges of victims, such as transportation to a safe location, temporary housing, restraining orders and participation in victim assistance programmes. Furthermore, 'although not guilty, an abuse victim who has been arrested may waive legal rights and plead guilty in order to speed up the legal process and minimize potential danger to self and children' (Hirschel and Buzawa 2002: 1459 citing the National Clearinghouse for the Defense of Women). Battered women who use violence may be those women whose physical and mental health is most at risk. In reviewing the literature, Sullivan *et al.* (2005: 292) found that 'high rates of childhood abuse, the witnessing of parental aggression, being victimized by partners in adulthood, posttraumatic stress disorder (PTSD), suicide attempts, and substance abuse were documented in women mandated to anger management programmes for their use of interpersonal aggression, including intimate partner violence'.

Categorizing women who use violence

Understanding women's use of violence requires an analysis of the role of gender in the use of IPV. One of the more important contributions in this area is Johnson's (in press) conceptualization of IPV as 'intimate terrorism', which is use of the violence to control, perpetrated primarily by males, 'violent resistance', which is used primarily by women in response to intimate terrorism, and 'situational couple violence', which is not part of a general pattern of control. Johnson applies gender theory to all three, recognizing the role that patriarchal social structures, gender socialization and individual sex differences play in all these types of violence. Using data from the National Violence Against Women (NVAW) study (Tjaden and Thoennes 2000a, 2000b), women experiencing intimate terrorism were compared with women experiencing situational couple violence (Johnson and Leone 2005). Women experiencing IPV were attacked and injured more frequently, experienced violence that was less likely to stop, exhibited more signs of post-traumatic stress disorder (PTSD), were more likely to leave their husbands, used painkillers more often and missed more work.

In an effort to examine the differences among women who use violence, a number of scholars have categorized women into groups based upon whether they were primarily aggressors, victims or engaging in mutual violence (Swan and Snow 2002); violent only against their partners or violent toward other people in general (Babcock and Siard 2003); or responding out of frustration, defending themselves or because they were generally violent individuals (Miller 2005). Women's lives, however, are complicated, and placing them neatly into categories is a challenge for both researchers and practitioners alike.

During two group sessions with mostly court-order women, the author and her colleagues explored with women whether they viewed themselves as mostly the aggressor, mostly reacting to aggression from their partner, or viewed their violence as being equal in terms of its frequency, severity and harm to others. Most of the women placed themselves in the reactive category, relatively fewer in the equal category and very few in the primary aggressor category. In exploring the life circumstances of women who placed themselves in the primary aggressor category, their extensive histories of victimization, as well as aggression, emerged. While these women initiated dangerous levels of violence, they also experienced coercive control by their partners. These women seemed to interpret their use of aggression as meaning that they had not allowed themselves to become victims, however, their stories seemed to tell otherwise. For example, one woman was virtually homeless, having been relocated with her husband for his work, isolated from others, and then evicted by him from their home. He did not use violence to control her, but her violent acting-out behaviour actually allowed him to increase his control over her because of the criminal justice intervention that resulted. Another woman, who reported that she was always the primary aggressor, came to the group with visible injuries, leading group leaders to doubt whether she had the upper hand as she claimed. These anecdotes are used here to illustrate how a woman's aggression is connected to her own victimization even for those women who are viewed by themselves and others as the primary aggressor. The lines between victim and aggressor categories become blurred when we examine gender differences and other contextual factors in greater depth.

Implications for practice

Practitioners in the field of domestic violence should recognize that battered women who use violence do so in response to the victimization and oppression they are experiencing in their lives. In working with a battered woman who has used violence it is important to understand the contextual factors that have shaped her response to her particular situation. Contextual factors include: her partner's use of violence and coercive control; the economic, social and spiritual supports available to her; the needs of her family and children; her physical and emotional health; her behavioural skills; her level of commitment to maintaining the relationship; and the social and cultural conditions that limit the options available to her. Once a clearer understanding of these contextual factors is achieved, we can work collaboratively with her to identify ways that she can enhance her safety and well-being without using violence.

Practitioners should not use the term 'female batterers' to describe women they come into contact with who have been violent toward their partners. Most women who are arrested and court-mandated to group counselling are victims of battering themselves (Miller 2005). In the words of Susan Osthoff (2002: 1540), 'If you are battered, you are not a batterer. You may use violence against your partner, but it takes more than mere violence to be a batterer'.

An intervention priority should be to address immediate safety issues. Factors such as the use of drugs and alcohol, the presence of weapons in the home, past injuries, increasing levels of violence, sexual abuse and obsessive behaviour are indicators of serious levels of risk and proactive steps should be taken to connect women with advocacy services. Women using violence may be at a greater risk of becoming victims of severe violence. Battered women who use violence need the services that other victims require, such as safe housing, education and empowerment, and civil orders for protection. Women may be surprised that they were arrested for what they believed to be self-defensive and justifiable behaviour. A lack of knowledge about the criminal justice system and the desire to put the incident behind them can put women at a disadvantage when dealing with abusive partners who may know more about how the system works. Providing women with information about the criminal justice system and what is considered self-defence can help them to make realistic choices.

Interventions to address violence used by battered women should be part of a coordinated community response, whereby agencies collaborate to develop policies and procedures that recognize that all acts of violence in intimate relationships are not the same and which provide guidelines that assist practitioners in sorting out the differences. One model is the Crossroads Programme in Duluth, Minnesota, USA (Asmus 2004). Working with key stakeholders, the Duluth City Attorney's Office has developed a programme to defer prosecution in cases meeting certain criteria. In order to be considered, candidates must have been the victim of physical abuse by the complainant in the current case, have no prior assault charges, nor been charged with violent behaviour toward law enforcement officers. After the initial eligibility requirements are met, a more in-depth evaluation takes places of the defendant's history of criminal and violent behaviour, victimization history, the severity of the incident, the nature of the defendant's admission to the offence, the views of the complainant, the circumstances surrounding the use of violence, the motives for the use of violence and the defendant's willingness to participate in recommended education and counselling programmes. Prosecution is deferred for candidates meeting the eligibility requirements and who agree to attend group sessions that address issues confronting battered women who have used violence (Asmus 2004).

Whether battered women should be court-mandated to participate in counselling groups when they are arrested for using violence presents a dilemma for domestic violence practitioners. It holds the potential for re-victimizing women and sending the message to partners, family members and the community at large that women's use of violence is the same as battering. Just as 'anger management' programmes have sanitized the issue of battering in many communities, women's groups can be used as one way to minimize the gendered nature of battering or intimate terrorism. Still, some women have exceeded the legal limits of self-defence and must face legal consequences. A court order to group counselling can be helpful to women who have been reluctant to seek help on their own or who have been blocked from seeking help by their abusive partners. It may diminish their isolation, connect them with needed resources and help to reduce their own harmful use of violence.

In a curriculum manual designed for women who abuse in intimate relationships, Hamlett (1998) recommends that women be carefully screened and those women who are clearly the victim should be referred to other resources with recommendations made when necessary to probation officers for more appropriate services. While this is desirable, it does not appear to be happening in many parts of the USA. Practitioners may not be adequately prepared to make this distinction, particularly as women's use of violence does not always fit into neat categories. The challenge is to find approaches that hold women accountable for using violence, but which do not re-victimize them for seeking to defend themselves.

The dilemma posed by mandating that battered women receive services for their use of violence has led to the reluctance of advocates to contribute to the development of effective methods of intervention. The lack of advocacy involvement may lead to the development of models that are not well grounded in the experiences of battered women. Women are being court-ordered to attend programmes that have been designed for men (Butell 2002). Applying programme models designed for male batterers to work with women who have used violence, such as the widely used Duluth curriculum (Pence and Paymar 1993), is ill advised. While women benefit from learning about the use of battering to maintain power and control in relationships, the Duluth model, which is based on male privilege and power, is not applicable to women's use of violence. The theory of planned behaviour change, another approach that guides the treatment of male batterers, has been found to be moderately predictive of male behaviour (Tolman *et al.* 1996), but not female violent behaviour (Kernsmith 2005b). This approach addresses the components of attitudes toward violence, normative beliefs about the acceptability of violence and perceived behaviour control, all of which are heavily influenced by issues of gender.

Some intervention approaches have been developed for work with battered women who have used violence. Miller (2005) describes a group programme that uses a feminist philosophy to empower and educate women while focusing on accountability, choices and options. Other approaches include the use of cognitive-behavioural and solution-focused approaches to address issues such as safety planning, anger management, substance abuse, mental health, assertiveness, stress, communication, accountability, effects of violence on children, developing support systems and accomplishing goals (e.g. Loy *et al.* 2005). The field lacks outcome data on these programmes. One study by Tutty *et al.* (in press) of a group programme that combines an unstructured, psychotherapeutic component and a structured educational component to teach skills for making responsible choices, found that women reported statistically significant improvements in five areas: non-physical abuse of partner; self-esteem; general contentment; clinical stress; and adult self-expression. The women had low rates of physical abuse to start with and no statistically significant improvements were found in this area or in marital satisfaction or family relations.

Intervention guidelines

Practitioners from different disciplines can use the following intervention guidelines:

- The label 'female batterer' should be avoided because most women who use violence in heterosexual relationships do not engage in a pattern of coercive control that is typical of male battering.
- It is important to address issues of victimization because violence is primarily used by battered women in response to abuse they experience in their intimate partner relationships.
- The context in which violence has taken place must be explored, including an examination of the actual incident, as well as the women's individual life circumstances that shape the choices available to them.
- An intervention priority should be to address safety issues for women and other family members.
- Women should be held accountable for their use of violence, while being offered support and resources for promoting change in their lives.

Conclusions

Critical reflection, discussion, and evaluation must occur on an ongoing basis as we seek to understand and address the use of violence by battered women. Our efforts can result in unintended outcomes that we must address as we work together to end domestic violence. Ultimately, the best way to prevent the use of violence by battered women is to stop the violence by their abusive partners.

12 The role of health care professionals in preventing and intervening with intimate partner violence

Patricia O'Campo, Farah Ahmad and Ajitha Cyriac

Introduction

Over the past few decades, health care professionals have systematically taken on the issues of intimate partner violence (IPV). Both the magnitude and health sequelae of IPV result in high levels of health care system involvement in terms of service utilization and cost of health care. While the health care system has acknowledged the importance of addressing IPV, the response has been varied. In this chapter we will discuss the current focus of IPV within the health care system, which is mainly on screening and referral. We will place the discussion of all proposed interventions, including screening, within the context of IPV as a chronic condition, since the majority of survivors do not experience single episodes or even short-term exposures to IPV. While we also cover emerging literature on more comprehensive interventions and recommendations for expanded services to address IPV within the health care system, we note up front that this literature as a whole lacks a strong evaluative component and most recommendations cannot be supported by evidence demonstrating their efficacy. Nevertheless, these recommendations form the foundation of an urgent research agenda that can improve the current state of health care related services for survivors of IPV.

Health care utilization for victims of IPV

IPV is highly prevalent, with 25 to 54 per cent of women reporting exposure in their adult lifetime, varying by the population sampled, definitions of IPV used, and data collection methods (Hegarty and Roberts 1998; Jones *et al.* 1999; Coker *et al.* 2000a; Tjaden and Thoennes 2000a, 2000b; Thompson *et al.* 2006). IPV has long-term negative health consequences for survivors, even after the abuse has ended (Koss *et al.* 1991; Jones *et al.* 1999). These effects can manifest as poor health status, poor quality of life and high use of health services (Campbell *et al.* 2002).

Abused women often utilize health care services for reasons other than injuries (Dearwater *et al.* 1998; Tjaden and Thoennes 2000a). Physical health consequences include a 50 to 70 per cent increase in gynecological, central nervous system and stress-related problems compared to women who have never experienced abuse (Campbell 2002b; Campbell *et al.* 2002). Mental and emotional health issues include: depression, anxiety, suicide tendencies, post-traumatic stress disorder (PTSD, mood and eating disorders, substance dependence, antisocial personality disorders and non-affective psychosis (Danielson *et al.* 1998; Roberts *et al.* 1998; Sutherland *et al.* 1998; Golding 1999b). Co-morbidity with other health conditions or risky health behaviours such as substance abuse are also common (Martin *et al.* 2003; Testa *et al.* 2003; Burke *et al.* 2005; O'Campo *et al.* 2006). Women may access health care settings before they present to criminal justice or social service settings, and if IPV is appropriately recognized and managed within the health system they can receive interventions that increase their well-being and possibly improve their health (Campbell 2002b).

Women's disclosure of abuse

Despite negative health consequences and frequent health care visits, abused women refrain from spontaneous disclosure of IPV to health care providers. Feelings of shame, embarrassment, failure, guilt, confidentiality concerns and a fear of the physician's reaction and/or rejection often comprise a significant segment of these women's propensity to disclosure (Rodriguez *et al.* 1996; Bauer *et al.* 2000a, 2000b; Plichta and Falik 2001). Moreover, mandatory reporting laws, found in selected US states, that require physicians to report to the police when a patient's injury *may be* linked to IPV (Warshaw and Ganley 1996), have been found to be a barrier to disclosure (Rodriguez *et al.* 2001a), contrary to their original intent. However, asking women about IPV in a sensitive manner gives them permission to communicate (Titus 1996; Rodriguez *et al.* 2001b). In 2001, Rodrigeuz and colleagues found that 85 per cent of the abused women disclosed when asked, while only 25 per cent disclosed in absence of asking (Rodriguez *et al.* 2001b). Further, several surveys in primary care and emergency settings report that more than two-thirds of women patients approve of routine screening for IPV (Bradley *et al.* 2002; Richardson *et al.* 2002).

Screening for IPV in health care settings

While screening for IPV is intuitively appealing, it is an area of current controversy. Because of the magnitude of the problem and the potential for health care profession-als to intervene on IPV, myriad professional organizations have recommended IPV screening in health care settings – for example, the American Medical Association, the American College of Obstetrics and Gynecology, the Society of Obstetricians and Gynecologists of Canada, the American Academy of Family Practice, the American College of Emergency Physicians and the American Academy of Nurse Practitioners, to name a few. The specific activities that physicians are expected to implement are wide ranging and include, but are not limited to: conducting routine screening for IPV; enquiring about child abuse and abuse history; identifying coping mechanisms; validating patients' experiences; assessing safety; developing safety plans; document-ing the abuse (sometimes with photos); referral to appropriate resources; reporting to law enforcement agencies; and creating a care coordination and follow-up plan for the patient (Gerbert *et al.* 2002). While this suggests that physicians must act as both mental health professionals and advocates for victims of IPV, a smaller and clearly defined role for physicians has been suggested by many (Titus 1996; Alpert *et al.* 1998; Gerbert *et al.* 2002). For example, Gerbert and others have noted that the role of the physician should be limited to manageable tasks that overcome documented barriers and fit within the realities of the health care visit (Gerbert *et al.* 2002). The four components of the AVDR recommendation include: (1) *Asking* about abuse; (2) providing *Validating* messages which acknowledge that abuse is wrong, not the fault of the victim and confirm the patient's worth; (3) *Documenting* the abuse; and (4) *Referring* the patient to appropriate services and specialists (Gerbert *et al.* 2002) (see Table 12.1).

Table 12.1 Screening, identification and referral of IPV victims in the health care setting (Gerbert *et al.* 2002)

Step	Examples of the activities within each step
ASKING	All patients should be asked at each visit about IPV in a private and confidential setting Questions about IPV should be asked using non-judgemental language Questions about IPV can be included along with other routine questions on safety such as seat belt use and gun safety
VALIDATING	Providers must offer validating messages, acknowledge that the abuse is wrong and confirm patient worth Validation can be provided even if the patient does not disclose violence
DOCUMENTING	Document the presenting signs and symptoms of the abuse in a non-judgemental way and perhaps include specific information such as names, locations and even witnesses The patient's own words can be used in the documentation

Step	Examples of the activities within each step
REFERRAL	Victims should be referred to IPV specialists such as trained advocates or dedicated staff on site who are available around the clock
	Specialists can take a complete history of the abuse, assess for safety and develop a safety plan
	Specialists can explain and comply with any mandatory law reporting requirements

Since these calls for action on the part of the health care provider, an enormous amount of data has been collected to assess the effectiveness of various strategies to promote and implement screening in health care settings. In summarizing this body of research, two national task forces in the USA and Canada have concluded that the literature does not yield sufficient evidence to recommend *universal* screening for IPV by physicians (Wathen and MacMillan 2003; Nelson *et al.* 2004). One major point of contention that still remains is whether health professionals should ask 'all' women about domestic violence (universal screening) or 'target' diagnostic assessments on suspicious cases (case-finding) (Taket *et al.* 2004). Nevertheless, the US Task Force states that inclusion of a few direct questions about abuse as part of the routine history in adult patients may be recommended because of the substantial prevalence of undetected abuse (Nelson *et al.* 2004).

The support of having a health care professional enquire about the socially stigmatized issue of partner abuse is growing and has been shown to have potential therapeutic effects. Gerbert *et al.* (1999a) showed that women who contacted advocacy services reported that concerned nurses and physicians motivated them to seek help by improving their feelings of self-worth and decreasing their sense of isolation. Warshaw (1989) concurred that just talking about the abuse is therapeutic as it may decrease the sense of isolation that many victims feel. In a focus group study by Zink *et al.* (2004), abused women from shelters and support groups encouraged physicians to affirm the abuse on disclosure and educate the patient, provide information about local resources, make appropriate referrals and document abuse history. These women perceived that providers' screening for IPV was important even for women in 'early' phases of victimization, in order to raise awareness.

Effectiveness of screening

Health care screening interventions aim to improve early detection of victims and the consequences of IPV. Some of these initiatives have focused on provider education in schools (Centres for Disease Control 1989; Alpert *et al.* 1998; Short *et al.* 1998) and clinical settings (Lo Vecchio *et al.* 1998; Abraham *et al.* 2001; Glowa *et al.* 2002), while others have focused on screening instruments and methods (Abbott *et al.* 1995; Norton *et al.* 1995; Rhodes *et al.* 2001; Coker *et al.* 2002b; Krasnoff and Moscati 2002; McNutt *et al.* 2002; Bair-Merritt *et al.* 2006). In 2002, Waalen and colleagues conducted a critical appraisal of relevant literature and concluded that educational interventions for providers had no significant and sustainable effect on IPV screening, but inclusion of specific strategies (e.g. screening questions) improved the screening and identification rates (Waalen *et al.* 2000).

In 2004, inclusion of IPV screening questions was systematically reviewed by Nelson *et al.* This review demonstrated that some valid and reliable instruments are now available to screen and detect cases of IPV, such as the Abuse Assessment Screen (McFarlane *et al.* 1992), the Partner Violence Screen (Feldhaus *et al.* 1997), HITS (Sherin *et al.* 1998) and the Ongoing Abuse Screen (Ernst *et al.* 2002). The authors also identified a dearth of rigorous studies on the various methods of administering the screening tools. Addressing this knowledge gap, some randomized controlled trials have compared face-to-face interviews and/or patient self-administered methods of screening (e.g. written, audiotape or computer-based surveys) (Gerbert *et al.* 1999b; Bair-Merritt *et al.* 2006; MacMillan *et al.* 2006). The results of these trials converge about the potential advantages of patient-administered IPV screening methods. However, others have found that the implementation of screening protocols leads to an initial rise in IPV screening but the rates decline over time (McLeer *et al.* 1989). Thus, IPV screening interventions should be effective in multiple ways: identification of IPV risk, acceptance by patients, feasibility for providers and sustainable use.

Physicians' barriers to screening and post-screening interventions

An area requiring greater attention is the issue of barriers to screening. Physicians report barriers to screening for IPV such as discomfort, fear of patients' negative reactions, lack of time, the priority of the acute problem, and a lack of familiarity with resources (Rodrigues *et al.* 1999; Garimella *et al.* 2000; Waalen *et al.* 2000; Bradley *et al.* 2002). In a recent survey of physicians and nurses, lack of preparedness was identified as a key barrier to screening. Provider training would help remedy this situation, at least to some extent, as over 60 per cent of those in the study reported no training on methods for screening and referral (Gutmanis *et al.* 2007).

Currently, a minority of physicians routinely screen for IPV, although they feel professionally obliged to detect cases (Ferris 1994), with a belief in their role to assist the victims (Garimella *et al.* 2000). Recent assessments of IPV screening practices among physicians and midwives yielded rates between 2 and 11 per cent (Rodriguez *et al.* 1999; Elliott *et al.* 2002; Carroll *et al.* 2005). Consequently, it is clear that abused women are likely to visit clinicians without being identified as victims of violence (Caralis and Musialowski 1997; Thomas 2000). Even if screening itself was addressed via patient-administered IPV screening methods, providers still require greater comfort with discussing such a sensitive topic.

Screening and identification alone within the health care setting are not sufficient. Providers must refer women to appropriate services to increase short- and long-term safety of the IPV survivor as well as to address the health and psychological consequences of IPV. While numerous programmes exist for such referral, such as shelters, counselling, housing programmes and other community-based services, data to support the effectiveness of such interventions in promoting short- or long-term safety is weak as very few studies have demonstrated effectiveness in addressing subsequent IPV and IPV sequelae.

There is only preliminary evidence on the benefits of advocacy counselling post-shelter (Sullivan and Bybee 1999), individual counselling by a professional counsellor (Tiwari *et al.* 2005) and community-based services for employment and social support (Bybee and Sullivan 2005). A clinician's referral to such community-based services or to a social worker is important after identification of at-risk patients, in addition to acknowledgement and empathy. Yet, such programmes are scarce. There is an urgent need for the development of programmes with demonstrated effectiveness to ensure the safety and well-being of IPV survivors.

IPV as a chronic condition and the continuum of care

Assessment and management of IPV within the health care system that focuses on acute problem identification and immediate resolution is insufficient for the majority of IPV survivors. Data suggest that the majority of women experience IPV episodes repeatedly and that their relationships involving IPV typically last several years (Tjaden and Thoennes 2000a, 2000b; Nicolaidis and Touhouliotis 2006). Experiences of IPV vary in terms of severity, chronicity, comorbidities and sequelae. Moreover, while many, but not all, victims have histories of prior abusive relationships or child abuse, many existing programmes and interventions just focus on the current relationship, leaving historical issues unresolved. Services should match the varying needs of IPV victims.

The appropriate health care response, therefore, is to treat IPV as a potentially chronic condition which often involves multiple health issues (e.g. depression, anxiety, PTSD, substance abuse, HIV, acute or chronic injury) and social issues (e.g. need for housing, job training, social support), all needing a coordinated response. This response should include (1) screening and identification of IPV victims and (2) comprehensive assessment of the related multiple health and social issues at all follow-up visits. This loop of care calls for proactive roles by multi-disciplinary professionals such as physicians and/or nurses performing screening and identifying the victims, and social workers and/or trained advocates meeting the specific needs of the referred victims as a team. Currently, coordination within the health care system or between the health care and social or community service systems to serve women who are IPV survivors is rare to non-existent.

A number of useful frameworks have been proposed to promote the perspective that IPV is a chronic condition requiring long-term attention and intervention on the part of multiple sectors within the health care system. This perspective includes the recognition that victims may have a history of child or adult abuse and also recognizes that women need assistance to address their vulnerabilities with regard to IPV once the victim has disclosed. Moreover, the frameworks tailor referral, service, coordination and follow-up within a context of the IPV process and experience. For example, there needs to be recognition that follow-up appointments may be missed *because* of IPV (e.g. partner control) and that special attention may be required to ensure that women stay connected to necessary services. Two such frameworks are the Critical Pathway for IPV across the continuum of care, for use across health care settings and the Chronic Care Model for IPV survivors (Dienemann *et al.* 2003; Nicolaidis and Touhouliotis 2006). In describing this comprehensive approach to the health care delivery system for IPV survivors, Nicolaidis and Touhouliotis (2006: 106) note that:

> Care managers could provide ongoing support and communication to otherwise isolated patients; decision support systems could alleviate providers' fear of addressing violence with patients; self-support tools could improve patients' self-efficacy in regards to safety planning or their self-management of other co-morbid conditions; formalized collaboration with community agencies could lead to higher use of resources; and information systems could systematically track risks and outcomes.

Integrated health care interventions

An example of a successful integrated programme that emphasizes both screening and identification as well as incorporating elements of a continuum of care model is the WomanKind programme located in Minneapolis, Minnesota, USA. It was designed to address noted barriers to IPV identification and referral within the health care setting – namely that providers have little or no training in recognizing abuse, that intervening on IPV is uncomfortable for providers, that providers may not see intervention as their responsibility, and that providers' time and resources for assisting victims of IPV are limited. The components of the WomanKind programme therefore include specialized training for all hospital staff and a protocol for universal screening as well as an in-house system of paid professional staff and volunteers who are available 24 hours a day. The training covers numerous topics including challenging myths about IPV, providing background on the incidence of IPV and the cycle of violence, discussing the approach to and methods for routine screening and assessment, discussing health care and community resources for IPV, and discussing the process of behaviour change for victims of IPV (Short *et al.* 1998). Evaluation of the programme, which included an evaluation of comparison hospitals in the area, showed impressive results. For example, in the hospitals with the WomanKind programme, 1719 IPV victims were identified and referred to the programme; the comparison hospitals had only 27 referrals to trained social workers during this period. Providers at WomanKind hospitals demonstrated higher knowledge, attitudes, beliefs and behaviours for appropriate responses to IPV than staff at comparison hospitals. Identification and referrals included those previously identified (54 per cent of those identified were repeat contacts), suggesting that this programme has the potential to address IPV on the continuum of care.

Other means of strengthening the health care response have been identified. These are briefly mentioned inTable 12.2. While large-scale health care responses are required to address this growing problem, it will be important to develop effective approaches, based upon solid research evidence, for each of the areas described in the table. As yet, few programmes have been evaluated.

Table 12.2 Improving the health care system's response to IPV: selected activities

Area	Activity (examples)
EDUCATION	Conduct awareness campaigns on IPV Offer continuing education on IPV regularly Create and include comprehensive curriculum on IPV in health professional schools and clinical training programmes
STANDARD OF CLINICAL CARE	Create and strengthen clinical care guidelines for IPV Increase integration and coordination of services for IPV victims
POLICIES FOR ADDRESSING IPV	Create incentives and accreditation requirements for institutions to comprehensively respond to IPV Support the protection of confidentiality of victims' health records Create reimbursement mechanisms to provide appropriate services to IPV victims

Effective provider education and training about IPV is a critical component of the health care provider response, and has gained greater attention in recent years (Davis and Harsh 2001; Frank *et al.* 2006; Stinson and Robinson 2006). Yet, few medical or nursing schools implement a curriculum that comprehensively trains providers in the identification and management of partner violence. Given the complexity in managing the risks associated with domestic violence, current training modules are inadequate. Also, there is a need to enhance provider sensitivity to variations in patient readiness to take action when experiencing domestic violence. Fortunately, greater attention is being given in the curriculum and continuing education on assessing provider readiness to counsel patients about IPV, addressing provider sensitivity, designing curricula which include survivors' perspectives, and using web-based modules (Alpert *et al.* 1998; Nicolaidis *et al.* 2005; Short *et al.* 2006).

Future research

While numerous efforts are underway to address IPV within the health care context – screening and identification, statements from professional organizations calling for increased and routine screening for IPV, and even a few studies that have attempted to evaluate clinic-based intervention programmes – strong evidence that documents the positive impact upon IPV and the short- and long-term well-being of victim's is non-existent. This is not to suggest that such efforts should be stopped, as the nature of IPV requires intervention at any and all possible points of contact with the health and social system. However, data needed to design the most effective screening and intervention programmes are lacking. In part, the lack of evidence may be due to the evaluation challenges of assessing complex problems and interventions. For example, systematic reviews are excellent tools when interventions are narrow, but IPV interventions, when properly designed, are complex. Certainly, future efforts to evaluate IPV programmes might consider methods of synthesis that accommodate more complex interventions (Pawson *et al.* 2005). However, the limitations of the current evaluation data on IPV interventions extend well beyond the issue of evaluation of complex programmes for IPV. The fact of the matter is that few IPV interventions implement evaluations. Consequently, the field is left with little evidence, and virtually no strong evidence, to support calls for specific programmes such as screening or more complex interventions.

Thus, an enormous amount of research is yet required before evidence-based interventions can be designed and promoted. Given the magnitude of IPV and its far-reaching health and social consequences, an accelerated research agenda is urgently needed which includes strong partnerships between policy-makers, providers, IPV survivors and researchers. Data are needed to inform the design of programmes that can be appropriately tailored to the numerous settings that victims of IPV access within the health care arena, such as primary health care settings, community health care settings, specialty health care settings and emergency services, to name a few. Moreover, this future research agenda should include primary prevention approaches to address IPV within the health care setting in the same way that advocacy around the top killers such as cardiovascular disease has prioritized provider messaging about smoking, diet and exercise for all patients regardless of risk.

Conclusions

The health care system plays an important role in assisting victims of IPV; not only do IPV survivors have high health care utilization rates, but health care providers, professional agencies and institutions are increasingly recognizing the need for formal programmes to address the myriad concerns of those experiencing IPV. Ideally, an appropriate response to IPV would include not only coordinated systems to address secondary and tertiary prevention but also primary prevention of those at risk of IPV.

The good news is that there is political will to take action on prevention and treatment of IPV within the health care setting, as evidenced by the numerous calls by professional organizations, advocates and institutions to implement system changes to accommodate IPV programmes. Funding to support such programmes and, perhaps at this stage, greater research efforts to generate the evidence to support the most effective programmes to address IPV, are urgently needed.

13   Multi-disciplinary working

Karel Kurst-Swanger

Introduction

Domestic violence is a complex social problem that must be understood within the context of social, cultural, religious, political and socioeconomic factors. The consequences of such abuse are enormous, not only for individual victims and their families, but for communities as well. The physical and emotional well-being of victims is profoundly affected amid other concerns such as homelessness or economic insecurity. Children are particularly vulnerable to the negative effects of intimate partner abuse, often with consequences to their psychological, cognitive and physical development (Lehmann and Rabenstein 2002). Even beloved family pets can be maltreated within the context of violent relationships (Kurst-Swanger and Petcosky 2003). Employers face challenges as result of chronic absenteeism, reduced work performance and increased health care costs. Violence which spills into the workplace places additional security burdens on employers who seek to keep their employees safe.

Also, domestic violence presents as a complex social problem because it is often inextricably linked to other multi-faceted social issues such as underemployment, drug and alcohol abuse, mental illness and community-level violence. Additionally, the tendency of domestic violence to be transmitted from generation to generation (e.g. Gelles and Straus 1988) creates a circumstance in which abusive behaviours are deeply rooted within the histories of families. Tragically, domestic violence can also end in death.

Thus, the intervention and prevention of domestic violence requires approaches which are multi-dimensional and address the full range of concerns facing victims, perpetrators, their families and the community at large. These concerns span the obligations of many different types of professional discipline within the matrix of the helping professions, such as teachers, nurses, doctors, police officers, judges, lawyers, therapists, animal welfare officials, child welfare workers, victim advocates, faith leaders etc. Thus, leaders from these various professional groups have much to gain by working together, in a coordinated fashion, to impact the problem of domestic violence in their communities. What can result is a coordinated continuum of services which address the various dimensions of domestic violence. This chapter will present a multi-disciplinary planning group as a model to consider toward this end.

The benefits and challenges of such a planning group are discussed as well as some specific strategies that can help to alleviate difficulties.

Multi-disciplinary planning groups

Although the problem of domestic violence has received attention worldwide and intervention strategies have begun to evolve internationally, there is still much work to be done to develop appropriate public policy and effective intervention strategies for victims and perpetrators (Burton *et al.* 2000). Even in jurisdictions where domestic violence intervention is well defined, planning can be disjointed and fragmented, and thus may lack the type of comprehensive coordinated response that would be most beneficial. The benefits of multi-disciplinary coordination and collaboration are infinite, whether a community has a well established continuum of services or is just beginning to address the issues of domestic violence. Although working in a multi-disciplinary environment can be achieved in a number of different ways, I would suggest that the establishment of a multi-disciplinary planning body is a critical core method to effectively plan for the creation of new intervention strategies, to identify gaps in current services, or to resolve issues that surface in the various systems that interact with victims, perpetrators and their families. Also, multi-disciplinary planning groups can effectively advocate for important legislative reform and can jointly ensure appropriate funding is in place to support critical programmes and services. Social, political and legal change can be spurred on by the inherent power that can exist as a result of the joint efforts of a multi-disciplinary work group. In the case of domestic violence, practitioners and researchers have begun to recognize the importance of coordinating planning bodies to impact on such violence (e.g. Cranwell *et al.* 2004).

Additionally, it is important that such a planning group consists of the leaders from the various sectors. It is vital that key decision-makers be involved since they have the authority to make the type of sustainable changes that are necessary to reduce the incidence of domestic violence and to create a system of response that is amenable to the needs of victims and their children. Although effective planning can occur with mid-level or front-line staff, it is important that leaders play an active role. Leaders possess the power to make short-term and long-term programme planning decisions and to ensure implementation is successful. This is especially important in communities that desire systemic reform.

It is also important that such planning groups develop a way in which to seek ongoing representation or input from consumers and the community at large. Families should be viewed as a part of the solution, rather than solely being defined as the problem (Schorr 1998). An issue as complex as domestic violence requires that we work to build upon the established strengths of individuals and families, as opposed to solely focusing on the deficits (Kurst-Swanger and Petcosky 2003). In addition, survivors can often serve as a much needed 'reality check' to keep professionals honest about what changes are required in their specific community.

Establishing a multi-disciplinary planning body, whether it be considered an ad-hoc task force associated with another broader based planning group or a new group which has convened to combat domestic violence, should include as wide a representation of leaders from different disciplines as possible. As Kurst-Swanger and Petcosky (2003) note, there are numerous large and cumbersome systems that may play a role in domestic violence intervention in any given community. These systems span the professional disciplines of behavioural health, medicine, child welfare, animal welfare, geriatrics, criminal justice and civil legal services. In addition, the business and religious sectors have an important role to play in any comprehensive planning effort. The key feature of a multi-disciplinary planning group is that its membership is intentionally diverse to ensure that the problem of domestic violence can be approached from a number of different perspectives. Representatives who intervene in cases of child abuse and neglect, as well as elder abuse, sibling violence and parental abuse should also have a presence in domestic violence planning.

Multi-disciplinary planning groups enjoy a number of different benefits, and these include the following.

Reduction of system fragmentation

Certainly one of the biggest systemic concerns lies with the fact that service providers tend to concentrate on solutions only to the specific problems within their immediate domain. Health and human services are administered by many different types of organization, each with its own particular mission and purpose, source of funding, regulatory requirements and guidelines. Separate, and often conflicting, eligibility standards and rules governing the expenditure of funds create concrete boundaries which often work against holistic approaches to service delivery. For example, health care workers must be concerned with the physical health of their patients, and although the emotional health of their patients may also be considered, health care workers can generally do very little to impact other concerns such as legal, housing and overall safety issues.

Even communities rich with a myriad of health and human service programmes can experience fragmented, exclusionary and, in some instances, duplicative services. This is, at least in part, due to the fact that health and human service programmes have evolved as a series of systems that correspond to discrete problems and/or specific populations of people. As a result, many communities have an environment in which many organizations, functioning autonomously in many diverse areas, can produce unintended and contradictory results. In the case of domestic violence, it is imperative that the problem be approached from a variety of perspectives to reduce the possibility of unintended consequences. Thus, a multi-disciplinary planning body can help to organize and coordinate the divergent goals of various organizations toward one common purpose.

Creative problem-solving

Intentional multi-disciplinary planning can help to alleviate specific systemic problems which may exist in a given community. Planning processes which include a wide range of professional interests, from different sectors of the community, can effectively and creatively impact on social problems if there is a structure or venue in which to jointly discuss issues and potential solutions. Since different professional disciplines are concerned with different aspects of a problem, the consideration of specific issues from such divergent perspectives should ultimately yield more sustainable change and can work to solve systemic problems as they arise.

Improved communication across agencies/systems

One of the downfalls of the evolution of sophisticated professional disciplines in the helping professions has been what I would refer to as the 'disciplinary divide'. This is an artificial boundary which segregates the various disciplines from one another through differing ideologies, paradigms and guiding principles. The divide is cemented by occupational sub-cultures, which help to define the values and modes of operation of various disciplines. These occupational sub-cultures are marked by things such as language, customs and rituals which are specific to particular disciplines. As a consequence, professionals from one discipline may have a difficult time understanding the behaviours and decisions of professionals from another.

A multi-disciplinary planning body can substantially improve the communication between the various professional groups that engage with victims and/or perpetrators, and their families. This in turn helps to bridge the disciplinary divide. Enhanced communication between professionals can enhance the day-to-day interaction between staff and improve their ability to access services for individual victims or perpetrators. Improved communication between and among the various sectors and/or disciplines can help to remove barriers and create opportunities where divergent agencies and programmes can work together toward a common purpose, despite their unique and often conflicting goals. A common agenda, which crosses the boundaries created by differing ideologies and paradigms, can work to facilitate policy-makers, bureaucrats and service providers in looking toward a common vision. Targeted efforts to communicate across the disciplinary divide can help communities achieve systemic and programmatic reform. Multi-disciplinary planning groups, by their very nature and structure, can help bridge these gaps.

Strengthened knowledge base of staff

Another benefit of multi-disciplinary planning groups is the continual professional development opportunities that are created when professionals from different disciplines gather to engage in joint community planning. Health officials can learn from police officials and vice versa. This benefit is enhanced when multi-disciplinary planning groups sponsor training opportunities that may be discipline-specific, but deliberately involve professionals from different disciplines and/or community members. We all have much to gain by learning more about the issues that surround domestic violence, especially given the fact that our specific role with victims or perpetrators is likely to be limited by our professional discipline.

Reduction of the burden on victim service advocates to seek solutions on their own

In some communities, domestic violence advocates have had to struggle on their own to facilitate necessary changes in their community. It is through their advocacy that many prevention and intervention policies and programmes have evolved. Multi-disciplinary planning groups, which involve domestic violence advocacy organizations and victim service providers, but also actively involve others, can attend to the needs of families across the disciplinary divide, thus making the advocacy goals of the victim support programmes that much easier to achieve.

Provision of a venue for garnering resources

Multi-disciplinary planning groups can create a circumstance in which resources can be pooled and redistributed. Also, since different disciplines have access to different funding streams, there is the potential that an agency or programme could benefit from gaining access to a wider range of prospective funding sources which can be garnered through the multi-disciplinary work group. In fact, in the USA, it is not uncommon for government or private foundations to require multi-disciplinary planning groups to be established in order to receive grant funding.

Managing a multi-disciplinary planning group

As I have been arguing, multi-disciplinary work groups offer many benefits for both the professionals in the field and the community at large. Yet, as you might imagine, managing such a group brings with it its own unique set of challenges. These challenges include: negotiating conflicting goals or paradigms; dealing with personality conflicts among members; jurisdictional issues which arise when agencies or programmes are in competition for limited resources; and tensions that arises when all the members are not in agreement about what types of reform are necessary. Additionally, differing views about the causes and factors associated with domestic violence can add a further layer of discord.

Thus, working in a multi-disciplinary work group can be very trying; in fact, sometimes it can be down right painful. Yet, groups can overcome these tensions if they remain committed to the process and take the time to carefully resolve their differences. The following is a list of recommended strategies to assist in the management of a multi-disciplinary planning group.

Seek a skilled facilitator to run meetings

It is imperative, especially when a new group is being established, that a person with excellent facilitation skills be asked to run the meetings. Skilled facilitators can help to deal with conflicts in an open and honest manner and keep key professionals at the table, even during difficult periods. They can also play an important role in keeping a group focused and helping a group to prioritize its goals and objectives. Good facilitators can translate the concerns of individual members into group action, know when and when not to push a group, and can effectively gather diverse points of view to ensure all group members are heard. Also, skilled facilitators can keep meetings and projects moving forward by helping to organize realistic agendas, minimizing distractions and keeping track of interesting ideas that should be saved for discussion at a later date. It is important that facilitators remain neutral, so it is helpful if a person who has no immediate claim to the possible plans that will be initiated in the future is assigned to facilitate.

Establish ground rules

Establishing ground rules for the operation of the planning group is a helpful strategy to keep tensions at bay. This is especially important in multi-disciplinary groups that are likely to have members with different occupational norms and expectations. Thus, agreeing up front on operational issues, such as how and when the meetings will run, or defining the procedures for how decision-making will occur, will help meetings to run smoothly. Additionally, a formal or informal set of written bylaws may also assist the group to set boundaries for its operation. Provisions should be made to address problem behaviour, conflicts or what to do if members do not attend critical meetings. If ground rules are agreed upon shortly after a group is assembled, it is easier to act on operational problems further down the road.

Conduct a multi-disciplinary self-study

A strategy to assist divergent professional groups to come together to work on a particular social problem is a self-study. A self-study is a process by which group members learn about each other's organizations, programmes, services and goals in relation to domestic violence. A self-study can help to identify the availability of intervention and prevention efforts regarding domestic violence. This is especially important in large communities where many different kinds of agencies and organizations exist.

In addition, it is critical that a planning group go deeper than merely listing available services. A group should take the time to explore the varying paradigms which shape their discipline and the key terms they use to describe various aspects of the issues presented. It is important that group members come to understand the different philosophies and language that guide the provision of various services. Group members should each report their conceptual views on domestic violence, sharing what they believe to be root causes and what they believe needs to be done to reduce violence in their community.

In this vein, a multi-disciplinary planning group should have a theoretical discussion regarding domestic violence and explore the commonly-held assumptions and perceptions of each discipline's unique approach to the problem. Members should be encouraged to raise insightful and provocative questions so that they can fully appreciate the demands, barriers and challenges facing each discipline or organization. Coming to a common understanding of how each discipline approaches the problem and what their unique issues are in service provision can go a long way to reduce conflict in the future.

Also, groups would be well served if they also evaluate the membership of the group and determine whether or not all the appropriate disciplines or organizations are represented. Training and skill sets should also be evaluated. Groups can then determine what future training or expertise will be required to move the group's planning efforts forward. It is always a good idea to culminate the self-study process with a written document for future use. Once a self-study is completed, a group is more likely to be ready to engage in planning for the future in a more coordinated fashion. Extensive self-studies also serve to promote teamwork and get group members in the right frame of mind to work collaboratively.

Understand the process of collaboration

Engaging a multi-disciplinary planning group to impact on an issue as complex as domestic violence will be a long and difficult process. It is important that partners understand that such collaboration is likely to exist on a continuum in which there are different stages (Austin 2000). Acknowledging that such a group effort is a *process* is important. Groups, especially when they involve members from different occupational worlds, need time to develop trust and respect before true integration can occur.

Deal with conflict in an open and honest manner

Groups will inevitably experience some conflict. Dealing with whatever conflicts arise, when they arise, in an open and honest manner can help to diffuse problems early. This requires group members to attend to what is going on within the group process and to openly attempt to diagnose conflicts. Groups should first distinguish between *debates* and *arguments*. Disagreements can make some group members feel uncomfortable, while others seem to flourish when there is conflict. Since members are likely to have different 'conflict comfort zones', determining individual comfort levels can help a group adopt an effective procedure or process for resolving issues as they arise. It is also helpful if a group comes to understand that conflict, when managed properly, can actually result in very positive outcomes. Groups should not be disappointed when conflict arises, but rather be proactive by preparing processes so that conflicts can be embraced as a strategic tool to move a group toward common ground. There are some strategies that groups can use to help diffuse conflicts:

- *Small group exercises*: one strategy involves breaking the multi-disciplinary work group into smaller groups (of three to four people) to discuss issues. Give each small group time to discuss the difficult issue and document their findings/solutions. Once each group has had an opportunity to discuss the issue openly in their small group and document their results, the large group should reconvene to explore the common themes. A skilled facilitator can help the large group find common ground among the small groups. Individual members' conflict tends to get diffused, since their concerns can be fully aired and validated in the small group session.

- *Writing exercises*: another strategy is a written exercise. This is especially effective when conflict appears to dominate the group process. Prepare an open-ended questionnaire which contains questions pertinent to the conflict. Ask group members to comment, anonymously, on the issues at hand. One helpful question is to ask members to consider how they or their organization has contributed to the conflict. Have a neutral third party review the responses and report to the group their analysis of the results.
- *Use a round-robin approach*: a round-robin approach involves going to each and every person in a group to see what their thoughts are on a particular topic. This strategy is especially helpful when it is unclear what the level of conflict is in a group. Sometimes dominant individuals can portray a problem as being worse than it really is and the round-robin approach helps to clarify the extent of a particular problem among group members.
- *Structure a debate*: structuring a formal debate on an issue can help a group with a difficult decision. Assign different group members to debate the various sides to an issue. Assign other group members to evaluate the debate itself. After the conclusion of the debate, ask the group to process the results.
- *Meet privately with specific group members*: conflicts which erupt between individual members because of personality differences are another matter. These are best dealt with by discussing the problem with the individual parties in private. It is important that they understand the impact their behaviour might be having on the rest of the group.
- *Role playing*: another strategy to deal with group conflict is role playing. Asking group members to take on specific roles or perspectives and discussing the issue from that viewpoint can help members see things in a different way.

Celebrate accomplishments on a regular basis

Another positive strategy to working in a multi-disciplinary environment is to celebrate the achievements of the planning group. This can be done in a number of different ways, but groups tend to be re-energized when they remind themselves how much they have accomplished over the course of a particular period of time. If a group has not be able to accomplish anything, then it would be helpful if the group examined its processes to determine what is working well and what needs improvement. Groups which attend to group processes and dynamics have a better chance of creating and sustaining social change.

Encourage joint training

Multi-disciplinary planning groups should encourage as much training across disciplines as possible. Cross-training helps partners better understand domestic violence from a broader perspective than their immediate domain and helps to bridge barriers between agencies and organizations.

Conclusions

In summary, multi-disciplinary planning groups can help communities achieve positive change with regard to domestic violence and can assist service providers in developing integrated, coordinated responses that more adequately meet the needs of victims and perpetrators. Challenges and conflicts are inevitable and should be embraced as mechanisms of social change.

Part three
Involvement

14 Treatment and alcohol

Julie A. Schumacher

Introduction

Alcohol use disorders have been identified as frequently co-occurring problems for both perpetrators and victims of domestic violence. Efforts to provide integrated treatments for these two important public health issues are increasing, but remain limited. This chapter presents information on the co-occurrence of alcohol use disorders and intimate partner violence (IPV) perpetration and victimization, assessment strategies, and treatment options and considerations.

Prevalence estimates

Available evidence indicates that both perpetrators and victims of IPV are at significantly and substantially elevated risk of substance use disorders, particularly alcohol use.

Perpetration

The association between alcohol problems and IPV perpetration in men is well established in the literature. The association has been found in both community and clinical samples (e.g. Leonard 1993). Established annual prevalence estimates in the USA for IPV perpetration among men enrolled in individual or couples-based alcohol treatment programmes range from approximately 44 to 66 per cent (e.g. O'Farrell *et al.* 1999). These figures, typically based on female partner reports, are approximately four to six times higher than established population prevalence estimates for male partner violence perpetration (Straus and Gelles 1990a, 1990b). Within samples of men enrolled in treatment programmes for partner violence, the prevalence of reported problem drinking or alcohol use disorder diagnoses ranges from 17 to 56 per cent (Stuart *et al.* 2003). These figures contrast with population estimates of heavy drinking of approximately 6.8 per cent (Substance Abuse and Mental Health Services Administration 2004).

Much less information is available about female-to-male IPV, including risk factors and correlates. However, available research suggests that alcohol problems are associated with similarly heightened risk for engagement in IPV for women. This similar risk has been identified in, or is suggested by, findings from a large nationally representative survey in the USA (Caetano *et al.* 2001), court-referred IPV perpetrator treatment samples (Stuart *et al.* 2006), and substance abuse treatment samples (Chermack *et al.* 2000). For example, Chase *et al.* (2003) found that approximately two-thirds of a sample 103 women seeking couples-based alcohol treatment had engaged in violence toward their male partners in the year before treatment. Importantly, although these perpetration rates appear roughly similar to those established for men in couples-based alcohol treatment programmes, the negative consequences associated with female-to-male IPV are typically much less severe (Cascardi *et al.* 1992).

Victimization

Alcohol use disorders have also been linked with partner violence victimization. In a meta-analysis examining the co-occurrence of IPV with a variety of psychiatric diagnoses, Golding (1999a) identified ten studies examining the prevalence of alcohol abuse and dependence in samples of women identified as victims of IPV. These samples were drawn from battered women's shelters, emergency rooms, psychiatric populations and the general population. The mean prevalence of alcohol use disorders across the ten studies was 18.5 per cent. Importantly, the prevalence of alcohol use disorders in the shelter samples was significantly higher than the mean prevalence estimate (32.6 per cent) suggesting women in this population may be in particular need of interventions for alcohol abuse. Although the mechanisms under-lying this heightened prevalence are not clear, factors such as greater overall alcohol consumption and a diagnosis of alcohol abuse or dependence do appear to be significantly associated with drinking during victimization (Lipsky *et al.* 2005b). Comparable studies of male victims of IPV could not be identified.

There is also evidence that women who are involved in substance abuse treatment programmes report significantly higher rates of intimate partner victimiza-tion than women recruited from the community (e.g. Miller *et al.* 2000). For example, in a study comparing women in alcohol treatment programmes to community women without alcohol problems, differences in lifetime reports of partner violence victimization were pronounced. Eighty-seven per cent of women in the alcohol treatment sample reported a history of moderate partner violence victimization, and 40 per cent reported severe victimization. In contrast, the lifetime victimization prevalence estimates in the comparison sample were 28 and 8 per cent, respectively.

There is also evidence that men in alcohol treatment are also more likely to experience partner violence from their female partners than men in community samples. For example, O'Farrell and Murphy (1995) found that 53.4 per cent of the female partners of men seeking couples-based alcohol treatment reported engaging in one or more acts of IPV in the year before treatment, and 27.3 per cent reported engaging in one or more acts of severe aggression. Less information is available about acts of partner violence experienced by men enrolled in other types of alcohol treatment programme. Nonetheless, these findings suggest that relationship conflict may be an important treatment target for men involved in alcohol treatment programmes, even for men with no history of perpetration of IPV.

Although the co-prevalence studies reviewed in these sections do not generally speak to the nature of the relationship between alcohol use disorders and IPV perpetration and victimization (e.g. cause, effect, mediation, moderation), two very important conclusions can be drawn from this literature. First, it indicates that individuals identified as victims or perpetrators of IPV are at elevated risk of alcohol use disorders and should be appropriately assessed so that substance-related treatment needs can be established. Likewise, individuals with alcohol use disorders are at elevated risk of intimate partner perpetration and victimization and these issues should be assessed during substance abuse treatment so that appropriate services can be offered.

Assessment

Current assessment practices

Although there is limited research on the partner violence assessment practices of substance abuse treatment facilities, existing research on the issue suggests that despite repeated findings about the elevated rates of IPV among individuals seeking alcohol treatment, most men and women enrolled in treatment for alcohol-related problems are never asked about violence in their relationships. For example, a survey of 249 substance abuse treatment programme staff and 139 domestic violence treatment programme staff providers employed by substance abuse and domestic violence agencies across the state of Illinois, USA, revealed that screening for IPV perpetration and victimization in substance abuse treatment programmes tended to be haphazard. Furthermore, only a small minority of programmes formally screened all clients for IPV (Bennett and Lawson 1994). A more recent study examined almost 1500 married and cohabiting male clients at several outpatient alcohol treatment sites in the north-east of the USA (Schumacher *et al.* 2003). Forty-four per cent of the men in the study reported perpetrating one or more acts of partner physical aggression in the year before treatment on a self-report measure collected for research purposes. The policy at all sites was to refer men who reported partner violence to additional treatment, yet review of treatment records indicated that only 17 per cent of the men who reported IPV on the research instrument received referrals. This suggests that the assessment either did not occur regularly, was ineffective, or was not followed up with appropriate referrals.

In the survey of treatment agencies described previously, Bennett and Lawson (1994) found that programmes for female victims of IPV provided even less screening for substance use disorders than substance use programmes did for IPV. The authors noted anecdotally that some agencies reported avoiding assessment of substance abuse issues because the providers at battered women's shelters did not have appropriate training to assess or treat substance use. Based on available prevalence estimates for alcohol use disorders in shelter populations (e.g. Golding 1999a), as many as a third of women seeking such services might benefit from referrals to substance abuse treatment programmes. A promising finding of the Bennett and Lawson survey was that programmes for IPV perpetrators did include formal alcohol screening tools in their assessment protocols.

Special considerations

To improve cross-assessment practices within substance abuse and IPV treatment agencies, it is important to understand the realities of the contexts in which such assessment is expected to occur. Examination of these contexts reveals important barriers to cross-assessment. First, available evidence suggests that few substance abuse treatment facilities have in-house programmes to address the treatment needs of IPV victims or perpetrators, and that similarly few IPV programmes, particularly victims programmes, have in-house substance abuse treatment (Bennett and Lawson 1994). As such, assessment will result in the identification of a problem which many programmes are not equipped to address.

Second, many batterer treatment programmes were developed and designed to provide treatment to court-referred men and women, who were referred to treatment subsequent to an arrest for IPV. This means both that programmes may be somewhat or completely unwilling to accept 'walk-ins' or referrals from other treatment facilities, or that the treatment they provide may not be well-suited for men who are not court-referred. This leaves alcohol treatment providers with the same problem noted above – an identified problem with no accessible or appropriate solution. There may be similar heterogeneity among victims of violence, and not all individuals who have been victims of partner violence may be ready or willing to leave their relationship, which is typically a primary goal of agencies providing services to battered women.

Third, with few exceptions, acts of physical IPV are considered crimes. Reporting laws vary by jurisdiction, and in some jurisdictions treatment providers may be mandated by law to report acts of physical partner violence to the authorities (Easton and Sinha 2002). Providers may hesitate to ask questions about partner violence because they desire to protect clients from prosecution or because they do not wish to undermine an individual's substance use disorder treatment by involving outside authorities. Additionally, both victims and perpetrators may prefer to avoid police or social services involvement, leading to under-reporting. Similarly, use of certain substances constitutes a crime in many jurisdictions, and depending upon a particular client's circumstances, disclosure of illicit or even licit substance use may result in legal consequences. For example, programmes for perpetrators of domestic violence, which often serve a primarily court-referred population, may be required to report substance use to the referral source or other legal officials.

Although the barriers to cross-assessment are outlined above and raise important concerns, the public health significance of both IPV and substance use disorders suggests that these barriers must be overcome. Importantly, many of the barriers are not universal and reflect policy decisions within certain legal jurisdictions or treatment agencies. As such, removal of many of these barriers will rely on (1) political advocacy to ensure that laws are more sensitive to the heterogeneity among individuals impacted by the laws, and do not have significant, unintended, adverse impacts; (2) a willingness among treatment providers to critically and objectively evaluate current practices in their agencies and make changes if necessary to ensure the treatment needs of the individuals and the communities they serve are met; and (3) continued research to enhance understanding of relevant issues. While social, political and organizational change will occur slowly over time, as will acquisition of research findings, a few practical guidelines and considerations for providers currently working with both populations are provided below.

Overcoming assessment barriers

As noted by Bennett and Lawson (1994), providers at IPV treatment programmes may have limited knowledge of substance use disorders. Brief screening tools for alcohol and other substance-related problems might be used to guide and enhance referral practices in domestic violence agencies that do not have substance abuse treatment providers on site. Numerous screening measures for alcohol-related problems are currently available, and detailed descriptions of many existing measures, including the items, psychometric properties, scoring and interpretive criteria, and appropriate target populations, are available from the National Institute on Alcohol Abuse and Alcoholism (2003). Similarly, self-report measures of IPV can be utilized in substance abuse treatment settings to provide a relatively brief assessment of IPV that is more thorough, and perhaps more likely to yield accurate reports than a more general enquiry about problems in a relationship (O'Leary *et al.* 1992), or a single behaviorally non-specific enquiry about IPV (e.g. 'Has there been any violence in your relationship?'), which may be more typical of intake interviews (e.g. Schumacher *et al.* 2003). Importantly, the assessment of IPV also raises several important ethical issues about which practitioners should be aware (e.g. Rathus and Feindler 2004).

Treatment

Referrals

If assessment strategies are successful, the next step is to make sure that appropriate treatment is provided. Available evidence suggests referral is the most common approach to addressing these cross-problems (Collins *et al.* 1997). The degree to which individuals follow through on cross-problem referrals is largely unknown. An evaluation of an experimental programme involving a combined treatment approach for IPV and substance abuse indicated that 45 per cent of men referred to substance abuse treatment from a partner violence treatment programme never attended a single session of substance abuse treatment (Goldkamp 1996). In another study examining follow-through on referrals from substance abuse treatment to domestic violence treatment, only 13 per cent of men enrolled in substance abuse treatment programmes who received referrals to programmes for domestic violence followed through on the referral (Schumacher et al. 2003). Identifying and implementing practices to enhance follow-through on treatment referrals will be important in enhancing treatment outcomes for individuals struggling with both issues.

Additionally, incompatible philosophies and goals of domestic violence and substance abuse treatment programmes may prevent referrals from being made (Collins *et al.* 1997). Many established clinical intervention programmes for IPV perpetrators are based on feminist psychoeducational approaches, which heavily emphasize personal accountability for men who are violent toward their female partners (Healey and Smith 1998). In contrast, many common substance abuse treatment programmes, such as Alcoholics Anonymous, are based upon a disease model of addiction, which emphasizes the role of alcohol in behavioural problems, including violence, that occur during the active disease state. In the above described statewide survey, 65 per cent of the domestic violence programme staff and 45 per cent of the substance abuse programme staff surveyed viewed philosophical differences as a possible reason for limited cooperation between the two types of treatment programme (Bennett and Lawson 1994).

Substance abuse treatment

It is important to note mounting evidence suggesting that substance abuse treatment may directly impact IPV. Although the exact role that alcohol and other substance use disorders play in partner violence perpetration remains controversial, there is mounting evidence that successful intervention for alcohol use disorders should be an integral part of treatment for domestic violence perpetrators with alcohol problems. Although the prevalence of IPV perpetration is elevated in samples of male alcohol treatment-seekers, several studies indicate that completion of a partner-involved (e.g. O'Farrell *et al.* 2004) or individual (Fals-Stewart 2003) alcohol treatment programme is associated with reductions in the prevalence of IPV. An important caveat to these findings is that men who experience lapses or relapses during the post-treatment period (i.e. non-successful programme completers) are still at elevated risk for IPV. This caveat is not trivial, given that a sizeable percentage of clients who complete an alcohol treatment programme will experience some return to alcohol use following treatment (Connors *et al.* 1996). It is also important to note that the degree to which substance abuse treatment might reduce violence for men referred or ordered to partner violence treatment (as opposed to men who are referred or ordered to substance abuse treatment) is unknown.

Post-traumatic stress disorder

In treating victims of domestic violence, it is important for providers to be aware that victims of serious violence, as with victims of other serious traumatic events, are at elevated risk of post-traumatic stress disorder (PTSD) (Kubany *et al.* 2000). An important, but often overlooked, association between PTSD and partner violence perpetration has also been documented many times in the literature (e.g. Beckham *et al.* 1997). Although batterers' treatment programmes increasingly assess and provide treatment or referral for substance use disorders, other forms of psychopathology may well be overlooked.

The relevance of PTSD to this chapter is that PTSD and substance use disorders are frequently co-morbid conditions. For example, in a sample of individuals seeking treatment for substance abuse, 40 per cent met diagnostic criteria for current PTSD (Dansky et al.1997). Conversely, among community samples of individuals meeting diagnostic criteria for PTSD, co-occurring substance use disorders were 3.1–4.5 times more likely (Kilpatrick et al. 1997). Moreover, there is emerging evidence that untreated PTSD may interfere with recovery from substance use disorders, diminishing substance use disorder treatment outcomes and leaving individuals more vulnerable to relapse following treatment (e.g. Brown et al. 1996). Although additional research is needed, evidence is increasing that combined treatment for PTSD and substance use disorders will result in superior treatment outcomes, which in turn should result in superior IPV perpetration outcomes.

Motivational issues

Many of the men and women who seek substance abuse treatment are court-referred to such treatment, and those who are not legally coerced into these types of treatment may be coerced to enter treatment by a spouse or other family member, employer or friends (Weisner 1990). Therefore, it is not surprising that many clients entering alcohol treatment report limited motivation for treatment and limited readiness to change their drinking (e.g. DiClemente and Hughes 1990). Similarly, typical male clients in partner violence perpetration programmes demonstrate very limited motivation to reduce their interpersonal violence (e.g. Daniels and Murphy 1997). Even legal involvement does not necessarily result in treatment follow-through. In one study, approximately half of all first-time referrals to partner violence treatment, the vast majority of which were court referrals, did not complete even a single session of partner violence treatment (Kennerley 2000). Given that many individuals in substance abuse and partner violence perpetration treatment may be ambivalent about therapy, it is unlikely that clients who are offered additional treatment for another, perhaps seemingly unrelated problem, will respond favorably to the additional treatment.

Referral to existing treatment programmes for cross-problems represents the most feasible means of linking existing partner violence and alcohol treatment programmes, in that it makes use of pre-existing resources in the community. However, as previously pointed out, the effectiveness of this approach is logically limited by the small number of individuals who are likely to follow through on such referrals. Motivational interviewing is a preparatory approach designed to help individuals resolve ambivalence and prepare for behaviour change (Miller and Rollnick 2002). This approach has shown great promise for alcohol use disorders (e.g. Dunn *et al.* 2001) and might also enhance follow-through on referrals treatment recommendations for the combined problems of IPV and alcohol use disorders. Motivational interventions may also enhance the effectiveness of cross-treatment following referral. There is some evidence that confrontational approaches heighten resistance to change in clients who are ambivalent about change (e.g. Miller *et al.* 1993), and some traditional programmes for both substance abuse (Broekaert *et al.* 2004) and partner violence perpetration (e.g. Healey and Smith 1998) are fairly confrontational. Hence, reduction of ambivalence during the referral process may enhance client capacity to benefit from subsequent interventions. Further, motivational interviewing can be particularly effective for clients with high levels of anger, which has been associated with IPV perpetration (Project MATCH Research Group 1997).

Coping skills training

A recent study suggests that targeting the partners of individuals with alcohol use disorders with an intervention may provide another avenue for reducing partner violence in this population. Rychtarik and McGillicuddy (2005) found that provision of a group coping skills training programme to women who reported being distressed by their partners' untreated alcohol use disorder resulted in reductions in partner violence victimization. The coping skills training included teaching participants to conceptualize their distress according to a family stress and coping model, which incorporated basic cognitive behavioural principles, and to use a problem-solving approach to address distressing situations. The researchers found that coping skills training was as effective as a 12-step facilitation intervention, which encouraged participant engagement in Alcoholics Anonymous aimed at reducing symptoms of depression and partner drinking. Interestingly, and important for the present chapter, among women reporting pretreatment partner violence victimization, partners' drinking improved across follow-up for women in the coping skills treatment, but worsened for women in the 12-step facilitation intervention. Moreover, women in the coping skills treatment reported less partner violence victimization across the follow-up period than women in the 12-step facilitation treatment. Although additional research is needed to understand the mechanism of action in the coping skills treatment, this study suggests that providing women with skills to cope with the negative effects of their partners' drinking may help reduce the heightened risk of victimization associated with their partners' alcohol use disorder. This study represents a significant advance in the field, because, as Rychtarik and McGillicuddy note, previous research examining the effectiveness of interventions for the partners of alcoholics excluded couples with a history of IPV. Although careful assessment and referral to battered women's shelters when appropriate is essential, as the researchers note, these findings suggest that instead of being candidates for exclusion from skill training interventions, women who have been victims of partner violence may benefit significantly from them. A willingness to consider alternatives to traditional treatment approaches for individuals who come into contact with providers in non-traditional ways (e.g. seeking support in dealing with a loved one's substance use disorder) is particularly important as evidence continues to emerge for the heterogeneity of IPV (e.g. Holtzworth-Munroe 2000) and the need for treatment approaches that reflect this diversity.

Social, historical and political considerations

A number of historical, social and political factors influence current dialogues about IPV and alcohol use disorders, as well as treatments for each of these issues, individually and combined. For example, the gendered nature of much of the partner violence literature and the treatment community significantly influences the types of treatment made available to both victims and perpetrators of IPV. Although there are several important social, historical and practical reasons for a gendered view of, and patriarchal theorizing about, victims and perpetrators, this approach has created gaps in the literature that may adversely impact several categories of people, including gay and lesbian individuals involved in violent relationships, women who have been arrested and court-mandated to batterer treatment, and women who are involved in a relationship characterized by mild to moderate partner violence but who do not wish to leave that relationship. Far less is known about how to address the needs of these sub-populations. Another example is the widespread etiologic models of substance abuse and domestic violence that easily lead providers from the two treatment communities to believe that cross-assessment and treatment is not necessary or that the two problems are very unique and unrelated, requiring separate and specialized intervention approaches.

Conclusions

Providing the most effective treatments to the greatest number of individuals impacted by alcohol or other substance use disorders and IPV will rely on the willingness of providers and researchers to move beyond tradition to develop and implement new and innovative strategies for these combined problems. The problems of referral, attendance and the effectiveness of programmes will all need to be addressed if we are to progress in alleviating IPV.

15 Domestic violence myths

Jay Peters

Introduction

> 'She must like it if she doesn't leave.'
> 'Women can avoid physical abuse if they give in occasionally.'
> 'Hey, he just lost control for a second.'
> 'He was probably abused as a kid.'
> 'Domestic violence only happens in poor/problem families.'
> 'Domestic violence usually just involves pushing and shoving.'

Among domestic violence workers, advocates, victims and some family members, the statements above are instantly recognizable as domestic violence myths. These myths are analogous to rape myths: statements that usually shift the blame for the attack from the perpetrator to the victim. On internet sites sponsored by domestic violence advocacy groups, almost every site has its own list of myths, often contrasted with the facts. Yet myths about rape and domestic violence can be – and often are – defined as false statements which persist *despite* ample evidence of their falsity and *despite* the contradictory facts and experiences offered up by friends, family members and professionals. Thus, despite good empirical evidence that battered women are *not* masochistic and that batterers are not 'out of control' but rather retain exquisite control while psychologically and physically attacking their partners, the myths that the battered woman must have an unconscious wish to be battered and that the batterer 'just lost control' persist.

In this chapter I contend that if the myths persist despite evidence that they are false, those myths must be serving some important psychological or social purpose, or perhaps both individual psychological *and* social purposes. To be specific, I will argue that the myths listed above and all their kin serve a defensive function for individuals whereby they reduce the threat of harm for females and reduce the sense of guilt and blame for males. At the same time I will also argue that the myths serve a larger social function of supporting patriarchy by trivializing the abuse and marginalizing victims and with them the whole social problem of domestic violence.

These conclusions about the functions of domestic violence myths are based both on the theoretical literature and on two empirical studies which I conducted while developing and validating a new measure, the Domestic Violence Myth Acceptance Scale (DVMAS; Peters in press). Discussion of the development of the DVMAS is beyond the scope of the present chapter except to say that the 18-item scale has excellent reliability and good preliminary indications of several forms of validity. The DVMAS thus appears to measure what it sets out to measure and to produce consistent results.

The functions of domestic violence myths

In this discussion I will attempt to answer some of the questions raised in the introduction. Why do people endorse domestic violence myths despite evidence that they are false? What individual (psychological) and social functions might such false beliefs serve? And how might the DVMAS be useful for health care practitioners? I turn first to an examination of the individual functions of domestic violence myths.

Individual functions

Social psychologists studying how people reacted to accounts of trauma arrived at the conclusion that when faced with credible reports of serious accidents (Walster 1966) or victimization (e.g. Thornton 1984) we all engage in some form of *defensive attribution* whereby we defend ourselves psychologically from the threat of harm by making attributions about the character or behaviour of the victim. These characterological and behavioural attributions blame the victim in order to differentiate them from us so that we may reassure ourselves that 'that would never happen to me'.

Research with the DVMAS revealed that women engaged primarily in character and behavioural blame of the victim rather than exoneration and minimization as the males did. The character blame myths reinforce the notion that the victim is at least partially to blame for the violence because of a flaw in her character whereby she 'chooses' to stay and therefore be battered. Behind all the statements such as 'Victims bring it on themselves because they stay with the batterer' is the tacit statement 'But I would be out of there so fast it would make your head spin'.

In addition to blaming the abuse on the victim's character, the myths also promote the view that the victim causes the abuse by her (bad) behaviour through nagging, making the batterer jealous, through acting provocatively with other men, or arguing with her partner when she should 'know better'. These myths are defensive in that they allow women to say to themselves, 'But I'm much smarter and I would never do that'. Females thus blame victims' character (e.g. they are masochistic and seek out the abuse) or behaviour – or both – for causing their partner to abuse them.

For males, the function of the myths appears to be somewhat different. Males tend to agree most strongly with myths which exonerate the perpetrator and minimize the seriousness of the abuse. Males appear therefore to be invested in myths which say, 'It was just an accident and it's no big deal anyway'. For example, when compared with women, men more strongly endorse myths which state that the perpetrator 'just lost control of his temper' or 'just lost control for a second'. Second to this group, men then most strongly endorse items which minimize the seriousness and extent of the abuse with statements which imply the abuse does not happen often and does not affect many people. For males, the motivation of endorsing domestic violence myths appears to be blame avoidance. Interestingly, in the second study I conducted, males grouped these minimization statements together with myths which said women had an unconscious desire to be abused. Males therefore appear eager to avoid collective blame by minimizing the extent and seriousness of behaviour which they view as 'just' a momentary slip – and which the victim unconsciously wanted (and probably provoked).

To return to our first question, domestic violence myths may persist despite their obvious falsity because they serve important psychological functions. Specifically, they help women feel safe in an unsafe (relational) world, while helping men avoid feeling blamed for a social problem which often hits uncomfortably close to home. In addition to these individual psychological functions, domestic violence myths also serve powerful social functions, which I will examine next.

Social functions

In analysing the techniques used by individuals and groups that seek to deny the reality of the Holocaust, Deborah Lipstadt (1994) uncovered a set of techniques which cleverly reversed the labels of victim and perpetrator. These techniques begin with manipulations of fact and logic aimed at convincing people that 6 million Jews were not, and could not, have been murdered in the Holocaust. In fact, deniers assert, fewer Jews were killed than were members of other groups. They were not really victims of anything except the harsh living conditions of a continent at war. Having thus stripped the Jews of the status of victim they then begin the reversal. Here they point out that Jews have been largely responsible for creating and perpetuating Holocaust history. They then stretch this claim to assert that the Jews were not the victims of the Holocaust but rather the *perpetrators* of what the deniers call the hoax of the Holocaust' (Lipstadt 1994: 70). To complete the reversal, the Holocaust deniers then confess that, like you and me, they also were *victims* of this hoax. The reversal is now complete: the Jews are perpetrators of a massive hoax, of which we are the victims.

This elaborate gerrymandering of historical fact and logical reason is driven by the desire to strip the victims of the 'moral authority' which our society accords victims of genocide (Lipstadt 1994). I would go further and suggest that the goal is to strip that authority from the victims and *then* bestow it on the deniers who cleverly assert, 'No, no, *we* are the true victims here; listen to us, take us seriously, hear our grievances – and side with us'. Judith Herman (1992) argues that this inclination to side with the perpetrators is at the heart of the battles which have waged for the last 100 years and continue today concerning the reality of trauma and the credibility of victims. Even a cursory examination of the literature from the False Memory Syndrome Foundation (FMSF 1994a, 1994b, 1994c) reveals that they too argue that there cannot possibly be as many victims of child sexual abuse as are claimed, that the victims, under pressure from therapist-perpetrators (termed 'therps') make false accusations, and that innocent families are the 'true victims' of an 'epidemic' (Peters and Goodman 1997). While I have argued above that domestic violence myths serve an individual psychological function, I will here argue that they also serve a social function which is to support patriarchy by transforming the victim into the perpetrator in order to make her and the reality she confronts us with go away. As Judith Herman notes, 'Repression, dissociation, and denial are phenomena of social as well as individual consciousness' (1992: 9).

While not deliberately propagated by any one group, domestic violence myths deftly accomplish the reversal of victim-perpetrator status noted above regarding the Holocaust and the False Memory Syndrome Foundation. First, most domestic violence myths imply or state that the victim *caused* the abuse by her behaviour. If you cause an action, can you also claim to be the victim of that action? I think not. But the myths go further by stating or implying that the victim actually *wants*, seeks out and unconsciously gets pleasure or satisfaction from the abuse. If you want something to happen and then cause it to happen, you most certainly cannot be considered a victim.

To complete the reversal, however, requires exonerating the perpetrator. Domestic violence myths accomplish this in several ways. First, by stating that the victim unconsciously wanted the abuse and caused it through her nagging or other bad behaviour, the perpetrator is rendered almost blameless. How can he be responsible if he was thus set up? He is further rendered blameless by myths which say that he 'just lost control'. If he had no control then the damage he caused was not caused with malice or forethought. To complete the exoneration, the myths minimize the seriousness and extent of the abuse. These latter myths reduce the credibility of the victim and her allegations: if domestic violence happens rarely then what, realistically, are the odds that it *really* happened to her? And finally, through minimizing the seriousness of domestic violence, the myths exonerate the perpetrator by saying, 'Even if he did what you allege, it is such a rare occurrence that it is certainly not something which warrants the intervention of society within the sacred private sphere of the family'.

The effect of this victim-perpetrator reversal is insidious. If, as the myths suggest, the victim brought the abuse on herself for her own 'warped' psychological reasons, then she no longer deserves the caring and compassion usually accorded by society to victims of violence. Domestic violence myths may thus reduce the support available to battered women who are no longer seen as deserving victims. This lack of support may then limit the options of individual battered women. Cross-cultural studies of domestic violence indicate that in cultures where women are actively supported by their families, domestic violence is rare (Smuts 1996). In contrast, when women live in proximity to their husbands' families and out of touch with their own, the rates of domestic violence are dramatically higher. Thus the lack of support for victims engendered by domestic violence myths may have a real and measurable effect in that victims' families, to the degree they endorse the myths, may blame victims for the violence and therefore be less supportive. Anecdotal evidence from my own clinical practice indicates that this lack of support was often a factor in the decisions of battered women to remain with the batterer. Repeatedly, women told me that they stayed because their family blamed them exclusively for any marital difficulty and sided with the batterer in all matters.

On a wider social level, to the extent that the general public endorses domestic violence myths, the myths may reduce social (and financial) support for programmes to end domestic violence and to aid domestic violence victims. If, as the myths suggest, domestic violence victims actually seek out, desire and precipitate violence against themselves, then this is an individual and psychological problem, not a social one. If domestic violence is an individual problem then there is no call for taxpayer support of domestic violence advocacy or prevention programmes. If it is an individual problem it should be addressed on an individual, not social, level. Uniting the individual and social analyses presented above, it is possible to see that domestic violence myths institutionalize our personal, defensive needs for psychological safety by providing ready-made ways to blame the victim, exonerate the perpetrator, and minimize the whole problem, thus relegating domestic violence to a remote corner of our social conscience.

Implications for practitioners

In this final section of this chapter we (finally) turn to the impact of domestic violence myths on health care professionals and, perhaps more importantly, to an examination of their training needs. In this section I take a strengths-based approach which assumes that people endorse the myths for a good reason and that change will occur when that reason is illuminated and people are encouraged to find even better ways to meet the underlying need. First, however, we must be willing to admit that we and our colleagues all engage in some degree of blaming domestic violence victims, often through endorsement of the domestic violence myths we have discussed. For example, who among us has not, at least fleetingly, thought 'Why doesn't she just leave?' I would argue that the question is victim-blaming because inherent in it are two assumptions: that the abuse would end if a woman left and that the abuse is somehow the woman's fault if she stays and 'takes it'. Rationally we may know that leaving often increases the risk of violence (including lethal assaults), may place the woman in a dire financial condition, may force her to leave her job and relocate to a new area, and may jeopardize her custody of her children – yet we all occasionally ask ourselves that victim-blaming question. In this chapter I have argued that we continue to ask the question because it helps us psychologically: we blame victims because it helps us feel safe and secure in a threatening world.

As we have seen, on the individual and social levels, this endorsement may then affect the behaviour of health care providers. For example, health care providers who more strongly blame victims (as evidenced through endorsing the myths) may be less inclined to follow protocols regarding screening and intervention in suspected domestic violence cases. On a more subtle level, providers who endorse domestic violence myths may follow the protocols, but still communicate a victim-blaming attitude while so doing. Anecdotally, domestic violence advocates repeatedly report myriad ways in which the message that the woman was at fault and ought to 'give him another chance' was delivered to their clients by emergency room, primary care and other health care providers. While such acts might be termed unprofessional and deplorable, I instead see them as manifestations of the professionals' defenses against and internalization of socially accepted messages regarding domestic violence. Clearly if I, after many years of education and training, *still* engage in victim-blaming, then I cannot simply recommend that we eliminate domestic violence myths among health care professionals through staff education and training.

Instead I recommend that we engage in training which helps health care providers to be aware of which myths they do and do not endorse. We may simply encourage them to think in terms of keeping a finger on their psychological pulse, watching for any changes in rhythm or tempo. With their finger on this psychological pulse they may realize that they make distinctions based on socioeconomic status, race, class, ethnicity or sexual orientation. For example, many workers blame upper-class victims more than poor women; women of colour more than white women, and women who are dissimilar rather than similar to themselves. With this awareness firmly in hand we can next encourage health care providers to figure out what it is that those particular myths, deployed at those particular times, are protecting. This awareness leads directly to the positive, adaptive function of myth endorsement: how it helps them psychologically. While health care providers often want to engage in some sort of exorcism to get rid of this 'bad' part of their psyche, I instead encourage them simply to seek out other, even more elegant, ways of defending themselves psychologically. Repeatedly, in both my clinical and teaching work, I am surprised by the results of this rather vague intervention: students, professionals and clients all report an increase in their ability to 'sit with' uncomfortable thoughts and feelings (such as the awareness of domestic violence) without resorting to their previous defences. In this sort of psychological environment, where the positive intent of even quite negative (e.g. victim-blaming) behaviour is honoured, change occurs easily and often largely outside of conscious effort or teaching. Awareness and a desire to change seem to be enough; specific teaching and training are not needed and may, in fact, inhibit the uniquely creative solutions of individuals (Bandler and Grinder 1979).

Conclusions

To summarize: in this chapter I have discussed the individual and social functions of domestic violence myths as they were illuminated by two empirical studies I conducted while developing a new measure of such myths. The research supported both the defensive attribution and radical feminist theorizing regarding myths. In particular, the studies indicated that females appear to use the myths to defend against the threat of being victimized while males use them to reduce the threat of blame by minimizing the seriousness and extent of the problem of domestic violence, while shifting the blame to the woman whom the myths characterize as provoking and in fact desiring the abuse – or at least not stopping it.

While the research supported theorizing about these individual functions of the myths, it also supported a broader critical appraisal of the gendered nature and function of those myths. In this portion of the study it was shown that domestic violence myths are moderately to strongly correlated with negative attitudes toward women. These attitudes all 'suggest' that the roles and rights of women should be limited. Domestic violence myths thus appear to be conceptually related to a number of restrictive views of women. Myths thus appear to serve the social function of keeping women 'in their place' through reinforcing patriarchal attitudes towards the use of force and coercion towards women.

Combining both the defensive and social functions that were explored in these studies, I have speculated that endorsement of domestic violence myths may reduce support for individual battered women in health care settings as well as reduce support on the social level for programmes to support battered women generally. It is my hope that these ideas will be empirically supported through further research using the DVMAS. In addition, I have suggested that using the DVMAS in staff training may provide a way to create both discussion and change related to the very myths it measures.

The Domestic Violence Myth Acceptance Scale (DVMAS)

Below is the complete DVMAS (Peters 2003). Information on scoring and psychometric properties follows. The scale may be freely copied and used in research and evaluation without permission. I would, however, love to hear about your research with this instrument!

Domestic violence attitudes

The questions below ask about common attitudes toward domestic violence. While we all know the politically or socially correct answer, please answer how you truly think and feel. To answer, put a number on the line before each question indicating how strongly you agree or disagree with each statement

1	2	3	4	5	6	7
Strongly Disagree						*Strongly Agree*

1 _____ Domestic violence does not affect many people.
2 _____ When a man is violent it is because he lost control of his temper.
3 _____ If a woman continues living with a man who beats her, then it's her own fault if she is beaten again.
4 _____ Making a man jealous is asking for it.
5 _____ Some women unconsciously want their partners to control them.
6 _____ A lot of domestic violence occurs because women keep on arguing about things with their partners.
7 _____ If a woman doesn't like it, she can leave.
8 _____ Most domestic violence involves mutual violence between the partners.
9 _____ Abusive men lose control so much that they don't know what they're doing.
10 _____ I hate to say it, but if a woman stays with the man who abused her, she basically deserves what she gets.
11 _____ Domestic violence rarely happens in my neighbourhood.
12 _____ Women who flirt are asking for it.
13 _____ Women can avoid physical abuse if they give in occasionally.
14 _____ Many women have an unconscious wish to be dominated by their partners.
15 _____ Domestic violence results from a momentary loss of temper.
16 _____ I don't have much sympathy for a battered woman who keeps going back to the abuser.
17 _____ Women instigate most family violence.

1	2	3	4	5	6	7
Not at all						*Entirely*

18 _____ If a woman goes back to the abuser, how much is that due to something in her character?

©2003 Jay Peters. May be freely copied and used for research and evaluation.

DVMAS scoring

Add all items and divide by 18 for mean score.

DVMAS means and reliabilities

Study	Mean, SD	Mean, males	Mean, females	Alpha
Peters (2003)	M = 2.3 SD = .85	M = 2.6, SD = .89	M = 2.09, SD = .76	.88
Peters (ND)	M = 2.5, SD = .84	M = 2.8, SD = .82	M = 2.3, SD = .79	.865

DVMAS validity

Convergent Validity Correlations (a)

	DVMAS	ATW	RMA	SRS	AWA
DVMAS	1				
ATW	.47(**)	1			
RMA	.65(**)	.57(**)	1		
SRS	.51(**)	.69(**)	.54(**)	1	
AWA	.37(**)	.49(**)	.44(**)	.42(**)	1

A Pearson's correlation coefficient, 1-tailed

** Correlation is significant at the 0.01 level (1-tailed)

Attitudes toward women (ATW), rape myth acceptance (RMA), sex role stereotyping (SRS), attitudes towards wife abuse (AWA)

DVMAS factors and item numbers by sex

Females	Males
Character blame: 3, 5 7, 10, 14, 16, 18	Exoneration: 2, 5*, 9, 14*. 15, *18
Behavioural blame: 4, 6, 12, 13, 17	Character blame: 3, 7**, 10, 16
Exoneration: 2, 8*, 9, 15	Behavioural blame: 4, 6, 12, 13, 17
Minimization: 1, 11	Minimization: 1, 7*, 8*, 11

Factors listed in descending order of strength

* Item loading is different from theoretical expectation or other sex

** Secondary loading > .40

Note: factor solution was not stable across studies even within the same population; therefore factors should be used with caution

Comparison of mean factor scores for men and women (factor scores = mean of items loading on that factor)

Factor	Sex	
	Female	Male
Char	2.66	2.42
Beh	1.59	1.59
Exon	2.66	2.84
Min	2.09	2.52

Please feel free to contact the author with questions or comments at jpeters@maine.edu.

16 Offenders' experiences of interventions

Dana DeHart

Introduction

An important consideration in any systemic response to family violence is that offenders carry with them a history, a future and intimate or familial relationships beyond their current romantic partner. Establishing safety for victims and linking them with services is insufficient in itself as a response to violence. Rather, an effective multi-systemic response necessitates addressing offenders' use of power, control and aggression in close relationships. Unless offenders are held accountable for their behaviour and prevented from recidivating, family violence will continue its detrimental impact on the perpetrator and those around him (National Research Council 1996). In this chapter, we discuss common approaches to batterer intervention, ranging from criminal-legal sanctions and psychoeducational groups to community intervention programmes. We describe basic considerations of each, including participant impressions, quantitative data on outcomes, and implications for health care providers.

Criminal-legal sanctions

Perhaps the most commonly employed method of formal intervention with batterers involves reporting the violence to law enforcement. Yet, victims tend to call the police only after violence has escalated over time, become frequent or unpredictable, or created concerns regarding the safety of their children (Fischer and Rose 1995; Erez and Belknap 1998a, 1998b; Erez 2002). Even when the police are called, arrest of the batterer may not occur. The responding officer may exercise discretion based on ideological beliefs or judgements about the case's merit, or the officer may fail to identify a primary aggressor in the assault, leading to dual arrest of both batterer and victim (Ferraro 1989). A recent study of domestic violence reports in San Francisco found that, while more batterers are being arrested than in the past, for every 100 felony incidents reported to the police, on average only 32 are fully investigated, and only 14 result in criminal charges (Shields 2006). Contributing factors extend beyond officer training to include unavailability of pertinent information in records reviewed by prosecutors (e.g. primary aggressor, offence history), as well as failure of the system to provide adequate protection or resources to victims throughout processing, resulting in victim reluctance to continue out of fear or personal and economic dependence upon offenders.

Thus, the criminal-legal system faces significant challenges in holding offenders accountable for their actions, and researchers have not found consistent deterrent effects of arrest on reoffending among batterers (Tolman and Edleson 1995). Shields (2006: 23) has concluded 'that the law enforcement and criminal justice systems afford little protection to families experiencing domestic violence despite the thousands of police responses to crisis situations and the laudable efforts of advocates, officers, inspectors and attorneys who care deeply about the protection of domestic violence victims and their children'. Indeed, there exist many dedicated professionals within the justice system, and these people continue to work toward an improved response. Increasingly, such responses are carried out through cooperative partnerships with community-based service providers.

Psychoeducational groups

A widely used community-based intervention for family violence offenders is the group batterers' intervention programme (BIP). Although BIPs vary in philosophy and duration, they typically consist of a series of weekly sessions, often working in conjunction with victim-service programmes to ensure women's safety and with the courts for men who have been mandated to attend (Kivel 1992; Pence and Paymar 1986; Gondolf 1999; Sullivan 2006). BIPs are generally recognized as more appropriate in cases of battering than alternatives such as couples' counselling, which – without careful screening and implementation – may inappropriately assign blame to, or endanger, victims (Bograd and Mederos 1999; Goldner 1999; Scuka 2006). Individual therapy for batterers, with its ethical foundation of privacy and confidentiality, has also been deemed a problematic alternative to BIPs by those who contend that battering, as a crime, is not a private matter (Kaufman 2001).

In contrast, BIPs are said to challenge men to take responsibility for their actions, keeping the reality of violence for other family members (not just the batterer) at the forefront of the intervention. BIPs also may alleviate the batterer's exclusive dependence on the victim to meet his social and emotional needs by requiring group participants to call one another regularly, go over safety plans and homework together, and call on others for support during 'red flag' situations. These programmes are often framed in an educational format to promote the idea that men can change by accepting personal responsibility for violent behaviour and learning attitudes and skills for non-violence (Edleson and Tolman 1992; Kaufman 2001).

Programme users' perceptions

At the present time, there is little published data regarding users' perceptions of BIPs. Gondolf and White (2000) conducted an exploratory study requesting programme recommendations from batterers and their partners, but fewer than 15 per cent of those contacted made suggestions about programme structure. Among these were men's calls for supportive counselling as a supplement or component of BIPs and women's recommendations pertaining to enhanced safety and information from BIPs. Austin and Dankwort (1999) found that women appreciated the 'respite' that BIPs offered from sole responsibility for providing social or emotional support to their partners. Mandel (2006), in a study of 546 men from 23 different programmes, found that a majority believed that their children were exposed to the violence and were being negatively affected in their behaviour, relationships, mental health and school performance; this data indicates that BIPs may be enhanced by integrating more information on parenting and related issues.

There are a few published studies examining participant ideas about BIPs' influence on their own behaviour. Gondolf (2000a) asked 443 men from multiple BIPs how they avoided violence following programme participation, with potential methods including *do nothing*, *interrupt* (e.g. stop arguments, leave the room), *discussion* (e.g. talk about feelings, call a friend), *respect* (e.g. respect women's point of view, empathize), and *other* (e.g. move out, less drinking). A narrow majority of men relied on interruption methods, followed by about 1 in 5 men using discussion, and 1 in 20 men using respect. Men in longer programmes were more likely to use discussion, and their partners were more likely to rate these men as having changed to a greater extent.

A small qualitative study of men who maintained behaviour change over a six-month period identified four key factors in their reduced violence: recognizing and taking responsibility for past abuse; developing empathy (e.g. understanding effects of fear on the relationship); reducing emotional dependency on their partner; and improving communication skills around feelings and other difficult topics. The authors suggest that these findings support interventions geared toward improving healthy relationship skills (Scott and Wolfe 2000).

Research on batterers' partners' perceptions of BIPs indicates that women felt they experienced positive changes following their partner's participation, but that the women's sense of 'safety' was somewhat subjective (i.e. some felt safer despite continued violence). Study findings indicate that some women's positive feelings toward the programmes may result from perceived increases in well-being due to emotional validation and informational support received through BIPs (Austin and Dankwort 1999).

Outcome-based evaluation

Given variability in BIPs' duration, curricula and implementation, as well as high batterer dropout rates and relocation of victims, objectively evaluating the ability of these programmes to reduce the use of violence has been difficult. Although early studies indicated that BIPs may contribute to short-term cessation of assault among a majority of batterers, more recent studies employing rigorous experimental designs indicate little or no reduction in the use of violence by programme participants

(Gondolf 1997; Dunford 2000; Feder and Forde 2000; Jackson *et al.* 2003). Further, researchers have found little variation in re-assault rates among men who attend BIPs of different types or durations (Edleson and Syers 1990; Gondolf 1999; Saunders 1996).

Some studies have found that BIPs may be more effective for men with a higher 'stake in conformity' (men who are employed, married, have higher incomes and own homes), and there is considerable evidence that ethnic minorities are more likely to drop out of BIPs than whites (Healey *et al.* 1998; Bennett and Williams 2001; Jackson *et al.* 2003; Sullivan 2006). Such findings indicate a need for greater exploration of cultural factors as influences in programme effectiveness. There are also concerns that reliance on measures of physical violence may overstate the effectiveness of BIPs as men learn to substitute psychological, economic or other forms of control over their victims (Bennett and Williams 2001).

Many community activists' attentions remain squarely focused on battering as a criminal offence. Research has indicated that programme compliance and court monitoring of attendance do appear to reduce re-assault among BIP participants (Gondolf 1997, 2000b, 2000c), prompting many to advocate the use of BIPs in conjunction with strict monitoring and legal sanctions for non-compliance. An emerging trend is for some programmes to discourage self-referral for non-mandated clients, arguing that batterers may use enrolment in BIPs to manipulate partners and that non-mandated participants do not face consequences for non-compliance (New York Office for the Prevention of Domestic Violence 1998). The ethical and practical utility of such policies, however, is debatable. An evaluation of four batterer programmes, including those with and without court review processes, found that batterers' perceptions regarding certainty and severity of sanctions for non-compliance did not predict dropout or re-assault (Heckert and Gondolf 2000).

All being said, perhaps a single point of agreement within research and practice communities is that methodological limitations of existing studies make it difficult to draw definitive conclusions regarding BIP effectiveness (Jackson et al. 2003).

Risk-reduction groups

Another psychoeducational model stems from the work of Steven Stosny and is geared toward a prevention or risk-reduction audience via its focus on healing 'resentful relationships'. Stosny argues that demonizing abusers will inhibit a full community response to violence because these abusers have friends, relatives, co-workers etc. living within the community. Thus, the Stosny Compassion-Based Model is presented as a method *for* loving, compassionate relationships versus *against* domestic violence (Geffner *et al.* 2006). The model is said to treat relationship violence and child abuse by organizing identity around the compassionate aspect of the self that does not want to be abusive. One study evaluated Stosny's Compassion Workshop (CW) against treatments offered through five other agencies. CW participants demonstrated lower rates of physical and verbal aggression as well as decreased anxiety and increased acceptance of responsibility for their own violence (Stosny

1995). Yet, the model is not without critics. Evaluations of the CW face design flaws similar to those for traditional BIPs, and Healey *et al.* (1998) note that the CW is controversial for a number of reasons. Among these are the CW's inclusion of men and women, gays and straights, batterers and victims, child abusers and others in a single programme, as well as the CW's philosophies of avoiding confrontation and allowing participants to postpone admission of abuse.

Community intervention programmes

There is a growing consensus among researchers and practitioners that a coordinated, community-wide response is needed to effectively establish batterer accountability and link both batterers and victims with resources that promote safe and healthy non-violent relationships. Sullivan (2006: 202) describes the combined justice and service responses of a typical community intervention programme (CIP):

> Under many different names across the [USA], these projects bring together multiple community partners to respond more effectively to domestic violence. The police agree to contact the CIP after responding to a domestic violence call, and perpetrators are held in jail for a set period of time ... The CIP then sends female volunteers to the survivor's home and sends male volunteers to visit the perpetrator in jail. Survivors are given information, referrals, and transportation to a shelter if needed, and perpetrators are encouraged to accept responsibility for their actions and to attend a batterer intervention programme. Prosecutors agree to pursue domestic violence charges aggressively, and judges agree to order presentence investigations and to mandate jail time or batterer intervention or both. Probation officers ... agree to incorporate the perpetrator's violent history and the survivor's wishes in the presentence investigation, and they sentence perpetrators to jail time if they do not attend their mandatory batterer intervention meetings.

Evaluation of such CIPs indicates increased arrests relative to number of calls received, increased success of prosecution, and an increased number of offenders mandated to BIPs (Gamache *et al.* 1988). Based on data from survivors, police reports and advocacy records, research findings indicate that arrest followed by mandated BIPs results in lower batterer recidivism relative to arrest-only or no-intervention conditions (Syers and Edleson 1992).

Tolman and Edleson (1995) have noted that modest and contradictory evaluation findings suggest that batterer intervention efforts should extend beyond criminal justice and psychoeducational programmes. Sullivan (2006), for instance, advocates educating the public and creating systems change in order to create a social climate that rejects family violence. Literature from the New York Office for the Prevention of Domestic Violence (1998, 2001, 2006) likens the response to family violence to that for *driving under the influence*, professing that programme groups or classes are 'one front in a pattern of consistent responses ... that indicate society deems it a serious offense' (New York Office for the Prevention of Domestic Violence 2004: 1). This type of social norm perspective has merit, although the New York model includes questionable elements such as eschewing outcome-based evaluation of BIPs because the programmes are 'agents of the courts' focused on batterer accountability. Conversely, Bennett and Williams (2001) note that evaluation is one component of accountability of the system to society as a whole, asserting that programmes that routinely conduct outcome-based evaluation are likely to be safer than those that do not. Similarly, Rosenbaum (Geffner *et al.* 2006) has argued that, because the legal system is not geared toward treatment, it is not the role of the state (e.g. the courts) to control treatment. He emphasizes that the intent of a coordinated response is not for different entities to do one another's jobs; rather, these entities must coordinate to allow each professional to practise within his or her own domain of expertise.

Conclusions

Orchestrating activities of multiple governmental, non-profit and private entities into a coordinated response is the essence of community intervention projects, and such projects can maximize their potential by expanding beyond justice and psychoeducational interventions to include health care providers, faith communities, schools, places of employment and so on. In this way, researchers, advocates, practitioners and policy-makers throughout communities can work with one another to ensure that both their distinct and collective goals and protocols contribute to a norm of non-violence. Specific actions that health care providers can take include:

- Developing a relationship with the domestic violence coalition in their state or region. The coalition can assist in linking health care providers with resources for batterer intervention and victim safety, as well as directing health care providers toward helpful contacts in the justice system.
- Learning about BIPs and related programmes in their area. Some programmes that focus more on anger management or work with couples may not be appropriate in domestic violence situations, so it may be helpful to find out if there are standards for BIPs in the area and which programmes comply with these standards.
- Offering to work with members of the BIP, victim service and justice communities to improve community responses to family violence, particularly around linkage of health care providers with other professionals. Collaborative efforts might include developing protocols for cross-referral, assessment and response to victimization.
- Providing opportunities for patients to learn about and discuss violence and healthy relationships. Strategies might include placing programme brochures in waiting areas or restrooms or including questions about violence on intake forms and in discussion of stressors.

Implementing such changes in day-to-day practice takes effort, but the strength of a coordinated community approach is that providers need not tackle these tasks alone.

Rather, research and outreach to existing community resources can greatly improve health care practice and policy regarding family violence issues.

17 Couples' approaches to treating intimate partner violence

Danielle M. Mitnick and Richard E. Heyman

Introduction

The treatment of intimate partner violence (IPV) in conjoint settings, although controversial (e.g. McMahon and Pence 1996), has seemingly gained more acceptability with the increasing recognition that the vast majority of couples using physical aggression (1) do not fit the classic 'male batterer profile' of patriarchal, power and control-based terroristic violence (e.g. Johnson and Leone 2005); (2) tend to report relatively low-level aggression and only within their relationships (Holtzworth-Munroe *et al.* 2000); (3) have female partners who are equally aggressive (e.g. Slep and O'Leary 2005) and who use physical aggression for reasons other than self-defence in the vast majority of incidents (e.g. Cascardi and Vivian 1995); (4) have two partners whose behaviours, attitudes and personality characteristics are predictive of violence (e.g. O'Leary *et al.* 2007); and (5) report that communication problems are the most common precipitant of aggression (e.g. Babcock *et al.* 2004a).

In this chapter we will discuss why and for whom conjoint treatment of IPV is appropriate, assessment and treatment planning for conjoint treatment, major treatment components and general guidelines for the dyadic intervention of IPV.

Why treat IPV conjointly?

The belief that IPV should never be treated conjointly is rooted in the notion that batterers and victims are distinct and that treating them together would at best be fear-provoking for the victim and at worst physically dangerous (e.g. McMahon and Pence 1996). This proscription is codified into policy in many US states and Canadian provinces (Dutton and Corvo 2006). However, efficacy trials indicate that conjoint therapy is often suitable and even desirable for treating IPV (e.g. Stith *et al.* 2004). Further, few women in intact relationships presenting for couples therapy are fearful of remaining with their partners or of participating in a treatment with them (O'Leary *et al.* 1999). Thus, research indicates that concerns about inappropriateness of conjoint treatment are unfounded for most intact couples presenting for relationship therapy.

Treating IPV within the context of the dyad seems to be a better match for how intact, distressed couples conceptualize their problems (e.g. Ehrensaft and Vivian 1996). Most couples enter into couples treatment with the primary concern not of partner aggression but rather of relationship problems such as conflict. Nevertheless, although only 1.5 per cent of husbands and 6 per cent of wives list physical aggression as a presenting problem, 71 per cent reported physical aggression within their relationship within the past year on an intake questionnaire (O'Leary *et al.* 1992). IPV is under-reported because it is not considered by couples to be as important, as frequent, or as negative as the communication problems, psychological aggression or lack of love in the relationship (Ehrensaft and Vivian 1996). Therefore, separating the dyad into individual gender-specific treatment that would solely focus on aggression reduction would likely lead to decreased motivation or compliance from the couple than would treatment that focuses on the dyad but prioritizes the reduction of physical aggression within that context. Indeed, couples report that conjoint therapy allows them to see things from a new perspective, renew togetherness and underscore teamwork in a way that individual treatment would be unlikely to do (Allen and St George 2001).

An additional benefit of treating IPV conjointly is that to reduce aggression effectively all possible determinants of that aggression ought to be addressed, and since a number of key determinants are interpersonal, it is beneficial to have the interpersonal system in the therapy office to make changes. For example, most incidents of couple violence occur during an argument between partners (e.g. Cascardi and Vivian 1995), in which conflict escalates until one or both partners strikes the other (Heyman and Schlee 2003). Furthermore, destructive couple conflict and mutual verbal aggression have been found through observational studies to be strongly associated with partner aggression (Weiss and Heyman 1997). In other words, the majority of IPV occurs within a particular context (i.e. problematic communication), not spontaneously due only to one person's actions. Johnson and Leone (2005) have labelled conflict-based IPV 'common couple violence' and power/control-based IPV 'intimate terrorism'.

Because each person's behaviour is not only a response to the partner's behaviour but also a stimulus for the partner's subsequent response (the systems theory concept known as 'circular causality'; von Bertalanffy 1976), both partners contribute to conflict escalation, and thus each can work to reduce that escalation (and thus, in turn, the risk of IPV), although each individual is ultimately responsible for his or her own use of physical aggression (Neidig and Friedman 1984). In fact, men's violence is least likely when both partners adopt a non-violent philosophy (e.g. Straus 1990b). Therefore, having the system within which the aggression takes place available during intervention allows for this circular causality to become apparent and for multiple points of intervention to be made. Furthermore, because each person's actions elicit certain thoughts, emotions and behaviours in the partner, having both people present allows for these raw materials, such as hot cognitions and negative affect, to be used therapeutically in conjoint sessions.

Another major advantage of treating couple violence in conjoint therapy is the possibility of a shared, transparent treatment plan. Because individuals are already working at cross-purposes and have separate goals and strategies, their attempts are ineffective and often misattributed as provocation (e.g. Bradbury and Fincham 1990). Thus, it is advantageous for both partners to be cognizant of what each is attempting to do to better the situation (e.g. Rosen *et al.* 2003). For example, if an individual is urged to utilize a time-out technique in the midst of conflict to control his anger, his partner, if blind to his aims, might misinterpret this technique as withdrawal, likely leading to an increased pursuance of the conflict and heightened conflict escalation (e.g. Rosen *et al.* 2003). Both partners in this case are left with hopelessness that conflict is consciously manageable. On the other hand, when both partners are aware of the strategies each will use to de-escalate conflict, they are more likely to attribute these attempts to neutral or even positive causes. Furthermore, because *both* individuals are encouraged in conjoint treatment to accept personal responsibility for their behaviour, the therapist is less likely to be met with the persistent resistance and partner-blaming that is typical in gender-specific treatment, in which a sole focus on the individual and the omission of discussion of the partner's responsibility can foster defensiveness.

One final benefit of conjoint treatment is that monitoring of aggression is more easily accomplished when both spouses are asked to report the instances of violence. In conjoint therapy, both partners are typically forthcoming about violence that may occur, and any discrepancies between husband and wife reports can be clarified and thoroughly examined. More accurate tracking of aggression allows for better assessment of progress, sharper conceptualizations and more appropriate treatment adjustment.

However, conjoint treatment is contraindicated under certain circumstances, such as when the wife is severely victimized (i.e. injured, fearful, feeling controlled) (O'Leary 1996). In these cases, the determinants of aggression seem to be less rooted in couple processes but more in intrapersonal power and control issues within the husband (e.g. Johnson and Leone 2005). Although there are no differences in power and control behaviours between distressed assaultive and non-assaultive relationships in general (e.g. Tolman 1999), in the individual cases in which attempts to exert power and control over the partner are the primary precipitants of IPV, conjoint treatment would not be appropriate. Furthermore, in these cases, the wife is more likely to be fearful of speaking out in therapy, which would certainly interfere with treatment. There are other couple attributes that might make conjoint treatment less effective and ideal. In some cases, if the degree to which the couple's conflict escalation is extremely volatile and poorly controlled, individual relationship therapy aimed at self-regulation (e.g. Halford *et al.* 1994) or anger control (e.g. Del Vecchio and O'Leary 2004) might be more appropriate at first, to lay the foundations on which conjoint treatment can then build. Another possibility that could interfere with conjoint therapy is that some individuals might be less willing to take direction in the presence of their partners, in which case flexible alternation between individual and conjoint sessions might be best. Finally, substance abuse (including alcohol) by either partner is a contraindication for conjoint therapy. Specialized therapy for the substance problem, followed by conjoint treatment, has been efficacious in reducing not only substance use and relationship distress, but IPV as well (Fals-Stewart *et al.* 2002; O'Farrell *et al.* 2004).

Assessment and treatment planning

Because IPV is ubiquitous but is rarely a presenting problem, thorough assessment of the couple and potential role of violence is crucial, both for proper treatment and for determination of whether conjoint treatment is appropriate. As a starting point for assessment, certain questionnaires provide an easy and efficient manner of obtaining information about relationship and individual variables of interest. To measure variables relating to the relationship, one could administer the Dyadic Adjustment Scale (DAS) (Spanier 1976) or Relationship Satisfaction Questionnaire (RSAT) (Burns and Sayers 1992) to assess relationship adjustment and satisfaction, the Areas of Change Questionnaire (ACQ) (Weiss *et al.* 1973) to assess the realms of discontent for each partner in the relationship, and the Marital Status Inventory (MSI) (Weiss and Cerreto 1980) to assess marital dissolution potential. The Alcohol Use Disorders Identification Test (AUDIT) (Babor *et al.* 1992) should be used to assess for alcohol abuse or dependence.

Questionnaires can also be used to begin the assessment of violence, and offer certain advantages, such as that they provide higher detection than interviews, can be completed outside of session, provide behaviourally specific definitions of abuse, offer a common language for the clinician and client, and make it easier to broach the topic for both clinician and client (e.g. O'Leary *et al.* 1992). A standard violence assessment battery might include the Revised Conflict Tactics Scale (CTS2) (Straus *et al.* 1996) and the Psychological Maltreatment of Women Inventory (PMWI) (Tolman 1989).

Although questionnaires are a good starting point for assessment, individual interviews will provide richer clinical information and some additional reports of aggression (O'Leary *et al.* 1992). In separate sessions, individuals should be asked to estimate the overall frequency of aggressive episodes in the past year and to discuss the most severe and several recent episodes of aggression in the past year (e.g. Vivian and Heyman 1996). Factors such as severity, chronicity, injury or potential for injury, need for medical attention, fear, police involvement, context and the inferred function of the aggression should be directly assessed. The assessment should aim to determine if a conjoint format is appropriate – that is, if the aggression is not extreme in frequency or severity, if neither partner has sustained injuries serious enough to merit medical care, if the aggressor(s) admits to and takes responsibility for the use of aggression and wants to stop, and if neither partner reports fearfulness of participating in conjoint sessions or of increased aggression as a result of participating. If conjoint treatment is indeed appropriate, the therapist might also have the couple discuss a problematic topic, to observe the strengths and weaknesses of communication patterns during conflict (Heyman 2001).

Finally, another aspect of assessment that affects treatment planning is the level of explosiveness of the violence. If the aggression is of low explosiveness, the dyadic approach is appropriate throughout, and the function of the aggression should be explored. If, however, the aggression is characterized by high lability, it may be difficult to ensure that conjoint sessions would be safe. Individual sessions for the partners would be desirable until there is demonstrable improvement in anger control.

Major components of treatment

This section will review the common components of conjoint cognitive-behavioural treatments for IPV (e.g. Geffne *et al.* 1989; Heyman and Neidig 1997; Stith *et al.* 2004; LaTaillade *et al.* 2006).

Goal-setting

To ensure that each partner and the therapist agree on the direction the therapy will take, clear goals should be set before the intervention starts. To emphasize the primary goal of aggression cessation, the therapist can review the couple's accounts that their arguments often escalate out of control, sometimes resulting in behaviours of which they are not proud (i.e. verbal and physical aggression). The therapist then offers concern about the out-of-control processes and asks if the couple would like to feel more in control and reduce the occurrence of such processes. Invariably, they say yes. The therapist then asks whether – considering the possible (often inadvertent) danger and hurt feelings that result from out-of-control escalation and the ways even the possibility of such incidents can interfere with discussing anything – they would feel comfortable making aggression and the volatile thoughts and behaviours that precede that aggression the first target of intervention. We have yet to have a couple who did not wholeheartedly endorse this goal. Systems therapist Jay Haley (1987) has written that the goal of the initial sessions is to provide clients with a different problem to the ones with which they came to therapy. In this way, we aim for clients who arrive typically blaming their partners for their woes but who do not think that physical aggression is a problem to leave agreeing that physical aggression, its precipitants, and *dyadic* (not individual) problems should be the primary focus of therapy.

To cement the no-aggression treatment goal, a no-physical-violence contract can be employed (Heyman and Neidig 1997). Additionally, therapists can help partners mutually construct and commit to other therapy goals, such as reducing verbal aggression, improving self-regulation and anger management, improving conflict resolution skills and enhancing positive interactions between partners (O'Leary *et al.* 1998). Therapists should enforce that individuals set goals for themselves and not their partners, highlighting the message of personal control and responsibility.

Anger management

Anger control techniques play a significant role in reducing aggression and allowing for better partner interactions. Clients should be assisted in identifying their own affective, behavioural and cognitive cues that their anger is escalating, and then taught anger management strategies to be used when those cues indicate that self-soothing strategies would be appropriate and helpful. One such strategy is the use of a time-out. This strategy should be employed by the couple when the conflict becomes risky (i.e. before anger builds to a destructive level). Couples should agree to separate to cool off – without drinking alcohol or driving – and return to the discussion at a later time. Therapists should help partners negotiate how to call for a time-out, how long they should wait before returning to the discussion, what each should be doing during the separation, and how to signal the end of the time-out. It is especially important that two things are highlighted: (1) that time-out is not a strategy to avoid discussion or to quiet a partner, but rather a strategy to promote better conflict resolution without debilitating anger; and (2) that simply removing oneself from the situation but persisting in rumination about the issue does not constitute a successful time-out. Effort should be made during the time to reduce anger (see section on cognitive restructuring). Rosen *et al.* (2003) emphasize the importance for the couple that the time-out be learned, negotiated and practised together, to avoid the abuse or misinterpretation of this technique.

Cognitive restructuring

Therapists should help clients understand the usually overlooked major role that cognition plays between triggering events and their own anger responses, and how this cognition can be a point of intervention and a means by which anger can be reduced. Clients can identify specific cognitions that are associated with their own anger and aggressive behaviour; these cognitions might involve negative attributions about their partners' intentions, beliefs and rules about how husbands or wives ought to behave, or cognitions that only focus on the short-term positive effects of aggression. Therapists should guide clients to uncover both the underlying distortions in these cognitions and the ineffectiveness of these cognitions in achieving their long-term goals, and then encourage clients to learn to challenge these cognitions.

Communication and problem-solving skills training

Once individuals have mastered the skills necessary to prevent aggression or anger escalation, they can benefit from learning how to adeptly communicate and problem-solve with their partners. Research on communication (as reviewed by Schumacher *et al.* 2001) indicates that couples who do not engage with this problem-solving approach are more likely to display more aversive behaviours such as negative communication, mutual blame, contempt, belligerence, anger, anxiety, and feelings of being attacked (complicated by dominant-submissive relationships across genders). Thus both partners deserve clinical attention in terms of their ability to comminicate with one another.

Distinguishing between constructive and destructive ways of expressing one's thoughts and feelings is key for proper conflict management, to combat popular beliefs that telling one's partner how one feels is always appropriate, regardless of delivery. This relates to the distinction between assertion – standing up for one's own rights without violating the rights of others – and aggression – enforcing one's own rights or will without regard of others. Once these distinctions are clear, basic communication skills such as asking permission, decision-making, request-making, talking about problems, and seeking and sharing information should be discussed and practised, and clients should be encouraged to see the differential outcomes of making conciliatory statements as opposed to reciprocating negativity. Couples should also be taught basic problem-solving steps such as behavioural problem definition, cooperative and non-judgemental brainstorming of possible solutions, evaluation of the advantages and disadvantages of each potential solution, choice of an initial test solution, and assessment of the solution after implementation. Partners should practise new expressive, listening and problem-solving skills with gradually increasingly difficult or contentious topics.

Relationship enhancement

Although anger and conflict management are crucial for reducing the destructive patterns in couple relationships, special effort should also be made to increase positive interactions. Many couples who present for treatment perceive their relationships to be entirely consumed with negative interactions; thus, increasing positive behaviours that had once made the relationship gratifying will help boost marital satisfaction, affection and support, and indirectly make compromise and conflict management more palatable.

Guidelines for conjoint therapeutic intervention

Find human qualities in each person

Considering popular images of male batterers and victimized wives, it is easy for therapists to designate individuals into roles such as perpetrator and victim, or even to get pulled into partners' appeals about who is right and who is wrong. However, as is applicable to any therapeutic situation, this approach will interfere with proper conceptualizations and formation of therapeutic alliances with both partners (Neidig and Friedman 1984). Instead, the therapist must view each partner as a flawed human responding to circumstances as he or she perceives them; this stance makes it easier to avoid judgement and instead to identify and address factors that maintain undesirable behaviour.

Aggression is not 'dysfunctional'

Although it's convenient to argue (or even 'psychoeducate') that aggression is a dysfunctional response in nearly every context, there are problems with that stance.

Most obviously, whether something is 'functional' technically refers to reinforcement and punishment of behaviour (Domjan 2003). That is, if a wife stops asking for change when her husband screams and looks threatening, then he is reinforced for screaming. Although perhaps not healthy in the long run, screaming is 'functional' in behavioural terms because it produces a reward (e.g. Patterson 1982). By not examining or at least hypothesizing about the rewards in the clients' natural environment, therapists put themselves at a disadvantage in targeting incompatible behaviours to reinforce. Many family environments either do not reward non-aggressive behaviour or even punish it, and therapists who expect that an individual's will and self-control will perpetually triumph over environmental contingencies are both overly optimistic and almost certainly will be disappointed. Therefore, therapists are encouraged to identify the function of aggression within the relationship and then attempt to modify the contingencies such that non-aggressive behaviour might be rewarded (Heyman and Slep 2007).

Join with each partner

Partners in highly contentious couples often attempt to pull the therapist into taking sides. However, any evidence that the therapist is working harder for one individual is bound to alienate the other partner and discourage attempts to change. Therefore, the therapist should be careful to gain each person's trust that the therapist is an ally and is working in his or her best interests (e.g. Minuchin 1974).

Amplify ambivalence

Many gender-specific treatments for IPV aggressively demand that the man changes; however, men often maintain equilibrium to such confrontations with defensiveness that frequently hinders therapy. Instead, therapists can encourage self-motivated change by drawing upon motivational interviewing approaches and amplifying ambivalence in the individual (Miller and Rollnick 2002). Comparing an individual's view of acceptable behaviour as a husband and role model to his children with current behaviours will likely elicit dissonance and motivate change for resolution. In other words, instead of forcing clients to accept the therapist's world view and solutions to the problem, the therapist should start where the clients are, and lead them to being open to new behaviours and strategies by empathically highlighting the differences between what the client wants and what is happening. This approach is more likely to make the client feel accepted and understood, and willing to take chances to change well-learned behaviours. ('Acceptance and commitment therapy' uses a similar approach, labelled 'creative hopelessness': see Eifert *et al.* 2006)

There is no such thing as unlearning

Converging neurobiological and behavioural research indicates that there is no such thing as 'unlearning'; instead, extinction involves new learning that coexists with the previously reinforced pairing (Bouton 2002). The longer and stronger a reinforced pattern (such as aggression) is, the harder it is to permanently eliminate its performance. This may be why many interventions for IPV find decrements in, but not permanent cessation of, aggression (e.g. O'Leary *et al.* 1999). Therefore, because bad behaviours cannot be unlearned, new behaviours must be practised and rewarded repeatedly to have any chance of replacing the bad ones. Therapists should expect individuals to need to practise new patterns of behaviour many times, and should make special efforts to ensure that those behaviours are rewarded.

Think dyadically, act individually

Halford *et al.* (1994) have argued that most skills-based approaches to couples treatment adopt the same problematic approach that produces couple distress: individuals trying to change their partners. In a self-regulation approach, intervention involves moving participants toward a self-focused, positive change orientation. This approach is empowering because individuals have no direct control over their partner's behaviour but do have control over their own. Halford *et al.* demonstrated the efficacy of a self-regulation approach to couples problems; and their approach is especially useful with IPV couples because it emphasizes modifying one's own behaviour to achieve positive relationship outcomes

Control sessions

Because conflict with aggressive couples can quickly become heated – derailing gains and affording the practice of coercive behaviours – it is especially important for the therapist to have a clear goal in mind for each session and to stop behaviours that interfere with those goals. When stopping escalating in-session conflicts and processing them, the therapist should consistently both empathize with each person's world view and work toward an understanding of each person's desired outcomes and their own thoughts/behaviours that are unwittingly thwarting achieving those outcomes (McCullough 2000). Following McCullough, we work with clients in identifying desired outcomes that are within their own control (e.g. calmly stating my point of view).

Conclusions

Although certainly not appropriate for all couples reporting aggression (e.g. psychopaths, those who use fear to dominate and control their partners), conjoint treatment is an appropriate format for most couples who present for couples therapy. This chapter has provided a brief overview of the rationale and enactment of such treatment. The efficacy of all interventions for IPV is low (Babcock *et al.* 2004b), so developers of all approaches have much work to do to improve the services that are offered to those experiencing IPV. Perhaps the modest effect is due to most studies being conducted with court-mandated samples, with the primacy of group treatment over individualized treatment, and with the one-size-fits-all approaches that predominate. Conjoint treatment appears to be a viable alternative, but one in which much work remains to be done.

Acknowledgements

Preparation of this chapter was supported by the National Institute of Child Health and Human Development (Grant R01HD046901).

18 Domestic violence: a family health perspective

Iona Heath

Introduction

Throughout this chapter, the masculine personal pronoun is used for the perpetrators of domestic violence and the feminine for the victims/survivors. This is not to claim that domestic violence is exclusively male abuse of women, but to give explicit recognition to the fact that such abuse accounts for the major proportion of domestic violence, particularly that which results in serious injury.

In most countries, primary medical care, provided by family doctors or general practitioners, serves as the point of entry to the health care system as a whole. Primary care physicians provide personal and continuing care to individual patients in the context of their family and wider social context (WONCA 2002). Effective care is built on mutual trust which, in most cases, is deliberately constructed over a series of encounters. The doctor must trust the patient to provide an authentic account of his or her subjective experience of illness. The patient must trust the doctor to take this account seriously and to apply his or her medical knowledge and skills for the benefit of each individual, in the context of that person's own life story, aspirations and values. This can only be achieved if the doctor cultivates a deliberate positive regard for each patient: an understanding that each is doing his or her best to cope with the challenges of life within the situation in which he or she finds themselves. Providing care for families and communities, primary care physicians see different members of nuclear and extended families – young and old – sometimes together, sometimes separately. They attempt to believe the best of each one and to act in his or her best interest. The ugly reality of domestic violence cuts right across this commitment.

The existence of family violence profoundly disrupts our notions of what both the family and the discipline of general practice/family medicine are meant to be. Not only is the family distorted by the experience of violence, but the attitudes and role of the doctor are also affected. As a result, numerous difficulties and dilemmas arise: practical, interpersonal and ethical. Nonetheless, at the same time, the primary care physician is in a position to make a positive and sometimes pivotal contribution to the challenge of domestic violence: its prevention, its early detection and the mitigation of its consequences.

Domestic violence:

Such a harmless term for people who don't know what lies behind it. Do you know what it is like, living in constant fear your whole life?

> Living with hatred every single day, it never stops no matter what you do, and you can never do anything to change it, until you lose your independent will and just wait and hope that the next beating won't be as bad as the one before.

(Indridason 2006: 227)

These are the fictional words of the now adult daughter of a woman subjected to years of domestic violence in Arnaldur Indridason's extraordinary crime novel published in English under the title *Silence of the Grave*. The words capture, with great imaginative power, the profound destructiveness of family violence.

Families are supposed to provide love, care and security for each member – and many do. However, too many are also, or instead, the setting for fear, hurt and violence: 'with the exception of the police and the military, the family is perhaps the most violent social group and the home, the most violent setting in our society' (Gelles and Strauss 1979: 15). The attitudes and aspirations of the family doctor are constructed for the first sort of family and they are severely tested by families which harbour violence.

At this point, it may be helpful to consider in more detail the effects of coercion and the use of force. In 1939, while in the process of extricating herself from occupied France, Simone Weil wrote a brilliant essay entitled 'The Iliad, or the poem of force'. It was published in Marseilles in 1940, while Weil and her parents were waiting for exit visas for America – waiting for an enforced exile. The essay begins with a definition of force: 'To define force – it is the *x* that turns anybody who is subjected to it into a *thing*. Exercised to the limit, it turns man into a thing in the most literal sense: it makes a corpse out of him' (Weil 2005: 3). The parallels between this description of the effects of force and Indridason's description of a survivor of domestic violence are, for me, astonishing. The person who is abused is not seen as a unique human individual but as a *thing*.

Yet families are meant to be built on bonds of love and love is evoked for a particular irreplaceable other: 'A loved one is … singular, distinct, separate. The more closely one defines, regardless of any given values, the more intimately one loves. The finite outline is proof of its opposite, the infinity of emotion provoked by what the outline contains' (Berger 1985: 105).

How can anyone who is 'singular, distinct and separate' become transformed into a thing? Yet, violence can only happen if this transformation occurs. Those who abuse others must first blind themselves to the full subjectivity and dignity of the one they hurt. It is this blinding that makes abuse within intimate relationships so shocking and so damaging. Given this context, it should not be surprising that sexual intercourse which, at its best, is the physical expression of love, should so often be forced and amount to rape within abusive relationships.

Martin Buber describes a relevant dichotomy between 'I-It' and 'I-Thou' relationships. 'I-It' relationships treat people as objects to be manipulated for individual or collective ends while 'I-Thou' relationships acknowledge the limitless subjectivity of the other and in so doing awake and engage the subjectivity of the I. Abusive relationships seem to represent an extreme example of 'I-It' interactions and it is possible that the abuser in such relationships is unable to acknowledge the full subjectivity either of the 'thing' he abuses or of himself (Buber 1923). Felicity de Zulueta (2003) has examined the relationship between violence and infant attachment behaviour. About two-thirds of 1-year-olds have formed secure attachments to their primary carers and these equip them with the capacity to form loving relationships. They are able to perceive the other as another human individual who also has needs and can initiate and sustain 'I-Thou' relationships. However, a fifth of infants have experienced rejection and have developed an avoidant pattern of attachment behaviour. Such children show no distress when their mother leaves them and ignores her when she returns. They have learnt to suppress their feelings of anger and fear in order to avoid further rejection. Such children grow up unable to acknowledge their own feelings and similarly unable to acknowledge the feelings and needs of others. They have little or no capacity for empathy. Their relationships will tend to remain 'I-It'. Primary care physicians have the opportunity to see these processes playing out in families as children grow and develop in both favourable and unfavourable family contexts.

Victim/survivor

The experience of those who have been subjected to force and abuse is of being treated as a 'thing'. When such a person seeks help, it is essential that her subjectivity and autonomy are fully acknowledged. In these circumstances, more than almost any other, the doctor has a responsibility to address the Thou rather than the It. Doctors need to be aware of the prevalence of domestic violence and the very real probability that many of their patients are being subjected to violence in a regular and recurring pattern. The first professional responsibility is to listen and through listening to validate experience – not to resort to hasty judgements.

As in the whole of medicine, no diagnosis can be made unless the doctor is aware of its possibility. Domestic violence is an issue that raises such a painful awareness of the enduring ugliness of human nature that it is very easy not to allow oneself to think of it – especially in relation to people with whom one has built a relationship of positive regard. To keep the possibility in mind demands determination and a sort of courage as well as an understanding of the serious health consequences of domestic violence, and an awareness of the range of symptoms and conditions which are known to be caused by it.

Clearly, domestic violence causes a whole range of physical injuries up to and including death. Injuries to the head, face, neck, chest, breast and abdomen, particularly in women, should be assumed to have been caused by domestic violence unless proved otherwise. Beyond physical injury, let us go back for a moment to Simone Weil's description of the soul: 'It was not made to live inside a thing; if it does so, under pressure of necessity, there is not a single element of its nature to which violence is not done' (Weil 2005: 5). This makes sense of the profound damage done to the psychological well-being of those who suffer repeated abuse. Women who have experienced domestic violence suffer a high incidence of psychiatric disorders, particularly depression and a range of self-damaging behaviours including drug and alcohol abuse, and suicide, both attempted and achieved. In this context, it is important to be absolutely clear that these conditions present after the first exposure to violence and must therefore be viewed as consequences of the violence rather than, as some perpetrators might have us believe, causes of it or even excuses for it.

Once the doctor has considered the possibility of domestic violence, once his or her suspicion is aroused, the next task is to pose a direct question: 'I fell down the stairs again, I told her – Sorry. No questions asked. What about the burn on my hand? The missing hair? The teeth? I waited to be asked. Ask me. Ask me. Ask me. I'd tell her. I'd tell them everything. Look at the burn. Ask me about it. Ask' (Doyle 1996: 164). These are the fictional words of Roddy Doyle's Paula Spencer, the woman who walked into doors. She is once again in a Dublin casualty department, behind the curtain, hoping to be asked a direct question about the cause of her injuries, convinced that if someone would just ask, she would tell them what was happening and her life would begin to change.

The family is meant to be a place of love, warmth, support and intimacy. The difficulty of admitting that one's own family is also a source of violent abuse should never be underestimated. Many women feel humiliated and ashamed of their predicament, and it is essential that a patient feels that her privacy will be respected. She should always be enabled to consult on her own and, if at all possible, she should be offered the chance to talk to a woman health care professional if she prefers to do so. She should be reminded that anything she chooses to talk about is confidential and that the only exception to this will occur if the doctor becomes aware that a dependent child is at risk of serious harm.

The concept of medical confidentiality may be unfamiliar, particularly to many first-generation immigrant women, and the protection it offers will need to be emphasized and explained. Provided the patient gives consent, the involvement of translators, advocacy workers or ethnic community link-workers can be very helpful to both patient and doctor.

Practitioners need to experiment with questions, to find the particular form of words that works reliably for them. Ones that work for me include:

- Did someone at home do this to you?
- Have you ever been in a relationship where you have been hurt in any way? Are you in such a relationship now?

In one American study, almost three-quarters of women subject to domestic violence were identified by answers to any one of the following three questions:

- Have you been hit, kicked, punched or otherwise physically hurt by someone in the past year? If so, by whom?
- Do you feel safe in your current relationship?

- Is there a partner from a previous relationship who is making you feel unsafe now? (Feldhaus *et al.* 1997).

Once answered in the affirmative, the doctor then has a responsibility to document carefully any physical injuries and to record any additional contextual evidence of abuse, such as torn clothing or damage to the home, if the patient is being seen on a home visit. The doctor should also ask about the whereabouts of any children at the time of the assault.

At this point, most doctors, certainly in UK general practice, will be feeling the pressure of time and the presence of other patients waiting to be seen. It is helpful to understand that the doctor cannot treat and solve the situation but two things must be done – first the safety of the immediate situation must be assessed and secondly the woman must be offered a choice of options as to how she might wish to proceed. Is she in immediate danger? Is he verbally threatening her or her friends or relatives? Has he threatened to use weapons? Does he have access to any? Are the children in danger? Where are they now? Does she have anywhere she could go now, other than home? She needs to be told unequivocally that *she is the victim of a crime*, that violence in the home is as illegal as violence on the street, and that she has a right to be protected from further assault. She should be offered support from the police, from Women's Aid and from any other appropriate local agencies. All those working in primary care should have the contact details for these agencies readily available.

In the context of a history of violence, often extending over many years, and all the while eroding and destroying self-esteem and self-determination, it is essential to understand that effective help must be directed towards enabling the woman to retake control of her own life. The aim should be to offer her realistic choices, while accepting that the decisions are hers alone and are always valid in her particular situation. No patient should ever be pressurized into following any particular course of action. Her autonomy should be encouraged and respected. Even if the patient decides to return to the violent situation, she is not likely to forget the information and care that she has been given and, in time, this may help her to break out of the cycle of abuse. There is, of course, one exception to all this which occurs when there are dependent children who are at present risk of serious harm. In these circumstances, the doctor must assess whether the non-abusing parent is able to act to protect her children from further harm. She should be offered any support necessary to make this possible. If she is unable to provide adequate protection, a referral to social services is essential.

Perpetrator

The discovery that a familiar patient is a perpetrator of domestic violence is often deeply shocking to the family doctor and presents probably the most difficult challenge to that doctor and, perhaps, especially if that doctor is a woman. From the moment of discovery, it becomes almost impossible to retain that unconditional positive regard which is the optimal basis for the imaginative sympathy required for the full execution of the role of doctor. Most commonly, the doctor will discover the status of the perpetrator from the account of the victim and the demands of confidentiality will mean that the perpetrator will be unaware of the doctor's new knowledge. The doctor needs to understand very clearly that any hint of disclosure may put the victim at increased risk of further violence.

All too rarely the perpetrator makes things much easier for the doctor by coming to seek help and by revealing an awareness of the damage that is being caused by his violence. The doctor is then in a position to make a referral to an anger management course or to a specialist domestic violence perpetrator programme, both of which are often in regrettably short supply.

Standard couple therapy or family therapy is never likely to be appropriate where family discord has spilled over into violence and become a crime. Such interventions may also serve to increase the risk of further violence by inviting the victim to confront her abuser. An exception to this general rule can occur when specialist therapy, most commonly on the Duluth model, is mandated by the court, with the perpetrator obliged to attend and the victim offered robust protection throughout. However, sadly, even these interventions appear to have a minimal impact on reducing further violence beyond the documented effect of being arrested (Babcock *et al.* 2004b).

Children

The abuse of women and the abuse of children are intimately connected. Roddy Doyle's Paula Spencer is very aware of this: 'I was going nowhere, straight there. Trapped in a house that would never be mine. With a husband who fed on my pain. Watching my children going nowhere with me; the cruellest thing of the lot. No hope to give them. They saw him throw me across the kitchen. They saw him put a knife to my throat. Their father; my husband' (Doyle 1996: 204). The effects of family violence on children can be imagined but remain relatively poorly documented. Children tend to make sense of the world by assuming that they themselves are in some way responsible for the situations in which they find themselves. As a result they may blame themselves for domestic violence or for being unable to prevent it happening. They may try to intervene and be injured themselves.

Children who suffer physical abuse are more likely to have mothers who have been subjected to domestic violence and the reverse is also true. More than half of the men who use violence against their partners also abuse their children (Gayford 1975). Children exposed to domestic violence are more likely to present with physical injuries (Braun *et al.* 2005). In an American study, at least 45 per cent of the mothers of abused children were found to be themselves battered, and these women had already presented an average of four injury episodes to the hospital. However, the battering clearly predated the child abuse, and the children of battered mothers are significantly more likely to be physically abused than neglected (Stark and Flitcraft 1988). Similar findings are now reported from the UK and the National Society for the Prevention of Cruelty to Children (NSPCC) has found similar levels of domestic violence towards the mothers of children who are known to have been abused. In another UK study, 27 per cent of abused mothers reported that their partners had also abused the children (NCH Action for Children 1994).

Despite these correlations, many UK general practitioners will have experience of women who have been held responsible, by social services departments, for their inability to protect their children from violence to which they are also being subjected:

> In contrast to battering, where sexist interpretations and practices confront a grass-roots political movement, in the child abuse field, stereotypic and patronizing imagery of women goes unchallenged. One result is that men are invisible. Another is that 'mothers' are held responsible for child abuse, even when the mother and child are being battered by an identifiable man ... the best way to prevent child abuse is to protect women's physical integrity and support their empowerment.
>
> *(Stark and Flitcraft 1988: 97–118).*

For just these reasons, the Statement of Aims and Principles of the Women's Aid Federation (England) defines domestic violence as 'the emotional, sexual or physical abuse of women and children in their homes by partners or known others, usually men' (Women's Aid Federation of England 1992). The Federation's guiding principle is that the safety and empowerment of the non-abusing parent (usually the mother) is the most effective form of child protection. This contrasts with the current policy rhetoric which seems to assume that the welfare of children can be detached and treated separately from the welfare of their mothers. Any health worker responsible for the care of families knows that this is not the case.

Male violence against women from ethnic minority communities

Women from ethnic minority communities face particular difficulties which include racism, language barriers and worries about what will happen to their immigration status if they attempt to leave their violent partner. The enduring pervasiveness of racism within society and the stereotyping of members of some communities mean that black women may be very reluctant to call the police or involve them in any way, feeling that by doing so they are betraying their whole community. Some women may be subjected to enormous pressure from their extended families to stay with a violent partner because of the stigma which is attached to the breakdown of family structures. Some whose first language is not English may have insurmountable problems in communicating their predicament to professionals or agencies who might be able to offer help. Other women may fear deportation if they leave a violent partner within 12 months of coming to the UK (Women's Aid Federation of England 1992).

Male violence against women with disabilities

> 'In attempting to address the specific problem of male violence against women with disability it is necessary to take into account the fact that all people with disability face a range of oppressive and discriminatory factors in their lives' (Strathclyde Regional Council 1995: 4).

There is some evidence to suggest that disabled women are at increased risk of violence (Strathclyde Regional Council 1995) and certainly the relatively increased dependency and isolation which so often accompanies disability can make it harder for disabled women to extricate themselves from violent situations. The abuser may be the woman's sole carer, and fears of continuing violence may be balanced by fears of being unable to cope alone, fears of becoming dependent on the inadequacies of statutory services and, perhaps at worst, fears of being obliged to accept institutional care. Others, including relatives and friends, may be unwilling to accept that the partner, who undertakes the additional burden of caring for a disabled partner, could be capable of violence. And this may all be compounded because the confidentiality of a disabled person is much more easily compromised by the, sometimes accustomed, presence of the carer.

To screen or not to screen?

Many have argued that all women presenting for health care should be asked routinely about their exposure to domestic violence, and that such an approach is justified by the estimated prevalence of domestic violence and by the huge toll that it takes on the physical and psychological health of so many women. Many women attending for health care support the idea of routine screening questions but, importantly, a significant minority of abused women do not (Ramsay *et al.* 2002). When questioning was combined with mandatory reporting, two-thirds of one study sample thought women would be less likely to tell their health care providers about abuse (Gielen *et al.* 2000). My view is that routine screening questions will never be appropriate in the very diverse setting of ordinary general practice consultations, where formulaic, protocol-driven approaches can so easily dominate the patient's own, often carefully planned, agenda for the consultation. Nonetheless, it is of course essential that all practitioners retain a high index of suspicion within all consultations, and are prepared to act on those suspicions as soon as they arise.

The problem is that standardized care using compulsory and standardized questions once again turns people into Simone Weil's 'things'. A potential Thou is turned into an unequivocal It. No account is taken of the particularities of the individuals involved or their contexts. Each becomes a cipher – either as doctor or patient. Such approaches have no place in general practice/family medicine which is predicated on continuing relationships between particular patients and particular doctors. For doctors, the imperative becomes that we treat our patients always as an end in themselves whatever else we seek to achieve, and also that we treat ourselves as doctors as an end and do not allow ourselves to be used simply as a means to someone else's end.

Conclusions

The push towards mandatory questioning treats both patients and doctors as the means to a greater good and neglects at the same time to treat them as ends in themselves. The greater good of seeking to reduce the suffering caused by family violence is crucially important, however, someone who has already been turned into a 'thing' by the effects of violence and who is then treated simply as a means to others' ends has that 'thingness' confirmed. If people are to be treated as ends in themselves, the relationship between the patient and the doctor has to be genuine. The conversation between them has to be authentic and it has to be a conversation that is generated by that particular dyad of people, not by others dictating the agenda from outside. Only by insisting on dignifying our patients with the fullness of their humanity can we hope to begin to mitigate the immense and horrifying damage inflicted by domestic violence.

Part four
Outcome

19 Partner homicide including murder-suicide: gender differences

Katherine van Wormer and Albert R. Roberts

Introduction

Intimate partner violence (IPV) is all too common throughout the world and takes many forms. The most serious of these is homicide by an intimate partner. The fear of being killed, in fact, is a major dynamic in male-on-female violence and oftentimes in motivating women to kill the perpetrator of abuse in desperation. Our concern in this chapter is with the extent and nature of such violence. Our sources are government reports from the UK Home Office, the US Bureau of Justice Statistics, the Violence Policy Center, and original data from New Jersey criminal justice records concerning demographic factors in domestic homicide and recidivism rates by the perpetrators of this crime. Personal narratives from interviews with 105 women inmates in a north-eastern US state penitentiary who had been convicted of killing their partners highlight the discussion. Derived from qualitative data from these interviews, this chapter provides a conceptual framework or continuum for evaluating battered women and improving risk assessments of dangerousness. A section on murder-suicide analyses the apparent motives behind this largely male-on-female form of domestic homicide. We conclude with a discussion of strategies of crisis intervention and risk reduction.

Overview

In Britain, as elsewhere, a woman is more vulnerable to violence in her home than in public. In the UK, domestic violence costs the lives of more than two women every week (Home Office 2005b) and in the USA, with a much larger population, estimates are that more than three women a day are killed by their intimate partners (Rennison 2003).

Homicide is a leading cause of traumatic death for pregnant and post-partum women in the USA, accounting for 31 per cent of maternal injury deaths (Family Violence Prevention Fund 2006). In the UK, pregnancy is a period of high risk as well.

Whereas in the USA females who are killed are most often killed by guns, in England and Wales, three times as many women are killed by a sharp instrument or by strangulation as by shooting. Over the past decade, about four times as many females who were killed as males were partners or ex-partners of the murderer (Home Office 2005a). As in the USA, far more males than females are victimized by homicide of a general nature; they are killed often in fights with other men.

Domestic violence is one of the US nation's most prevalent crimes, occurring in all types of communities – urban, suburban and rural. The victims of domestic violence come from all races, ethnic groups, religions and income levels. It is also a gruesome fact that domestic violence sometimes ends in homicide. According to the Bureau of Justice Statistics (Rennison 2003) 1247 women and 440 men were murdered by their intimate male partners or former partners in 2001. In the past, in the 1980s, these numbers were about even – in other words, about as many men as women were killed in domestic violence situations.

According to the Centers for Disease Control and Prevention document *Surveillance for Homicide Among Intimate Partners* (2001), in the USA the majority of domestic homicides during an eight-year period (1990–8) were committed by men or women who killed a spouse, former spouse, boyfriend or girlfriend. Approximately 50 per cent of the domestic violence victims of both sexes were killed by their *spouses*, while 33 per cent were killed by *girlfriends or boyfriends*.

An extensive search by Aldridge and Browne (2003) revealed 22 empirical research studies on risk factors for spousal homicide. In the UK, 37 per cent of all the women victims were murdered by their current or former intimate partner compared to 6 per cent of men who were killed. As previously mentioned, the most common cause of an intimate partner's death in England and Wales was being attacked with a sharp implement or being strangled. By contrast, the most common cause in the USA for spousal homicide was getting shot. Nine major risk factors are found that may help predict the probability of a partner homicide and prevent future victims (Aldridge and Browne 2003).

Women who killed their partners

In about three-fourths of intimate murders in the USA the woman is the victim (Rennison 2003). This still leaves a substantial number of cases, approximately 440, in which the woman killed her spouse or boyfriend. Since 1976 the number of male intimates killed decreased by around two-thirds while the decline in the number of female victims decreased by about one-fourth. Statistics Canada (1998: 2005) reveals a similar decline in the numbers of male domestic homicide victims but not of female victims of homicide. The increase in violence prevention programming and the availability of shelters or refuges is the generally stated explanation for the decrease in the numbers of women who kill their partners in self-defence.

Van Wormer and Bartollas (2007) explain the striking decline in female-on-male homicides by their partners in terms of avenues of escape. This theory holds that if a woman can escape from a dangerous battering situation, she will do so, and that if she cannot do so, the risk is that she will resort to using lethal partner violence. In any case, it is a paradox, rarely realized, that the proliferation of domestic violence prevention for which women and victims assistance advocates have fought so hard is saving the lives of battering men more than of female victims who are so often still stalked and killed in attempted break-up situations.

In an extensive study conducted by Roberts (2007), over 500 battered women were interviewed about their relationship to their batterer. Interviews were gathered from four sub-sets of battered women in New Jersey. Samples were obtained from three police departments, three shelters for battered women, a convenience sample of battered women in the community and, relevant to our purposes, a large sample of 105 women who had killed their partners and who were serving time in a state prison. From the total sample of women, Roberts developed a five-level continuum of severity of abuse:

- Level 1: short-term abuse.
- Level 2: abuse of moderate to severe injury lasting up to two years.
- Level 3: intermittent abuse punctuated by long periods that were violence-free.

Women in the survey at these first three levels tended to be middle class and well educated. These others were predominantly working class:

- Level 4: chronic and severe violence.
- Level 5: severe violence that lasted on average for eight years.

The 105 women who were classified at Level 5 were women serving time in prison for killing their abusers. The overwhelming majority (59.2 per cent) of these women lacked the skills to earn a decent income on their own (Roberts 2002). Almost half (47.6 per cent) of the inmate interviewees had been on public assistance for many years during the battering episodes.

Women from the prison sample had usually begun at Level 2 on the continuum, and then had escalated to either Level 4 or Level 5 for several years, after which the death threats had become more explicit and lethal. Also, in a number of cases, the victim had finally left the abuser and obtained a restraining order, which he then violated. Many of the women in this category suffered from post-traumatic stress disorder (PTSD), nightmares and insomnia, and some had attempted suicide. A smaller group of the convicted women indicated that at the time that they killed their batterer, they were delusional or hallucinating due to heavy use of LSD, metham-phetamines, cocaine or other drugs. The most significant finding related to these women is that the overwhelming majority (65.7 per cent) had received specific lethal death threats in which the batterer specified the method, time and/or location of their demise.

Although most perpetrators of domestic violence homicides are male, there is a considerable number of women who, following repeated acts of violence by their partner, lash out and kill him, sometimes accidentally or in self-defence. The women who were interviewed as part of this research project had all been convicted of murder or manslaughter and other charges, and women were sentenced to an average of 12 years in prison. Often, a specific death threat was made against their lives by their abusive partners in the 24 hours prior to the homicide – and sometimes the death threat occurred just prior to the homicide. Some batterers were very specific about their threats. Some of the deaths of the abusive men seemed to be accidental, or in self-defence, as the man and woman were fighting over a weapon; other deaths were caused by impulsive, violent retaliatory acts on the part of the women.

Of the 105 women in the study who killed their abusive husband or partner, Tamika's story is typical. Like the others, she described a painful and impoverished childhood, early childhood sexual abuse (in her case by her brothers), abuse of alcohol and other drugs, overwhelming anger, and mutual combat among both partners that resulted in lethal violence in which the woman who had been brutally victimized killed the abuser. Collectively, these interviews revealed frequent use by both parties of hallucinogenic drugs, and a much higher occurrence of attempted suicide than the women in the other groups.

Tamika's recollection of the worst incident is the argument that started when she became furious that her husband had used their rent money to buy drugs, and ended when they were fighting over his gun, and she shot and killed him.

> It was over drugs, when he took the rent money to buy drugs. I hid the money and he took it. I started hitting him, and then he started beating me. He held me down to keep me from hitting him. When I hit him, he started hitting me and kicking and slapping me ... Then he went for his gun and said he was going to kill me, but I got to it first.

As they were fighting for control of the gun, Tamika shot her husband and killed him. The judge sentenced her to serve 10 to 15 years in the women's prison.

An unexpected finding in this study was the very high rate of depression for the chronically battered women and for the women who killed their partners (67.5 per cent). In contrast to the community sample of battered women, the women in the prison sample frequently had a history of drug use. Other relevant factors that emerged in the interviews were reports of the batterer's extreme jealousy, emotional dependence and drunken episodes. Traumatization plus anger seem to have made for a volatile combination that spelled disaster for all of the women (and their families) in this category. Regrettably, none of these women had sought help from a shelter for battered women.

Male-on-female homicide

Domestic violence homicides take place in all regions of the USA, and in the majority of these murders the weapon used was a handgun. The national, non-profit Violence Policy Center, located in Washington, DC, prepared a state-by-state ranking on women who were murdered in the year 2000, and found that overwhelmingly the perpetrator was a husband, boyfriend or other close relative – rather than a stranger. The study found that 1689 (86.7 per cent) women throughout the USA were killed by a man they knew, compared with 137 (13.3 per cent) women who were killed by a male stranger (Violence Policy Center 2006). The states with the highest per capita number of women who were killed by men in 2000 were (in order of prevalence): Mississippi, Arizona, South Carolina, Tennessee, Louisiana, North Carolina, Arkansas, New Mexico, Nevada, Oklahoma, Alabama and Virginia.

Fascinating insights are provided by Kathryn Ann Farr (2002) in interviews with a sample of women who survived an attempted domestic homicide. Most typically, as described by these women and confirmed in police reports, the perpetrator was an alcoholic or drug addict, a gun owner and, if the victim had left him, her stalker. Interviewees described the attack that followed as terrifying in that they were certain they were going to die.

Situations of murder-suicide

Because government data in the UK and the USA providing national statistics on homicide that ends in suicide are hard to come by, other, less official and comprehensive sources, must be consulted. A recent development in the USA is a promising one, however, for future research. The emerging state-based National Violent Death Reporting System has recently begun providing data on murder-suicide for a sample of American states. The majority of the research that is available, however, is not focused on domestic homicide situations.

In the first epidemiological study of instances of murder-suicide in England and Wales, Barraclough and Harris (2002) studied death certificates for all murder-suicides over a four-year time span. They found that 3 per cent of male, 11 per cent of female and 19 per cent of child homicides were of this type. Similarly, of all suicides, 0.8 per cent male and 0.4 per cent female deaths occurred in murder-suicide incidents. The typical cases involved families of low socioeconomic status.

Data provided by the Home Office (2005b) for England and Wales give support for Barraclough and Harris's findings of a low instance of murders ending in suicide. One can determine that of the 659 murders that were committed in 2004, 19 individuals committed suicide before indictments could be issued. We do not know the nature of the murders, however. Regardless of whether or not these were acts related to domestic violence or other types of murder, the figures do seem to indicate only a small number of the murders in the Home Office crime reports are of the murder-suicide variety.

A rare find in the American literature is the research presented by Bossarte *et al.* (2006) who analysed data from the National Violent Death Reporting System (NVDRS). This active state-based surveillance system includes data from seven states for 2003 and 13 for 2004. Results reveal that within participating states, 65 murder-suicide incidents (murder rate = 0.230/100,000) occurred in 2003 and 144 incidents (murder rate = 0.238/100,000) occurred in 2004. Most victims (58 per cent) were current or former intimate partners of the perpetrator. Among all male perpetrators of intimate partner murder 30.6 per cent were also suicides. A substantial proportion of the victims (13.7 per cent) were the children of the perpetrator. Overall, most victims (74.6 per cent) were female and most perpetrators were male (91.9 per cent). A recent history of legal problems (25.3 per cent) or financial problems (9.3 per cent) was common among the perpetrators.

From Statistics Canada (2005) we learn that over the past 40 years, one in ten solved murders were cases in which the suspect took his or her own life following the murder. About three-quarters of these victims were killed by a family member. Virtually all of the incidents (97 per cent) involved female victims killed by a male spouse. And, as Easteal (1994) demonstrated in an earlier study, a third of *spousal* murders in the USA and Canada end in suicide. Few other varieties of murder end in this way.

Probably related to the availability of guns, the murder rate in the USA is much higher than the British rate, although the difference has diminished in recent years. According to an international comparative study, the murder rate in the USA is 0.04 per 1000 residents while in the UK the rate is 0.014 per 1000 residents (NationMaster.com 2007). The difference in murder rates between large American and British cities is even more pronounced.

Guns are by far the most common weapon used in these crimes (Violence Policy Center 2006). One could speculate that if you shoot someone, it is relatively easy to then turn the gun on yourself. If you stab or strangle someone, however, suicide becomes much more difficult. In any case, the high rate of spousal murder-suicides is consistent with the murder-as-extended-suicide hypothesis of Palermo (1994).

The *Journal of the American Medical Association* (*JAMA*) reviewed the epidemiology, patterns and determinants of murder-suicide and made a strong case for the need for systematic data-gathering so that prevention strategies can be developed (Marzuk *et al.* 1992). Extrapolating from the best statistics available, the report found that in the USA murder-suicide represents 1.5 per cent of all suicides and 5 per cent of all murders annually. In Denmark, on the other hand, 42 per cent of murders are of this variety.

According to the Violence Policy Center (2006), 591 murder-suicide deaths took place nationwide between 1 January and 30 June 2005. This averages out to ten murder-suicide events each week. Of those, Texas had 18 cases. Other statistics from the Violence Policy Center include:

- Male offenders: 94 per cent.
- Cases involving an intimate partner: 74 per cent.
- Occurred in the home: 75 per cent.
- Average age difference between offender and primary victim: 6.3 years.
- Involved a firearm: 92 per cent.

As reported by the Violence Policy Center (2006), the pattern of the murder-suicide is predictable: a male perpetrator, female victim, decision by the woman to leave the man, and a gun. The typical Florida pattern (Florida had the largest number at 35 of the 2002 total) involved an elderly male caregiver overwhelmed by his inability to care for an infirm wife.

As an example of *murder-suicide in the family*, we can consider war veterans such as soldiers who have fought in Iraq. These returning troops have a high rate of both murder and suicide, and sometimes both. A report from Washington State sees such events as a risk factor distinct to the military, in which armed men are trained to kill, and many later carry the invisible scars of war (*Seattle Weekly* 2005). It is impossible to tell whether the externalized aggression (murder) or internalized aggression (suicide) is primary. Consider these two cases from 2003:

- Army Specialist Thomas R. Stroh, 21, strangled his wife and son at their Fort Lewis home. He later committed suicide by driving head-on into a semi-truck. The soldier had a record of abusing his wife and being drunk on duty.
- Young Marine Renee Di Li Lorenzo was shot and killed by her boyfriend who had been discharged earlier from the Marines. He then turned the shotgun on himself (*Seattle Weekly* 2005).

Some researchers argue that murder is the primary motive in such cases. Certainly, the urge to kill is the overwhelming factor; the urge can be described as self-destruction including the destruction of people who were once loved. Regarding murder and suicide in such cases, it may not be a case of either-or but of both-and.

We are introducing the term *suicide-murder* to refer to killings, in whichever age group, that are suicide-driven. There are two basic types of suicide-murders. One is the elderly couple situation in which an elderly man kills his frail, usually dying, wife and then himself. The second and more common variety of suicide-murder is the case of IPV. The pattern that emerges in these cases involves intimate partners in the 20- to 35-year-old range. The man is abusive, psychologically and/or physically. Obsessed with the woman to the extent that he feels he can't live without her, he is fiercely jealous and determined to isolate her. Characteristically, suicidal murderers have little regard for the lives of other people; they would be considered, in mental health jargon, to be antisocial. So dependent are these men on their wives or girlfriends that they would sooner be dead than live without them. When the girlfriend/wife makes a move to leave, her partner is absolutely distraught.

Milton Rosenbaum (1990), of the Department of Psychiatry at the University of New Mexico, compared 12 cases of murder-suicide to 24 couple murder cases, through interviews with family members and friends. The most striking finding was that the perpetrators of murder-suicide were depressed and almost all of these killers were men, while the perpetrators of murder alone were not depressed and half were women.

Conclusions

Based on interviews with family members and friends of 220 female victims of domestic murder, compared to a control group of 343 victims of physical violence, Campbell *et al.* (2003) found that the strongest risk factor for such an outcome was an abuser's lack of employment compounded by a lack of education. Significant relationship variables are separating from an abusive partner and having a child in the home who is not the partner's biological child. Other factors that can help predict murder are an abuser's use of illicit drugs and access to firearms. Threats of use of a weapon were common in cases where the partner actually did so.

Our analysis in this chapter in terms of the lower rates of domestic murder and murder-suicide in the UK has implications related to the importance of the control of weapons. Tightening gun control laws and restricting the access to firearms by convicted batterers is a serious step in reducing rates of lethal violence. A further consideration relates to prevention of murder in connection with suicide. Since the suicide rate is much higher among perpetrators of intimate murder compared to murder in general, suicidal ideation in battering men might be considered a possible risk factor for murder-suicide.

Domestic violence is harmful, destructive of one's mental and physical health, and sometimes fatal. This chapter has focused on cases in which domestic violence ends in the death of one of the parties, most often the woman. In cases of domestic murder, the gender differences are pronounced. The overwhelming majority of the women who had killed their partners and who were serving time in prison for this act received specific lethal threats in which the batterer gave every indication that he would kill the woman, maybe then, maybe later.

It is important for all health and social work practitioners to document the duration and intensity of battering histories among clients in order to provide the best possible safety planning, risk assessments, crisis intervention and effective social services. All assessments should start with an evaluation of the psychological harm and physical injury to the victim, and the likelihood of the victim escaping and ending the battering cycle.

In knowing such facts about the dynamics of life-threatening situations that might end in the death of one or both of the partners, health care practitioners can be cognizant of the indicators that can serve as a basis for preventive intervention crisis and, in collaboration with the potential victim of domestic murder, the development of a safety plan at the earliest possible moment.

20 Relationship conflict and abuse outcomes

Christopher M. Murphy and Christina G. Watlington

Introduction

This chapter focuses on relationship conflict, most notably destructive means of coping with conflict or disagreement, and how conflict is important in understanding, preventing, and treating intimate partner violence (IPV). Relationship conflict refers to various forms of miscommunication, disagreement regarding tastes, desires, goals and values, and the means through which couples attempt to resolve these differences. Thus, relationship conflict involves both *content* and *process*. Content refers to the specific areas and topics of disagreement, such as finances, child-rearing practices, how to spend free time, roles and duties etc. Process refers to the manner in which disagreements are transacted, including communication behaviours such as outward expressions of discontent, partner blaming, conflict avoidance and acquiescence. Some level of disagreement and conflict is inherent to all significant interpersonal relationships, and therefore the manner in which conflict is transacted is usually of greater import than the specific topics of conflict for understanding relationship discord, abuse and violence (Fincham and Beach 1999).

Conceptualizing partner abuse from a relationship systems perspective

Given that relationship conflict implies multi-person dynamics, conceptualizations of partner violence that focus on relationship conflict intersect with relationship systems theories. From a systems perspective, partner abuse is the result of dyadic conflict escalation or mutual role enactments in which both partners help to stimulate and maintain aggressive interactions (e.g. Stith *et al.* 2002). Abuse is therefore seen as similar to other forms of relationship conflict, although unique clinical adaptations may be promoted to address safety concerns. In the extreme, systems theories challenge the notion of abuser and victim roles altogether through an emphasis on mutual aggression, or interpret these roles as elements of a complementary relationship system. Some systems theorists also highlight broader social influences on intimate relationships, including factors that support men's control over women in the domestic sphere (Hansen and Harway 1993).

The empirical support for the role of dyadic relationship conflict in understanding partner abuse is substantial. Most notable are studies in which couples are audio- or videotaped while attempting to resolve a prominent relationship difficulty, with subsequent coding of communication behaviours by trained observers. When compared to distressed but non-violent relationships, the average levels of critical, aversive, defensive and hostile communication behaviours are much higher in couples that have experienced husband-to-wife violence (e.g. Murphy and O'Farrell 1997). In support of the systems view, both husbands and wives in the violent couples tend to display high rates of negative communication behaviour. The partner violent samples also tend to reciprocate negative communication more reliably, responding to critical or negative comments in like fashion with a greater probability than seen in non-violent dyads (e.g. Murphy and O'Farrell 1997).

Negative reciprocity is further supported by high rates of bi-directional physical aggression in both community and marriage clinic samples (e.g. Gottman *et al.* 1995). Self-defence may partially account for mutual violence among women seeking treatment for abuse victimization (Saunders 1988). However, in community surveys, women report that they are equally likely as their male partners to initiate physical aggression during conflict incidents (Stets and Straus 1990). In addition, the collective evidence suggests that men and women perpetrate partner violent behaviours at roughly equal rates overall (Archer 2000), although negative consequences of aggressive victimization, such as injury and fear, are experienced more predominantly by women (e.g. Archer 2000).

Limitations of relationship systems theories

Dyadic process explanations of relationship conflict escalation have been criticized on several fronts. Most notable is the concern that by focusing on their putative role in conflict escalation, victims will be blamed or held responsible for their partner's abusive actions. Couples treatment may collude, inadvertently or explicitly, with abusers' tendency to blame the partner, or victims' tendency to blame themselves (e.g. Hansen 1993).

One very telling criticism of systems conceptualizations is that certain individuals will abuse anyone with whom they enter an intimate relationship, raising the prospect that individual factors are more important than system dynamics in understanding their abuse. For such cases, there may be nothing that any partner could do to prevent the escalation to abusive and violent behaviour. In so far as such cases exist, abuse is arguably more of a characterological than a relational problem (O'Leary 1993).

Most theories of partner violence, and their attendant intervention models, take an extreme perspective on these issues. Whereas some seek the causes of abuse entirely within the interpersonal dynamics of the relationship, others seek its causes entirely in factors that have nothing to do with the victim's behaviour, such as the abuser's personal characteristics or societal arrangements of gender and power (Margolin and Burman 1993). However, a more integrated explanation would suggest that mutual conflict escalation may play a large role in some cases of IPV, and a minor or non-existent role in other cases. Likewise, an abusive partner's individual problems, such as a negative developmental history, personality dysfunction or substance abuse may play a very large role in some cases, and a relatively minor role in others. This distinction has been viewed categorically by some scholars, for example in characterizing partner abuse as common couple violence versus patriarchal terrorism, which implies a systems conceptualization for one type of abuser and a sociopathological explanation for another type (Johnson 1995). Alternatively, abuse can be understood to fall along a continuum of severity and frequency. Relatively more contributing factors in both the individual dysfunction and relationship conflict domains are likely to be present at the severe end of the continuum (O'Leary 1993).

Relationship conflict in the origins of IPV

Empirical studies indicate that partner conflict is important in understanding the escalation to physical abuse in early relationship development. In a longitudinal study of newlywed couples, previous levels of psychological aggression by both partners significantly predicted subsequent instances of physical assault (e.g. O'Leary et al. 1994). These findings suggest that extensive verbally aggressive transactions typically precede the escalation to physical violence.

Relationship skills and the prevention of IPV

Relationship communication skills appear to be important not only in understanding the escalation to violence, but in preventing partner aggression as well. One notable study involved an intensive 15-week premarital programme designed to prevent relationship distress and divorce (Markman et al. 1993). The programme focused on communication skills, conflict resolution, values clarification and relationship enhancement. In comparison to a no-intervention control group, couples who received this intervention had significantly lower physical assault rates at follow-up assessments conducted three to five years into marriage. Although the programme was not specifically targeted toward violence prevention, the findings support the value of relationship conflict management skills in preventing abuse.

Wolfe et al. (2003) studied an intensive programme designed to prevent dating violence among high risk teenagers drawn from child protective service case lists. The prevention programme provided young people with consciousness-raising activities about abuse and extensive training in relationship skills designed to limit and prevent conflict escalation. Overall, the intervention was highly successful in preventing physical assault relative to a usual services control. Prevention group participants who became highly adept at active listening, in particular, had substantially reduced risk of physical assault. Listening skills have long been a mainstay of behavioural couples therapy (Jacobson and Margolin 1979), and are thought to diffuse conflict escalation by reducing the tendency to react on the basis of poor or distorted understanding of the partner's message, by imparting a sense of being heard or understood to the partner, and by slowing the pace of potentially volatile interchanges.

Relationship skills training in abuser intervention

Very little research has focused on the acquisition of relationship skills and conflict resolution within intervention programmes for abusive partners. Most notable is the dearth of research examining whether a focus on communication and conflict resolution skills is a productive component of abuser intervention, and whether increases in such skills predict violence cessation. One early investigation of a group programme for abusive men showed very promising effects on recidivism relative to an untreated control (Waldo 1988). This intervention was modelled after relationship enhancement approaches developed for the prevention of marital distress, with group sessions focused largely on training in communication skills through careful coaching and repetitive role-playing.

Couples therapy for partner violence

Despite the extensive evidence that communication problems and relationship conflict are involved in the initiation of partner violence and important targets for prevention of violence, studies to date have provided only limited and qualified support for the efficacy of couples interventions for partner violence. Such interventions are based on a variety of theoretical assumptions drawn from structural and strategic family therapies (e.g. Stith *et al.* 2002) and behavioural or social learning theories (e.g. Heyman and Neidig 1997).

Conjoint group couples therapy was one of four intervention conditions in a large-scale trial conducted with US Navy personnel who were charged with abusing their spouses (Dunford 2000). Treatment attendance was required by the abusive men, and their partners were invited and encouraged to participate along with the men in the conjoint condition. Session attendance by partners was quite low, with approximately two relationship partners attending couples group sessions for every five abusive clients who attended, on average. Violence recidivism during the year after scheduled completion of treatment was not significantly different for men assigned to the conjoint therapy condition as compared to men who were assigned to a more traditional gender-specific group programme, or those who received intensive monitoring or brief safety interventions. These findings highlight the practical barriers to partner involvement in legally mandated counselling for abusive individuals. Given that legitimate ethical and civil liberties concerns also arise from efforts to mandate services for victims of violent crime, couples interventions cannot be the sole, or even primary, modality used with legally mandated populations.

Studies of voluntary treatment-seeking couples, or couples recruited voluntarily from samples ordered to abuser intervention, have been more successful in securing programme attendance, but have not, as yet, provided convincing evidence of improved treatment outcomes from the use of couples intervention models. O'Leary *et al.* (1999) compared couples' group treatment to gender-specific groups for couples who reported husband to wife physical aggression. Participants were recruited from the community via newspaper advertisements. Both intervention conditions were based on a cognitive behavioural model of treatment, but the couples groups focused more on interactional dynamics and conflict escalation. The overall violence recidivism rates were not significantly different between treatment conditions. Although physical assault rates declined significantly from before to after treatment, recidivism rates were rather high in general, with about 75 per cent of men reported by one or both spouses to have engaged in at least one instance of physical assault during the year after treatment. Stith *et al.* (2004) studied multi-couple versus individual couple treatment formats. They found that aggression by both members of the couple decreased more substantially for those who received couples therapy in groups than for those who received couples therapy as an individual dyad. Relative to a small control group of couples who refused treatment, lower physical assault recidivism was found for those in the multi-couple group condition. Despite these encouraging initial results, as yet dyadic therapy for partner violence has not been shown to produce significantly better outcomes than approaches that do not use a dyadic intervention format.

The one area in which couples therapy has been superior to individual treatment in reducing partner violence outcomes is with substance abusing men (Brannen and Rubin 1996). One small-scale clinical trial with drug dependent men found that behavioural couples therapy, which uses contracts for a brief daily sobriety-affirming discussion and training in communication and relationship problem-solving skills, produced lower partner violence recidivism than standard individual substance use treatment that was equivalent in intensity of therapeutic contact (Fals–Stewart *et al.* 2002). These improved violence outcomes appeared to be partly explained by enhanced reductions in drug use for those receiving couples therapy, but not fully accounted for by drug abuse outcomes. It is likely that substance abuse treatment provides a powerful context in which to alter relationship communication and conflict dynamics, changes that have an important effect on risk for substance use relapse and violence recidivism (O'Farrell *et al.* 2004).

Conflict dynamics and intervention outcomes for partner-violent men

Surprisingly, despite extensive evidence on dyadic communication problems among partner-violent couples and the role of dyadic conflict in the escalation to partner violence in community samples, relatively little research has examined dyadic communication or conflict in samples seeking treatment services for partner violence. To some extent, ethical concerns have limited this work due to the potential dangers inherent in observations of conflict discussions for severely abusive clients. Perhaps more important, however, is the fact that the vast majority of intervention programmes for partner violence offenders focus on abuser accountability and individual responsibility, and downplay or ignore dyadic processes. Concerns about victim blaming, collusion with the abuser's externalization of responsibility and possible coercion of victims into couples treatment have directed attention away from explanations and interventions grounded in dyadic conflict theories and toward explanations and interventions grounded in sociocultural or individual psychopathological theories of partner abuse. However, such concerns may be taken to the extreme by denying any possible role or importance of the partner's behaviour in understanding and treating abuse. A high degree of variability in communication behaviour and aggression is likely to be present among the partners of men in treatment for partner-violent offending, and many questions remain as to whether such variability is important in understanding and predicting treatment outcomes.

In an unpublished masters thesis, the second author explored aggression levels by the partners of men in treatment for domestic violence, including the extent of dyadic correspondence in aggression levels and whether partner's level of aggression predicted treatment outcomes for abusive men (Watlington 2003). Baseline data were available on 77 couples in which the man participated in a 16-week abuser counselling programme. The men were predominantly Caucasian (58 per cent) and African American (31 per cent). Court mandates to treatment were in place for 70 per cent of the men, with 22 per cent self-referred and 8 per cent lawyer-referred with a court case pending. Their average age was 35.2 years ($sd = 8.3$) and they had an average of 13.4 years of formal education ($sd = 2.2$). Levels of psychological aggression and physical assault were measured with the Revised Conflict Tactics Scale (CTS2) at a pre-treatment assessment covering the six months before abuser counselling and a post-treatment assessment covering the roughly six month period of assessment and group treatment. Victim partners, who were interviewed by phone, completed the entire CTS2 with respect to the abusive client's behaviour, but a more limited sub-set of abusive behaviour items for reports about their own behaviour. Abusive behaviour scores for client and partner were computed by pooling the two reports for each person's abusive behaviour.

A high degree of dyadic correspondence was found in rates of psychological and physical aggression prior to treatment. The within-dyad correlations between men's and women's aggression levels at pre-treatment were 0.66 and 0.68 for physical assault and psychological aggression, respectively (both significant at $p < 0.01$). The associations at post-treatment diverged for the two forms of partner aggression. The within-dyad correlation was not statistically significant for physical assault at post-treatment ($r = 0.22$), but was highly significant for psychological aggression ($r = 0.80$, $p < 0.01$). Thus, with the exception of physical assault at post-treatment, these high correlations indicate that abusive clients with high levels of aggression tend to have partners with high levels of aggression, and abusive clients with relatively lower levels of aggression tend to have partners with relatively lower levels as well.

Prediction of abusive clients' post-treatment aggression levels from partner's pre-treatment aggression levels were explored first through simple bivariate correlations and then through multiple regression models which controlled for the abusive client's own pre-treatment aggression levels and whether or not he completed a credible dose of treatment (defined as attending 12 or more of the 16 scheduled group sessions). This latter analytic strategy represents a highly conservative test of the hypothesis that partner behaviour is an important predictor of treatment outcomes for abusive men, as it requires prediction from partner behaviour that was quite distant in time, and prediction above and beyond one's own past aggressive behaviour which may, in turn, have been influenced by dyadic processes.

The simple bivariate correlations revealed that abusive men's physical assault at post-treatment was significantly predicted by the partner's levels of both physical assault ($r = 0.29$, $p < 0.05$) and psychological aggression ($r = 0.29$, $p < 0.05$) at pre-treatment. Abusive men's psychological aggression at post-treatment was significantly predicted by the partner's level of psychological aggression at pre-treatment ($r = 0.46$, $p < 0.01$), but not by the partner's level of physical assault at pre-treatment ($r = 0.16$, not significant). Thus, at the level of uncorrected correlations, both physical assault and psychological aggression outcomes were significantly predicted by the partner's aggressive behaviour levels prior to treatment.

Using the more conservative multiple regression method controlling for abusive men's pre-treatment levels of physical assault and psychological aggression levels, and their treatment exposure, prediction of psychological aggression levels at post-treatment remained statistically significant, with the partner's pre-treatment aggression variables accounting for 8 per cent of the variance in abusive men's post-treatment psychological aggression (see Table 20.1). The partner's psychological aggression at pre-treatment in particular made a significant contribution to the prediction model.

Table 20.1 Multiple regression with female partner's pre-treatment psychological aggression and physical assault predicting abusive men's post-treatment psychological aggression

Variable	Beta	t	p
Treatment completion status	-.08	-.80	-.43
Client's pre-treatment physical assault	-.12	-.56	.58
Client's pre-treatment psychological aggression	.39	1.95	.06
Block 1: $R^2 = .19$, $F(3, 70) = 5.62$, $p < .05$			
Partner's pre-treatment physical assault	-1.89	-1.64	.12
Partner's pre-treatment psychological aggression	.37	2.46	02
Block 2: R^2 change = .08, $F(2, 68) = 6.52$, $p < .01$			

The men's physical assault at post-treatment, in contrast, was not significantly predicted by partner's pre-treatment aggression levels after control variables were included in the equation (see Table 20.2). The only significant predictor variable in this model was the abusive client's own pre-treatment physical assault level. Thus, when one's own prior abusive behaviour was included in the predictive model, assaultive behaviour in the recent past was the only significant predictor of assaultive behaviour at the post-treatment assessment.

Table 20.2 Sequential logistic regression with female partner's pre-treatment psychological aggression and physical assault predicting the male client's post-treatment physical assault

Variable	Beta	Wald stat.	p
Credible dose of treatment	-.59	.48	.48
Client's pre-treatment physical assault	.59	4.53	.04
Client's pre-treatment psychological aggression	-.11	.14	.71
Block 1: ^{2} (df = 3; N = 69) = 9.68, p <.05			
Partner's pre-treatment physical assault	-.76	.19	.66
Partner's pre-treatment psychological aggression	.25	1.08	.29
Block 2: ^{2} (df = 2; N = 69) = 1.08, not significant			

These results should be interpreted as preliminary given the modest sample size and limited data modelling strategies employed. Nevertheless, the findings have important implications regarding the potential relevance of dyadic conflict to treatment of partner-abusive men. First, abusive men's levels of psychological and physical aggression were highly correlated with their partners' levels of aggression prior to treatment. As with community samples, it appears that aggression tends to beget aggression in this clinical sample as well, as individuals with high levels of aggression tend to have partners with high levels of aggression. In community samples, women are about equally likely as men to report initiating physical aggression during conflict incidents (Stets and Straus 1990). However, the extent to which these clinical sample findings reflect self-defence, mutual combat, independent aggressive outbursts or some combination of these patterns cannot as yet be discerned, and should be an important focus for future investigations.

Second, the partner's aggression levels at pre-treatment were correlated with the abusive client's subsequent aggression levels at post-treatment. Thus, variability in aggression levels by the partner has some implication for the prediction of abusive men's treatment outcome. Once again, the reasons for this finding remain unknown, and should most certainly not be used to shift responsibility away from the abusive client for controlling his own behaviour, nor to infer that dyadic conflict is invariably present in recidivist violence. Nevertheless, it would appear that a high level of ongoing dyadic conflict is an important consideration in understanding risk of physical assault among men in partner violence counselling.

Third, abusive men's psychological aggression levels at post-treatment were both highly correlated with the partner's psychological aggression levels at post-treatment and significantly predicted by the partner's aggression levels at pre-treatment, even after controlling for the abusive man's treatment exposure and prior aggression. It appears that psychological aggression outcomes most clearly match the expectations of a dyadic conflict model of treatment response. This finding may reflect important differences between physical assault recidivism and psychological aggression as treatment outcome variables. In large-scale trials, the majority of men in treatment for partner violence do not engage in physical assault recidivism (Gondolf 1997). It appears that a substantial number of men manage to control their physical aggression in response to legal system intervention and counselling. However, ongoing rates of psychological aggression may be more closely intertwined with dyadic conflict processes, supporting a need for greater attention to communication and conflict resolution in abuser intervention, or for couples intervention to address dyadic conflict after an initial period of counselling to establish safety and non-violence. In any event, the findings as a whole indicate that the decision to ignore dyadic conflict altogether may be an important oversight in intervention programmes for partner-violent men.

Conclusions

Relationship conflict, mutual escalation of aggressive interchanges and poor communication are important factors in understanding IPV. Empirical studies support the notion that hostile dyadic interchanges predict the onset of physical assault in early marriage. Both partners in abusive couples typically display high rates of negative communication behaviour, and psychological and physical relationship aggression are most often bi-directional in nature. However, relationship conflict and systems explanations have important limitations as well. In the most severe and pernicious cases, partner violence is often perpetrated by individuals with serious personality, emotional and behavioural difficulties who appear likely to abuse any intimate partner regardless of the relationship dynamics involved.

A number of studies highlight the potential value of improving relationship communication and conflict resolution skills in efforts to prevent or end partner violence. Programmes emphasizing relationship communication and conflict resolution skills have been shown to prevent or reduce partner aggression among high-risk teenagers (Wolfe *et al.* 2003), newlywed couples (Markman *et al.* 1993), drug-dependent men (Fals–Stewart *et al.* 2002) and partner-violent men (Waldo 1988). As demonstrated with previously unpublished data from our partner violence research clinic, aggressive behaviour by the relationship partner is an important predictor of ongoing abuse by men in treatment for partner violence, particularly psychological aggression. Nevertheless, despite the strong apparent role of dyadic conflict in understanding and preventing relationship abuse, to date there is no compelling clinical trial evidence to support the notion that dyadic interventions for partner violence are more efficacious than other approaches.

One possible explanation for this state of affairs is that the communication and problem-solving dynamics in clinically violent couples are already so severely compromised that standard dyadic interventions are not sufficient to alter problem-atic relationship patterns for the majority of cases. If this is the case, then interven-tions aimed at early intervention and couples with very low levels of physical assault or only psychological aggression may prove to be more effective than efforts aimed at couples with more well-established patterns of aggression. It may also be the case that proper sequencing of individual and couples interventions could enhance outcomes. Clinically violent cases who habitually blame the partner for their own aggressive acts may need time to become personally responsible for their behaviour and invoke basic self-control strategies before they can be successful in conjoint treatment. At any rate, more research is needed to carefully examine relationship system dynamics and communication behaviour as it affects the outcomes of intervention for partner abuse. Finally, effective interventions may require greater screening and selection to identify couples for whom dyadic interventions are most likely to be safe and effective.

21 How female victims' responses affect the risk of future assaults by their male intimate partners

Marybeth J. Mattingly and Laura Dugan

Introduction

Statistics and news stories echo what many practitioners have known for a long time: partner violence is typically not a one-time event in a woman's life. Indeed, victimized women may be reassaulted either by the same violent partner or by another partner who becomes violent. Abusers may repeatedly attack their intimate partners for many reasons. Once violence is used it may be harder for the batterer to control himself in the face of relationship conflict, jealousies or the desire to control a partner's behaviour. Additionally, even when a violent relationship ends, previously victimized women may choose another violent partner. Repeated and severe violence seriously affect a woman's mental and physical health (For a discussion of how the health of severely victimized women differs from that of other women, see: Straus and Gelles 1990b), thus it is very important to understand what might help a woman end the cycle of violence in her relationships.

M.A. Dutton (1996) notes that 'The future of intervention with battered women and their families lies in better understanding battered women's efforts to resist, escape, avoid, and stop the violence against them and their children'. As practitioners, researchers and policy-makers, we cannot begin to end partner violence unless the victims have contact with interested others, outside of the home. This often means that a woman needs to take steps to secure her own safety. Yet, few understand which steps will effectively protect a victim from further partner violence. In this chapter we examine women's responses, during and following an attack, that may influence their risk of repeated attack by current or future partners. We have identified several actions that women may take to prevent future assaults, such as fighting back, notifying the police, seeking help at a shelter or other victim support agency, and getting medical help if injuries were sustained. By examining the current state of knowledge on the consequences of women's responses to intimate partner violence (IPV), we can better understand gaps in current practice and develop guidelines for improving interventions with assaulted women and their partners.

Following a review of the literature, we show findings from our own research that offer some insight into which factors are protective against repeat assault, and which are associated with increased risk. We discuss our findings in the light of the current literature and offer ideas for improving services for women victimized by an intimate partner. We limit our discussion and investigation in this chapter to violence perpetrated against women by their male partners. While research suggests the importance of considering IPV among same-sex couples (see, for example: Renzetti 1997), data limitations precluded our ability to do so. Additionally, we keep the focus of this chapter on violence perpetrated by men against women as evidence suggests the context and consequences of female perpetrated violence are different; Kaufman Kantor and Straus 1990; Kurz 1993; Morse 1995; Tjaden and Thoennes 2000). Further, men's responsive violence and help-seeking behaviours likely follow different trajectories than those of women.

Repeated exposure to IPV

Repeatedly being victimized by an intimate partner has deleterious effects above and beyond the consequences of single acts of abuse (see, for example: Walker 1984). The accumulation of violence is often associated with increased severity, and probably indicates higher conflict relationships in which partners are seeking greater control. Indeed, Johnson's (1995) categorization of IPV indicates that severe male violence used to control women is linked to future assaults escalating in severity. Such violence may erode the self-esteem of the victim (see, for example: Campbell and Soeken 1999b) and may make it harder for her to establish non-violent intimate relationships. Given these consequences, one must examine the extent of repeat assault in the population and identify the factors that increase or decrease the risk.

Although relatively little research has explored repeat victimization by an intimate partner, what evidence there is suggests that rates of re-victimization are fairly high, particularly for those with certain characteristics. Data from the 1975 and 1985 Family Violence Survey and Resurvey in the USA suggest that two-thirds of those reporting assault experienced more than one assault in the year prior to the survey (Feld and Straus 1990; Straus, Gelles, and Steinmetz 1980). Previous research using 1978–82 data from the National Crime Victimization Survey (NCVS) found that once a woman is assaulted by a partner, her chances of further assault within six months are relatively high (32 per cent) (Langan and Innes 1986). Further, 37 per cent of the married, divorced and separated victims who reported the incident to the police cited concerns about future violence. Lower rates of repeat assault were found by Rand and Saltzman (2003) who analysed recurrent IPV in more recent data collected through the same survey (the 1992–9 NCVS). Most victims (72 per cent) reported only one intimate partner victimization in the six months prior to interview. However, this figure ignores cases where women were unable to distinguish across repeated events, thus inflating the estimate of one-time victims.[1] Evidence also suggests that husbands are less likely to desist from aggression when the violence is more chronic or severe (Straus et al. 1980; Aldarondo and Kaufman Kantor 1997;

Campbell and Soeken 1999; Quigley and Leonard 1996). However, despite high rates of repeat assault, it is important to also remember that, for some couples, the violence ends. Feld and Straus (1990) found high rates of desistance (33 per cent of severely violent men in 1985 were non-violent at a one year follow-up), often without formal intervention. The authors note that this figure might be high because the follow-up period was short, and therefore less frequent but more violent perpetrators might appear as desisters. Finally, some evidence suggests that even when physical violence ends, men may continue to emotionally abuse their partners (Jacobson, Gottman, Gortner, Berns, and Shortt 1996).

One study directly addressed the correlates of repeat assault. Johnson (2003) analysed data from a nationally representative sample of Canadian women. Her findings 'suggest that a continuation of assaults on wives is predicted by the frequency of previous assaults, the youth of male perpetrators, living in a common-law relationship, the duration of the union [shorter unions imply greater risk], and higher education for female victims'. Further, she found that a partner's attempts to limit a woman's access to family income and restrict access to social networks elevated the risk that he later assaulted her.

Despite our knowledge that victims of repeated violence have the greatest risk of severe harm and that repeat victimization is relatively common, much of what policy-makers or practitioners can do first depends upon whether the victim initiates self-help or whether another intervenes. There are several things a woman can do during or following an assault that we might expect to decrease her chances of being victimized again. These include attacking her perpetrator during the assault, seeking legal or medical help following the assault, and seeking help through other agencies. We next review findings from the research literature for each of these actions.

Self-defence/responsive violence

First, let's consider who fights back. Research evidence has shown that women are equally violent in combative relationships (Moffitt, Caspi, Rutter, and Silva 2001; Straus and Gelles 1990a). Thus, much effort has been devoted to determine whether women really are equally combative or whether, instead, women attack as a reaction or response to violence precipitated by their partners. Even in cases where women are mutually combative with their partners, research suggests the violence was more likely to have been initiated by both parties or just the male, rather than only by the female. (see Kurz 1993; Morse 1995). Morse also found that women who had been assaulted were more likely than men to live in fear of their partners. These findings suggest that perhaps women, more often than men, act in self-defence when they are violent toward their intimate partners.

Some research challenges the claim that women's partner violence is more defensive than offensive. Specifically, work done by Moffitt *et al.* (2001) on the Dunedin Longitudinal Study in New Zealand finds very high rates of both male and female violence. This study suggests that while some women respond violently to male violence, an antisocial history also influences female (and male) violence regardless of whether the partner is violent. Further, factors such as individual attitudes toward aggression and involvement in other crime also predict partner violence.

Relatively little is known about how a woman's responsive violence influences her life and risk of continued assault. However, some research does suggest that responding violently is associated with more assaults (Gelles and Straus 1988). It is unclear whether women responding violently to their partners' assaults are at greater or lesser risk of health and lifestyle consequences. While self-defence could serve to stop a partner's violence, it might also incite retaliatory responses. Further, it is entirely possible that a woman's retaliatory violence could legitimize the use of violence within the relationship.

Help-seeking

Police/legal systems

Evidence strongly suggests that the legal system falls short of adequately protecting victims of partner violence (see Dworkin 1993; Martin 1995; Warshaw 1993; Stark, Flitcraft, and Frazier 1979). This seems particularly true for minority and poor women, given inherent race and class biases within the legal system (Ferraro 1993). In fact, findings by Dugan *et al.* (2003) strongly suggest that the criminal justice system responds to violent relationships in racially specific ways. Further, the legal system fails to adequately consider the gendered nature of assault. Ferraro (1993) notes that gender-neutral language ignores the differential context in which male and female violence tends to take place. She cites incidents where women who phoned the police wound up being the ones arrested, since officers ignored the gendered nature of family conflicts. Ferraro (1993: 169) notes: 'When police arrest women for defending themselves against battering, the abusers are provided social support for initiating and justifying violence'.

Researchers have specifically examined how arrest policies influence the continued risk of IPV. The most notable are a series of arrest experiments beginning with one by Sherman and Berk (Sherman and Berk 1984) who studied the effects of arrest on spouse assaults in Minneapolis. Their findings suggest that arrest was more effective in decreasing the prevalence of assault than were either offering advice or ordering the perpetrator away for eight hours. Similarly, after examining the police records of a southern California county, Berk and Newton (1985) concluded that arrests are associated with fewer new incidents of wife assaults, particularly among those most likely to be arrested. However, they were unable to determine whether this was because assaults went down or reporting declined. Further research in this area leaves us inconclusive about the effectiveness of arrest on partner violence. Replication studies of the Sherman and Berk arrest experiments in other cities found mixed and opposite results, particularly when looking at the unmarried and unemployed (see, for example: Berk, Campbell, Klap, and Western 1992; Pate and Hamilton 1992). Yet, Dugan *et al.* (2003), using the nationally representative files of the NCVS data, found evidence suggesting that mandatory arrest laws may actually reduce the number of spousal violent assaults (although they seem to have little influence on assaults by boyfriends or girlfriends).

Many feminist scholars express concern that an individual victim's needs are not adequately considered when developing arrest policies. Bowman (1992) critiques the decision to make arrest mandatory in domestic violence cases since there is insufficient evidence that arrest actually deters future violence, and it may not be the response that victims want. Ferraro (1993:173) also questions the effectiveness of mandatory arrest policies and emphasizes that ' ... women are the best experts on their own lives'. Bowman (1992) emphasizes the importance of the entire response to domestic assault, beginning with a call to police and extending through prosecution and aid to victims. While she realizes some women may find it empowering to have their abusers arrested, others may want a different response from the police. In fact, evidence shows that they may be reluctant to call the police if they fear their spouse will be arrested (see Dugan 2003).

Shelters and other victim support agencies

In their early monograph on partner violence, Straus *et al.* (1980: 224) highlighted the importance of shelters for helping women turn their lives around: 'Shelters do more than remove the woman from immediate danger. They also have tremendous potential for preventing further violence. This is because the woman is given the physical, economic, and psychological support needed to change the basis of the marriage'. However, the volume *Understanding Violence Against Women*, which compiles research in the area, acknowledges how little is truly known about the role of shelters in helping women end violent intimate partner relationships (Crowell and Burgess 1996). Most outcome studies are descriptive in nature, and include only small or biased samples that fail to compare shelter residents to those women who never seek shelter help. However, the evidence that does exist suggests that some women who enter shelters experience fewer repeat assaults and have improved psychological well-being, especially when follow-up services are provided (Sullivan and Davidson II 1991; Sullivan, Basta, Tan, and Davidson II 1992; Sullivan, Campbell, Angelique, Eby, and Davidson II 1994; see: Tutty 1996). Additionally, Berk *et al.* (1986) found that new cases of violence following a shelter stay decreased for women who also took other help-seeking actions. However, for those who only went to a shelter, the stay had either a neutral effect or sometimes incited retaliatory responses by their partners.

Given the wide array of services provided by different agencies, it would be unwise to assume that all shelters and victim support agencies offer the same benefits. In fact, some evidence suggests that not all women receive the same response from service providers. According to Dugan *et al.* (Dugan, Nagin, and Rosenfeld 2003), domestic violence services may systematically treat cases of partner violence differently depending on the victim's race and their marital relationship to their perpetrator.

Medical responses

Medical institutions can be an important intervention point for battered women. Yet, historically, many battered women have passed through medical services without notice. Detection and intervention were typically lacking and victims were often treated as if they were responsible for the abuse (Stark et al. 1979; Stark and Flitcraft 1996; see: Warshaw 1993). More recent literature acknowledges challenges faced by the health care system in developing effective policies and practices to respond to partner violence victims (Ross and Walther 2004; Allen, Lehrner, Marrison, Miles, and Russell 2007) and is suggestive of practices that may better serve assaulted women (see also: Campbell, Humphreys Kendall-Tackett 2004). While this research considers ways of improving detection and intervention, sometimes suggesting explicit strategies, it is clear that problems identified over 25 years ago are still not fully resolved (see, for example: Chamberlain and Perham-Hester 2002; Ernst and Weiss 2002). Despite great strides in developing screening protocols and educating health care providers about appropriate intervention and referrals, there are no universal standards. The assistance a victimized woman gets may largely depend upon the policies in place at the medical facility.

Regardless of policy, women who visit medical centres for other reasons will also benefit from routine screening (see: Campbell and Soeken 1999). Evidence suggests that speaking with a doctor explicitly about the abuse will increase a woman's chances of intervention, which may lead her to leave her abuser (McCloskey et al. 2006).

Many of these studies show inadequate consideration of victims' needs by service providers. Yet, they are limited to small geographic areas and/or only consider those who expressly seek help. Further, they fail to consider the role these interventions play in victims' lives. Our analyses presented below are designed to better understand the effects of victims' actions on repeat assault using a US nationally representative sample of females who were violently victimized at least once by a partner and were interviewed over time. This is one of the first times that nationally representative data following women over time have been used to evaluate the risk of repeat assault.

Other incident characteristics that might affect repeat assault

Clearly, other characteristics of the initial attack might also influence whether a woman is repeatedly attacked. Any indication of the perpetrator's instability during the attack, such as whether he used a weapon or was under the influence of drugs or alcohol, might suggest a higher risk to the victim. For instance, weapon use suggests that the offender is severely violent, perhaps representing a chronic problem. In any event, such incidents are likely to increase fear, impose more injuries, or lead to other detrimental consequences. A vast literature has linked chronic alcohol use to increased partner violence (Crowell and Burgess 1996)). The relationship between drug use and violence is likely to be similar, making these important aspects to consider when evaluating a woman's experiences. A final indicator of the severity of an attack is the victim's history of injuries.

Data

The NCVS is the largest nationally representative data set on criminal victimization in the USA. It is administered by the US Census Bureau, and is sponsored by the Bureau of Justice Statistics.[2] Its purpose is to gather information about criminal victimization directly from the victims. Thus, the data include incidents both reported and not reported to the police. The data are essentially a collection of individual interviews conducted with the residents of a sample of roughly 50,000 housing units who are interviewed every six months for three years. If a household moves, the new occupants of the housing unit are interviewed in the subsequent waves.

Because households are repeatedly interviewed, researchers can examine patterns of activity over time.[3] The NCVS includes information about the household, the respondents, and goes into great detail about all crime incidents reported to the interviewer. We use the only recent longitudinally linked NCVS data set constructed on behalf of the Bureau of Justice Statistics by the US Census Bureau. The Bureau used the identifiers from the confidential data to link information on the same respondents across interview periods, reducing possible error. By examining the actions and experiences of IPV victims, and estimating the trajectory of violence in their lives, we can see how such behaviours as responsive violence and help-seeking following the initial assault influence a woman's risk of repeat assault.

Although data collection began in 1973, additional probes were added in 1992 to better elicit responses about violence perpetrated within the family, thus making the survey better suited to study IPV (For discussion of the redesign, see Bachman and Taylor 1994). We use data collected from the second half of 1995 through to the end of 1999. Census Bureau changes in the survey design and sampling procedure preclude construction of a longitudinal file prior to this time (Bureau of Justice Statistics 2002) and longitudinally linked data are not available past 1999 due to budgetary constraints. Since there are currently no plans to release future waves of the data in a longitudinally linked format, these data offer a unique opportunity to examine the consequences of IPV.

In the following analyses, we include female respondents, age 16–49, who reported at least one violent victimization by an intimate partner.[4] This results in a sample size of 435 women. We omit 37 of these, who reported that their first incident was part of a series of victimizations.[5] Of the 398 remaining women, 52, or 14 per cent, reported more than one assault.[6]

Methods: how we use the NCVS to examine repeat assault

We used multivariate logistic regression analysis to estimate the effects of the variables described below on the probability that a victim who was violently attacked by a partner experienced a repeat assault before exiting the NCVS panel. All analyses were weighted with the person weight provided by the Bureau of Justice Statistics. Also, due to competing predictions, all statistical tests were two-tailed.

Primary variables [7]

The dependent variable, *subsequent IPV* is an indicator of whether or not more than one intimate partner assault was reported during a woman's NCVS interviews.

Intervening variables

Responsive violence used during the course of an assault was recorded through responses to two survey questions: 'Did respondent use or threaten to use physical force against the offender?' and 'Who was the first to use or threaten to use physical force – you, the offender, or someone else?' We coded an act of responsive violence in cases where the woman acted violently following her partner's assault during the first reported intimate partner assault. *Victim notifying the police* refers to when a victim reported that she herself contacted the police following the first intimate partner assault. *Police notification* describes when someone other than the victim contacted the police. *Arrest* refers to when the respondent reported that she knew of any arrests or charges brought as a result of the first reported intimate partner assault. *Agency* refers to when the victims had received 'help or advice from any office or agency – other than the police – that deals with victims of crime' (2002) after the first act of IPV. *Seeking medical attention* refers to when a woman injured received medical attention for any of her injuries. We also included *not injured* following violent crime, captured by responses to the survey question 'What were the injuries you suffered, if any? Anything else?' Combined, these two variables isolate those who are injured and seek medical help from those who are injured and seek no help.

Control variables

Weapon use was coded if the victim reports the perpetrator had ' ... a weapon such as a gun or knife, or something to use as a weapon, such as a bottle or wrench?' (Bureau of Justice Statistics 2002) for the first act of IPV. A perpetrator was considered to be *under the influence* if a victim reported that he was using drugs or alcohol at the time of the first reported assault. The model also controlled for minority status, educational attainment, household income (measured by $ value in the year 2000), public housing residence, age, marital status, employment status and family composition. Additionally, we included the number of NCVS interviews each woman completed to control for the time in the sample. Table 21.1 provides descriptive statistics for all of the variables. Note that we also included imputation and missing value flags, where there were sufficient cases to do so.

Table 21.1 Mean (standard deviation)/percentages for all variables

	All IPV victims – mean/% (standard deviation)
Subsequent assault	
First incident	13.72%
Responsive violence	11.65%
Notified the police	50.32%
Police notification by someone else	13.82%
Perpetrator arrested	25.07%
Medical attention for injuries	9.03%
Agency involvement	19.30%
Weapon use	15.54%
Perpetrator under Influence of drugs/alcohol	41.65%
Not injured	51.21%
Minority race	28.75%
Education*	
Less than 12 years	11.12%
12 years (reference/omitted category)	18.43%
More than 12 years	19.91%
Household income (year 2000 dollars)	$30,369.00 ($33,031)
Public housing resident	3.86%
Age in years	28.8 (8.28)
Marital status*	
Married	12.26%
Divorced	44.41%
Single	49.71%
Employed	66.73%
Household composition	
Lone adult	40.61%
Two adults (reference/omitted category)	26.01%
Many adults	33.38%
Number of children	1.08 (1.09)
Number of NCVS interviews completed	3.19 (2.13)
Sample size	**398**

* Categories will not sum to 100%, as missing cases are not shown. An indicator for missing cases is included in the model.

Presentation and discussion of findings

Recall that these analyses were designed to assess whether or not help-seeking behaviours reduce the likelihood that a victim of partner violence is victimized again. Our analysis produced a list of risk factors, protective factors and variables not associated with the likelihood of a repeat assault, which we present in Figure 21.1.

While control variables are included in this figure (in italics), our discussion will centre on those factors relevant to the victims' responses to violence.

Association	No association
Protective factors	Agency help
Arrest (marginally significant)	Any calls to police (by victim or someone
Number of children in the home	else)
Risk factors	Not injured
Responsive violence	Weapon use by perpetrator
Seeking medical care for injuries	Minority race
Perpetrator under the influence	Educational attainment
Never married/widowed	Income
More than two adults in the home	Public housing residence
	Employment
	One adult in the home
	Number of interviews

Figure 21.1 Variable association with repeat incident(s) of IPV

Surprisingly, none of the help-seeking behaviours acted as protective factors. The finding for arrest was marginal ($p < 0.10$), possibly suggesting a role for arrest. Further research is necessary to determine why police contact is not more effective in reducing the risk of repeat assault. Additionally, larger samples may discern whether arrest is truly effective at reducing risk.

Responsive violence during or following an earlier intimate partner assault is significantly associated with an increased risk of reporting a subsequent assault. This might diminish the hope that such actions would deter future violence. However, it is possible that responsive violence is part of a mutually violent dynamic in a relationship where violence is a normal form of conflict resolution. Future work is needed to disentangle self-defensive and retaliatory actions.

Our results show that those who seek medical attention have dramatically higher chances of being reassaulted. While it is tempting to assume that this means that seeking medical care is harmful, keep in mind that those women who sought medical assistance were more likely to be severely injured. This implies that violence in their households has already escalated and may also be characterized by repeated assault. This strongly suggests that health care practitioners need to take very seriously any suspicions of partner violence. Indeed, it is also possible that by seeking help, a woman has put herself in greater danger (should her partner retaliate). The chances of re-assault, however, appear to be unaffected if the police were contacted by the victim or a third party following an earlier intimate partner assault.[8]

Data limitations

These data are the best available for studying victimization; however, in using them one must keep in mind several limitations. First, we only have information on a woman's victimization history six months prior to the first interview and up to the last interview. Since there are no retrospective accounts of IPV prior to the survey reference period, it is entirely likely that many of the 'initial' victimizations actually represent repeat victimizations. Thus, there are respondents who are misclassified as one-time victims who were really experiencing a repeated assault. This type of measurement error makes it more difficult to distinguish between the two groups, thus biasing our estimates toward zero. In other words, our significant findings are valid despite this issue.

Additionally, several issues limit the generalization of our findings. First, because information about the first incident of a series is missing, we omit the 37 victims out of 435 whose first reported assault was actually a series of six or more incidents. Aside from underestimating the proportion of victims with repeat assault, our sample also only represents those victims who tend to not be victimized more than five times in a relatively short period of time. Second, institutionalized and homeless populations are excluded from the NCVS sampling design. We cannot assume that these groups share victimization patterns with other women. In fact, scholars suggest important differences for women residing on military bases and research evidence suggests different victimization patterns among incarcerated women (Dugan and Castro 2005; Richie 1996; McCarroll et al. 1999; Brannen and Hamlin II 2000; Heyman and Neidig 1999; Murdoch and Nichol 1995; Cronin 1995).

Conclusions and implications for research, policy and practice

Although we might like to think that any action a woman takes on her own behalf is better than doing nothing, our findings suggest this idea is problematic. Rather than reducing a victim's exposure to continued partner violence, it appears that contact with the medical establishment is associated with higher risk of repeat assault and contact with the police does nothing to protect a woman from being assaulted again. It is unclear whether women's efforts to seek help are ineffective because they are unable to reduce their exposure to their assailants or because their perpetrators retaliate after help is sought. This question was raised in earlier work (Dugan et al. 2003) that suggested a perpetrator is likely to retaliate if a woman seeks intervention but still has contact with her abuser. In fact, several scholars have indicated that men intensify their violence when women attempt to exit relationships, also suggesting that help-seeking can often hurt the victim (e.g. Riger *et al.* 2000). Thus, outside agencies and service providers must take extra precautions to protect victims (see Dugan *et al.* 2003 for a discussion of the potential lethal consequences to victims when adequate protection is not provided). At a minimum, the possibility for retaliation must be considered when developing intervention strategies.

While this work does not offer clear-cut policy recommendations, it suggests at least two important intervention points. First, because those women who seek medical help have the highest risk of repeated violence, if more resources are used to identify and assist battered women, repeated assault might go down. Second, since police contact appears ineffective against repeat assault, the criminal justice system can do more to protect women. Screening and intervention procedures can be further developed and evaluated for both medical personnel and the police. Finally, earlier research has stressed the importance of sensitive instruments that can address race and class differences.[9]

Our findings augment what the research literature had already indicated. First, and foremost, specific research is needed to better understand the motivations behind women's help-seeking and self-protective actions. Second, more qualitative analyses are essential to determine how different agencies and services are actually responding to partner violence victims. Third, there is evidence that the police and medical establishments are currently inadequate for meeting the needs of women violently victimized by an intimate. At best, both police and medical establishments have the potential to miss the opportunity to help battered women.

Acknowledgements

We appreciate the valuable comments and suggestions from members of the 2006–7 Family Research Laboratory Seminar. The work was supported by National Institute of Mental Health grant T32MH15161, and the University of New Hampshire. This research was initially funded by the National Institute of Justice and the Bureau of Justice Statistics.

Notes

1   These are referred to as *series incidents*, and they represent six or more victimizations in a six-month period that are similar and for which the respondent is unable to offer sufficient detail on each to report separately. In the Rand and Saltzman study (2003), a series incident was counted as only one victimization, leading to inherent undercounting of repeated incidents of violence.

2   Note that 'institutionalized' populations and the homeless are excluded, as discussed in the data limitations section.

3   Most NCVS files that are publicly available do not link respondents over time. The longitudinal nature of this data is a sampling convenience not meant for research purposes. Despite its intention, the longitudinal files can be linked properly, to be used for research with the help of the Bureau of Justice Statistics.

4   The age qualification is based on the respondent's age during the first interview.

5   Like earlier research with this data, omitting these cases will bias the sample toward less victimized women. While we would rather keep them in the sample, the coding strategy of the Bureau of Justice Statistics excludes key information for our analysis. When data is collected about series incidents, defined as six or more similar incidents about which respondents cannot distinguish enough detail to report separately, they only record information for the most recent assault. We require information on the circumstances of the first assault to assess what actions might influence the risk of a repeated victimization.

6   Percentage based on the weighted data.
7   Most variables are coded as 0 or 1. In these cases the variable is coded as 1 for the described condition and 0 for the absence of that condition. The names of the variables are in italics.
8   We also ran a model that estimated the effect of the police being informed regardless of who initiated contact. This finding was also null.
9   Unfortunately, the small sample size precluded us from identifying race-specific findings.

22 Conclusion

Tom Mason and June Keeling

Domestic violence is a particularly tragic affair for a number of reasons. First, it occurs between people who by and large love, or at least loved, each other at one time or another. It was probably not imagined as the relationship formed and not likely to have been included in early plans for the future. Of all the scenarios discussed in courtship, living together, saving, children, schools, holidays etc., what to do in the event of domestic violence probably did not feature. Thus, rooted in love, it appears the inverse of what was expected. As we have seen throughout this book, with many authors using the term 'intimate partner violence' (IPV), the tragedy resonates between these three words. The relationship is *intimate*, or at least was, which grounds it in trust, warmth and care. There is a *partnership* that issues forth such notions as honour, dependency, social contract and, again, trust. And, there is *violence* that shatters all the foregoing.

Second, violence towards any human being is inadmissible. However, violence between man and woman jars our sensibilities beyond this unacceptability. Although, as we have seen in many of the chapters, violence can occur between men, between women and between men and women in either direction, it is men being violent towards women that is the most common form in the domestic setting. We cannot evade the fact that men are usually the more physically powerful and that physicality is only one form of power. The physical force that can be applied may well cause injury and trauma, however, other factors feature large that accompany this. For example, fear, stress, stigma, shame and subjugation, to name but a few. To be dominated by physical force is also emotionally and psychologically damaging. Although bruises, wounds, burns and fractures may heal, albeit with scars, the trauma to the mind takes a different form. Psychological damage is slow to heal and its pain touches the soul. It scars the minds as well as the 'heart' and once crippled can manifest in nightmare scenarios. Although healing can, and does, occur in memory, the trauma remains.

Third, although intimacy involves various levels of analysis we have noted the close relationship between sex and power throughout the book. Without delving too deeply into a psychoanalytical interpretation of sex, suffice to say here that sex and power are intricately entwined. Although sex and power can be subtle and enticing, they can also be coercive and abusive. Furthermore, they can also be overwhelming and hateful in the form of rape. Thus, in intimate partnerships sexual pleasure and the power of enticement share an embrace rather than conflict with one another. As Michel Foucault stated 'pleasure and power do not cancel or turn back against one another; they seek out, overlap, and reinforce one another. They are linked together by complex mechanisms and devices of excitation and incitement' (Miller 1993: 263). Little wonder then, that history is replete with stories of women (and men) wanting to have sex with men (and women) in positions of power. However, when sex and power take the form of abuse, again, it shatters the enticement and turns to fear and hate. Arguably, once moved to this latter level there is no road back to the previous forms.

Fourth, we have seen that domestic violence damages the children in the family, which is a particular tragedy due to their youth and innocence. They may well be torn between their love for each parent and their desire to protect the victim. With such protection being difficult for the young child, fear becomes apparent. Although their love for their parents may be the starting point, this can quickly turn to hate for the father as perpetrator and can, in turn, cause further tension and conflict. Witnessing their (usually) mother being abused by their (usually) father, who in common understanding ought to care for and cherish her, creates a dilemma, if not a paradox, for the child. Within this common-sense understanding of the socially shared meaning of bonded love between mother and father, domestic violence creates a tension for the child who has great difficulty dealing with the dissonant themes. The child may come to blame themselves for the conflict and attribute the problem as theirs. This, again, can become internalized and create emotional problems for the child. Thus, caught up in a web of inner turmoil the child can become another victim of domestic violence: a dilemma for which a solution may be possible through prevention or intervention, or an undesirable paradox for which there is no solution.

The commonalities for survivors of abuse, such as the right to feel safe and protected from violence, have also been discussed. Within the chapters the authors have identified some of the complexities that require consideration in the provision of support for the people living with violence. These include individuals' lifestyle, ethnicity and cultural needs, all of which play a significant part in ensuring that the response to IPV is appropriate and effective.

On reading this book one could be forgiven for feeling an element of despair. Despair at the global prevalence rates of domestic violence and despair at the pain and suffering that it causes. In terms of unreported abuse we have only begun to scratch the surface, and screening for domestic violence remains contentious. In relation to treatment interventions and their efficacy we remain cautious and safe shelter approaches can be less than safe. Furthermore, the relationship between perpetrators, victims, significant others, professionals and the authority of the law can be a difficult one to balance. In all this, one can understand the turn towards pessimism. However, before we make that turn, note the contributors to this book, as well as the thousands of others throughout the world, who work tirelessly to understand and address these complex issues. Note too, those who help both victims and perpetrators in their difficult task to prevent further pain and suffering. Also note the research that is constantly being conducted in an effort to improve our knowledge of both preventative and interventive strategies. In the face of all the pain and suffering, we must have some degree of optimism.

References

Abbott, J., Johnson, R., Koziol-McLain, J. and Lowenstein, S. (1995) Domestic violence against women: incidence and prevalence in an emergency department population, *Journal of the American Medical Association,* 273(22): 1763.

Abel, E.M. (2001) Comparing the social service utilization, exposure to violence and trauma symptomology of domestic violence female 'victims' and female 'batterers', *Journal of Family Violence,* 16(4): 40–20.

Abraham, A., Cheng, T., Wright, J., Addlestone, I., Huang, Z. and Greenberg, L. (2001) Assessing an educational intervention to improve physician violence screening skills, *Pediatrics,* 107(5): 68.

Abyad, A. (1996) Elder abuse: diagnosis, management and prevention, *Medical Interface,* 9(10): 97–101.

Adelman, M. (2000) No way out: divorce-related domestic violence in Israel, *Violence Against Women,* 6: 1223–54.

Aggleton, P. and Chalmers, H. (2000) *Nursing Models and Nursing Practice.* Basingstoke: Palgrave.

Aldorondo, E. and Kaufman Kantor, G. (1997) Social Predictors of Wife Assault Cessation pp. 183–93 in G. Kaufman Kantor and J.L. Jasinski (eds) *Out of the Darkness: Contemporary Perspectives on Family Violence,* Thousand Oaks, CA: Sage Publications, Inc.

Aldridge, M.L. and Browne, K.D. (2003) Perpetrators of spousal homicide: a review, *Trauma, Violence and Abuse,* 4(3): 265–76.

Alexander, J. *et al.* (1994) *Midwifery Practice: A Research Based Approach.* New York: Palgrave Macmillan.

Allen, J.R. and St George, S.A. (2001) What couples say works in domestic violence therapy, *The Qualitative Report,* 6, retrieved 19 February 2007 from http://www.nova.edu/ssss/QR/QR6–3/allen.html.

Allen, N.E., Lehrner, A., Marrison, E., Miles, T. and Russell, A. (2007) Promoting systems change in the health care response to domestic violence, *Journal of Community Psychology,* 35(1): 103–20.

Alpert, E., Tonkin, A., Seeherman, A. and Holtz, H. (1998) Family violence curricula in US medical schools, *American Journal of Preventive Medicine,* 14(4): 273–82.

American College of Obstetricians and Gynaecologists (1995) Technical bulletin: domestic violence, no. 209, *International Journal of Gynaecology and Obstetrics,* 51: 161–70.

Anderson, K.G. (2006) How well does paternity confidence match actual paternity? Results from worldwide nonpaternity rates, *Current Anthropology,* 48: 511–8.

Andersson, M. (1994) *Sexual Selection.* Princeton, NJ: Princeton University Press.

Anetzberger, G.J. (1993) Elder abuse programming among geriatric education centers, *Journal of Elder Abuse and Neglect,* 5(3):69–87.

Anetzberger, G.J. (2001) Elder abuse identification and referral: the importance of screening tools and referral protocols, *Journal of Elder Abuse and Neglect,* 13(2): 3–22.

Anetzberger, G.J., Dayton, C., Miller, C.A., McGreevey, J.F., Jr. and Schimer, M. (2005) Multidisciplinary teams in the clinical management of elder abuse, in G.J. Anetzberger (ed.) *The Clinical Management of Elder Abuse,* pp. 157–71). Binghamton, NY: Haworth Press.

Anetzberger, G.J., Korbin, J.E. and Austin, C. (1994) Alcoholism and elder abuse, *Journal of Interpersonal Violence,* 9(2):184–93.

Archer, J. (2000) Sex differences in aggression between heterosexual partners: a meta-analytic review. *Psychological Bulletin,* 126: 651–80.

Archer, J. (2002) Sex differences in physically aggressive acts between heterosexual partners: a meta-analytic review, *Aggression and Violent Behavior,* 7: 313–51.

Asmus, M.E. (2004) *At a Crossroads: Developing a Prosecution Response to Battered Women who Fight Back.* Duluth, MN: Praxis International.

Astin, M.C., Ogland-Hand, S.M., Coleman, E.M. and Foy, D.S. (1995) Posttraumatic stress disorder and childhood abuse in battered women: comparisons with maritally distressed women, *Journal of Consulting Clinical Psychology,* 63: 308–12.

Atkinson, J. (2002) *Trauma Trails Recreating Songlines: The Transgenerational Effects of Trauma in Indigenous Australia.* North Melbourne, Vic: Spinifex Press Pty Ltd.

Austin, J.B. and Dankwort, J. (1999) The impact of a batterers' program on battered women, *Violence Against Women,* 5: 25–42.

Austin, J.E. (2000) *The Collaboration Challenge: How Nonprofits and Businesses Succeed through Strategic Alliances.* San Francisco, CA: Jossey-Bass.

Babcock, J.C. and Siard, C. (2003) Toward a typology of abusive women: differences between partner-only and generally violent women in the use of violence, *Psychology of Women Quarterly,* 27(2): 153–62.

Babcock, J.C., Costa, D.M., Green, C.E. and Eckhardt, C.I. (2004a) What situations induce intimate partner violence? A reliability and validity study of the Proximal Antecedents to Violent Episodes (PAVE) scale, *Journal of Family Psychology,* 18: 433–42.

Babcock, J.C., Green, C.E. and Robie, C. (2004b) Does batterers' treatment work? A meta-analytic review of domestic violence treatment, *Evidence Based Mental Health,* 7: 79.

Babor, T.F., de la Fuente, J.R., Saunders, J. and Grant, M. (1992) *AUDIT: The Alcohol Use Disorders Identification Test. Guidelines for Use in Primary Health Care.*

Geneva: World Health Organization.

Bacchus, L. *et al.* (2003) Experiences of seeking help from health professionals in a sample of women who experienced domestic violence, *Health and Social Care in the Community*, 11(1): 10–18.

Bachman, R. (2000) A comparison of annual incidence rates and contextual characteristics of intimate-partner violence against women from the National Crime Victimization Survey (NCVS) and the National Violence Against Women Survey (NVAWS) 1998, *Violence Against Women*, 6: 839–67.

Bachman, R. and Salzman, L. (1995) *Violence Against Women: Estimates from the Redesigned National Crime Victimization Survey.* Washington, DC: Department of Justice, Bureau of Justice Statistics.

Bachman, R. and Taylor, B. (1994) The measurement of family violence and rape by the Redesigned National Crime Victimization Survey. *Justice Quarterly*, 11(3): 701–14.

Bair-Merritt, M., Feudtnere, C., Mollen, C., Winters, S., Blackstone, M. and Fein, J. (2006) Screening for intimate partner violence using an audiotape questionnaire: a randomized controlled trial in a pediatric emergency department, *Archives of Pediatric Adolescence Medicine*, 160: 311–16.

Baker, A.A. (1975) Granny-battering, *Modern Geriatrics*, 5(8): 20–4.

Baker, R.R. and Bellis, M.A. (1993) Human sperm competition: ejaculate adjustment by males and the function of masturbation, *Animal Behaviour*, 46: 861–85.

Ballenger, J.C. *et al.* (2004) Consensus statement update on posttraumatic stress disorder from the international consensus group on depression and anxiety, *Journal of Clinical Psychiatry*, 65 (Suppl. 1): 55–62.

Bandler, R. and Grinder, J. (1979) *Frogs into Princes*. Moab, UT: Real People Press.

Barnard, G.W., Vera, H., Vera, M. and Newman, G. (1982) Till death do us part: a study of spousal murder, *Bulletin of the American Academy of Psychiatry and the Law*, 10: 271–80.

Barnett, O.W., Lee, C.Y. and Thelen, R.E. (1997) Gender differences in attributions of self-defense and control in interpartner aggression, *Violence Against Women*, 3(5): 462–81.

Barraclough, B. and Harris, E. (2002) Suicide preceded by murder: the epidemiology of homicide-suicide in England and Wales 1988–92, *Psychological Medicine*, 32(2): 577–84.

Basile, K. (1999) Rape by acquiescence: the ways in which women 'give in' to unwanted sex with their husbands, *Violence Against Women*, 5(9): 1036–58.

Bass, D.M., Anetzberger, G.J., Ejaz, F.K. and Nagpaul, K. (2001) Screening tools and referral protocol for stopping abuse against older Ohioans: a guide for service providers, *Journal of Elder Abuse and Neglect,* 13(2): 23–38.

Bauer, H.M., Rodriguez, M.A. and Perez-Stable, E.J. (2000a) Prevalence and determinants of intimate partner abuse among public hospital primary care patients, *Journal of General Internal Medicine,* 15: 811–17.

Bauer, H., Rodriguez, M., Quiroga, S. and YG, F.-O. (2000b) Barriers to health care for abused Latina and Asian immigrant women, *Journal of Health Care for the Poor and Underserved,* 11(1): 33–44.

Beaulieu, M. (1992) Elder abuse: levels of scientific knowledge in Quebec, *Journal of Elder Abuse and Neglect,* 4(1/2): 135–49.

Beckham, J.C, Feldman, M.E., Kirby, A.C., Hertzberg, M.A. and Moore, S.D. (1997) Interpersonal violence and its correlates in Vietnam veterans with chronic posttraumatic stress disorder, *Journal of Clinical Psychology,* 53: 859–69.

Bellis, M.A., Hughes, K., Hughes, S. and Ashton, J.R. (2005) Measuring paternal discrepancy and its public health consequences, *Journal of Epidemiology and Community Health,* 59: 749–54.

Beneke, T. (1982) *Men on Rape.* New York: St Martin's Press.

Bennett, L. and Lawson, M. (1994) Barriers to cooperation between domestic-violence and substance-abuse programs, *Families in Society,* 75: 277–86.

Bennett, L. and Williams, O. (2001) *Controversies and Recent Studies of Batterer Intervention Program Effectiveness.* Retrieved from www.vawnet.org.

Bergen, R.K. (1995) Surviving wife rape: how women define and cope with the violence, *Violence Against Women,* 1: 117–38.

Bergen, R.K. (1996) *Wife Rape: Understanding the Response of Survivors and Service Providers.* Thousand Oaks, CA: Sage.

Bergen, R.K. (1998) The reality of wife rape: women's experiences of sexual violence in marriage, in R.K.Bergen (ed.) *Issues in Intimate Violence.* Thousand Oaks, CA: Sage.

Berger, J. (1985) Modigliani's alphabet of love, in J. Berger (ed.) *The White Bird.* London: Chatto & Windus.

Berk, R.A. and Newton, P.J. (1985) Does arrest really deter wife battery? An effort to replicate the findings of the Minneapolis spouse abuse experiment, *American Sociological Review,* 50(2): 253–62.

Berk, R.A., Newton, P.J. and Berk, S.F. (1986) What a difference a day makes: an empirical study of the impact of shelters for battered women, *Journal of Marriage and the Family,* 48(3): 481–90.

Berk, R.A., Campbell, C., Klap, R. and Western, B. (1992) The deterrent effect of arrest in incidents of domestic violence: a Bayesian analysis of four field experiments, *American Sociological Review,* 57(5): 698–708.

Betzig, L. (1989) Causes of conjugal dissolution: a cross-cultural study, *Current Anthropology*, 30: 654–76.

Bever, E. (1982) Old age and witchcraft in early modern Europe, in P.N. Stearns (ed.) *Old Age in Preindustrial Society*, pp. 150–90. New York: Holmes & Meier.

Bhandari, M., Dosanjh, S., Tornetta, P. 3rd, Matthews, D. and Violence Against Women Health Research Collaborative (2006) Musculoskeletal manifestations of physical abuse after intimate partner violence, *Journal of Trauma*, 61(6): 1473–9.

Birkhead, T. (2000) *Promiscuity*. London: Faber & Faber.

Birkhead, T.R., Hunter, F.M. and Pellatt, J.E. (1989) Sperm competition in the zebra finch, *Taeniopygia guttata*, *Animal Behaviour*, 38: 935–50.

Bograd, M. and Mederos, F. (1999) Battering and couples therapy: universal screening and selection of treatment modality, *Journal of Marital and Family Therapy*, 25: 291–312.

Boldy, D. (2005) Addressing elder abuse: Western Australian case study, *Australasian Journal on Ageing*, 24(1): 3–8.

Bolstad, R. *et al.* (1992) *Communicating Caring: A Guide for Health Workers and Caregivers*. Auckland: Longman Paul Ltd.

Boone, E. (1985) *Developing Programs in Adult Education*. Upper Saddle River, NJ: Prentice Hall.

Boran, A. (2002) *Crime: Fear or Fascination?* Chester: Chester Academic Press.

Bossarte, R.M., Simon, T.R. and Barker, L. (2006) Characteristics of homicide followed by suicide incidents in multiple states, 2003–2004, *Injury Prevention*, 12: 33–8.

Boud, D. *et al.* (1985) *Reflection: Turning Experience into Learning*. London: Kogan Page.

Bouton, M.E. (2002) Context, ambiguity, and unlearning: sources of relapse after behavioral extinction, *Biological Psychiatry*, 52: 976–86.

Bowker, L. (ed.) (1998) *Masculinities and Violence*. Thousand Oaks, CA: Sage .

Bowman, C. (1992) The arrest experiments: a feminist critique, *The Journal of Criminal Law and Criminology*, 83(1): 201–8.

Bradbury, T.N. and Fincham, F.D. (1990) Attributions in marriage: review and critique. *Psychological Bulletin*, 107: 3–33.

Bradley, F., Smith, M., Long, J. and O'Dowd, T. (2002) Reported frequency of domestic violence: cross sectional survey of women attending general practice, *British Medical Journal*, 324(7332): 271.

Brannen, S.J. and Hamlin II, E.R. (2000) Understanding Spouse Abuse in Military Families pp 169–83 in J.A. Martin, L.N. Rosen, and L.R. Sparacino, (eds) *The Military Family: A Practice Guide for Human Service Professionals*, pp. 169–83. Westport, CT: Praeger.

Brannen, S.J. and Rubin, A. (1996) Comparing the effectiveness of gender-specific and couples groups in a court-mandated spouse abuse treatment program, *Research on Social Work Practice,* 6: 405–24.

Braun, P.A., Beaty, B.L., DiGuiseppi, C. and Steiner, G.E. (2005) Recent early childhood injuries among disadvantaged children in primary care settings, *Injury Prevention,* 11: 251–5.

Broekaert, E., Vandevelde, S., Schuyten, G., Erauw, K. and Bracke, R. (2004) Evolution of encounter group methods in therapeutic communities for substance abusers, *Addictive Behaviors,* 29: 231–44.

Bronfenbrenner, U. (1977) Toward an experimental ecology of human development, *American Psychologist,* 32: 513–31.

Brookfield, S. (1990) *The Skillful Teacher.* San Francisco: Jossey-Bass.

Brott, A. (1994) *Men: The Secret Victims of Domestic Violence.* Retrieved 15 January 2002 from www.vix.com/pub/men/battery/commentary/brott-hidden.html.

Brown, G. (2004) Gender as a factor in the response to the law-enforcement system to violence against partners, *Sexuality and Culture,* 8(3–4): 37–8.

Brown, P.J., Stout, R.L. and Mueller, T. (1996) Posttraumatic stress disorder and substance abuse relapse among women: a pilot study, *Psychology of Addictive Behaviors,* 10:124–8.

Browne, A. (1997) Violence in marriage: until death do us part, in A.P Cardarelli (ed.) *Violence Between Intimate Partners: Patterns, Causes and Effects.* Boston, MA: Allyn & Bacon.

Brownmiller, S. (1975) *Against Our Will: Men, Women, and Rape.* New York: Simon & Schuster.

Brownridge, D.A. (2003) Male partner violence against Aboriginal women in Canada: an empirical analysis, *Journal of Interpersonal Violence,* 18(1): 65–83.

Bryant, S.A. and Spencer, G.A. (2002) Domestic violence: what do nurse practitioners think? *Journal of the American Academy of Nurse Practitioners,* 14(9): 421–7.

Buber, M. (1923) *I and Thou.* London: Continuum International Publishing Group.

Burch, E.S., Jr. (1975) *Eskimo Kinsmen.* St Paul, MI: West Publishing.

Bureau of Justice Statistics (2002) *1996–1999 Longitudinally Linked National Crime Victimization Survey Data and Documentation.* Conducted by US Department of Commerce, Bureau of the Census. Data provided by Bureau of Justice Statistics, 2002. Documentation provided by ICPSR, Ann Arbor, MI.

Burke, J.G., Thieman, L.K., Gielen, A.C., O'Campo, P. and McDonnell, K.A. (2005) Intimate partner violence, substance use, and HIV among low-income women: taking a closer look, *Violence Against Women,* 11(9): 1040–61.

Burns, D.D. and Sayers, S. L. (1992) Development and validation of a brief relationship satisfaction scale. Unpublished manuscript. (Measure available by emailing Richard.Heyman@Stonybrook.edu).

Burston, G.R. (1975) Granny-battering, *British Medical Journal*, 3(5983): 592.

Burton, B., Duvvury, N. and Varia, N. (2000) *Justice, Change, and Human Rights: International Research and Responses to Domestic Violence*. The International Center for Research on Women and the Centre for Development and Population Activities. Retrieved 15 February 2007 from www.icrw.org/docs/domesticviolencesynthesis.pdf.

Buss, D.M. (1988) From vigilance to violence: tactics of mate retention in American undergraduates, *Ethology and Sociobiology*, 9: 291–317.

Buss, D.M. (1996) Sexual conflict: evolutionary insights into feminism and the 'battle of the sexes', in D.M. Buss and N.M. Malamuth (eds) *Sex, Power, Conflict*, pp. 296–318. New York: Oxford University Press.

Buss, D.M. (2000) *The Dangerous Passion*. New York: The Free Press.

Buss, D.M. (2005) *The Murderer Next Door*. New York: Penguin.

Buss, D.M. and Duntley, J.D. (1998) Evolved homicide modules. Paper presented at the Annual Meeting of the Human Behavior and Evolution Society, Davis, CA, 10July.

Buss, D.M. and Duntley, J.D. (2003) Homicide: an evolutionary perspective and implications for public policy, in N. Dress (ed.) *Violence and Public Policy*, pp. 115–28. Westport, CT: Greenwood Publishing Group.

Buss, D.M. and Shackelford, T.K (1997) From vigilance to violence: mate retention tactics in married couples, *Journal of Personality and Social Psychology*, 72: 346–61.

Buss, D.M., Larsen, R.J., Westen, D. and Semmelroth, J. (1992) Sex differences in jealousy: evolution, physiology and psychology, *Psychological Science*, 3: 251–55.

Butell, F.P. (2002) Levels of moral reasoning among female domestic violence offenders: evaluating the impact of treatment, *Research on Social Work Practice*,12(3): 349–63.

Butler, R.N. (1975) *Why Survive? Being Old in America*. New York: Harper & Row.

Bybee, D. and Sullivan, C. (2005) Predicting re-victimizaton of battered women 3 years after exiting a shelter program, *American Journal of Community Psychology*, 36(1/2): 85–96.

Caetano, R., Schafer, J. and Cunradi, C.B. (2001) Alcohol-related intimate partner violence among White, Black, and Hispanic couples in the United States, *Alcohol Research and Health*, 25: 58–65.

Camilleri, J.A. (2004) Investigating sexual coercion in romantic relationships: a test of the cuckoldry risk hypothesis. Unpublished masters thesis, University of Saskatchewan, Saskatoon, Saskatchewan, Canada.

Campbell, J.C. (1989) Women's responses to sexual abuse in intimate relationships, *Women's Health Care International,* 8: 335–47.

Campbell, J.C. (2002a) The health consequences of intimate partner violence, *The Lancet,* 359 (9314): 1509–14.

Campbell, J.C. (2002b) Violence against women and health consequences, *The Lancet,* 359 (9314): 1331–6.

Campbell, J.C. and Lewandowski, L.A. (1997) Mental and physical health effects of intimate partner violence on women and children, *Psychiatric Clinics of North America,* 20: 353–74.

Campbell, J.C. and Soeken, K.L. (1999a) Forced sex and intimate partner violence: effects on women's risk and women's health, *Violence Against Women,* 5(9): 1017–35.

Campbell, J.C. and Soeken, K.L. (1999b) Women's responses to battering over time, *Journal of Interpersonal Violence,* 14(1): 21–40.

Campbell, J.C., Woods, A.B., Chouaf, K.L. and Parker, B. (2000) Reproductive health consequences of intimate partner violence, *Clinical Nursing Research,* 9: 217–37.

Campbell, J.C. *et al.* (2002) Intimate partner violence and physical health consequences. *Archives of Internal Medicine,* 162: 1157–63.

Campbell, J. C. *et al.* (2003) Risk factors for femicide in abusive relationships: results from a mulitsite case control study, *American Journal of Public Health,* 93: 1089–97.

Canadian Panel on Violence Against Women (CPVAW) (1993) *Changing the Landscape: Ending Violence – Achieving Equality.* Ottawa: Ministry of Supply and Services.

Caralis, P. and Musialowski, R. (1997) Women's experiences with domestic violence and their attitudes and expectations regarding medical care of abuse victims, *Southern Medical Journal,* 90(11): 1075–80.

Carbone-Lopez, K., Kruttschnitt, C. and Macmillan, R. (2006) Patterns of intimate partner violence and their associations with physical health, psychological distress, and substance use, *Public Health Report,* 121(4): 382–92.

Carroll, J., Reid, A., Biringer, A., Midmer, D., Glazier, R. and Wilson, L. (2005) Effectiveness of the Antenatal Psychosocial Health Assesment (ALPHA) form in detecting psychosocial concerns: a randomized controlled trial, *Canadian Medical Association Journal,* 173(3): 253–7.

Cascardi, M. and Vivian, D. (1995) Context for specific episodes of marital violence: gender and severity of violence differences, *Journal of Family Violence,* 10: 265–93.

Cascardi, M., Langhinrichsen, J. and Vivian, D. (1992) Marital aggression: impact, injury, and health correlates for husbands and wives, *Archives of Internal Medicine,* 152: 1178–84.

Cascardi, M., O'Leary, K.D. and Schlee, K.A. (1999) Co-occurrence and correlates of posttraumatic stress disorder and major depression in physically abused women, *Journal of Family Violence,* 14: 227–50.

Catalano, S. (2006) *Intimate Partner Violence in the United States*. Retrieved 29 December 2006 from www.ojp.usdoj.gov/bjs/pub/pdf/ipvus.pdf.

Centres for Disease Control (1989) Education about adult domestic violence in US and Canadian edical schools, 1987–1988, *Morbidity and Mortality Weekly Report: 38*.

Centers for Disease Control and Prevention (2001) *Surveillance for Homicide Among Intimate Partners, US, 1981–1998*. Retrieved February 2007 from www.cdc.gov/MMWR/preview/mmwrhtml/ss5003a1.htm.

Chamberlain, L. and Perham-Hester, K.A. (2002) The impact of perceived barriers on primary care physicians' screening practices for female partner abuse, *Women and Health*, 35(2/3): 55–69.

Chambliss, L.R. *et al.* (1995) Domestic violence: an educational imperative? *American Journal of Obstetrics and Gynaecology*, 172(3): 1035–8.

Chang, J., Berg, C., Saltzman, L. and Herndon, J. (2005) Homicide: a leading cause of injury deaths among pregnant and postpartum women in the United States, 1991–1999, *American Journal of Public Health*, 95(3): 471–77.

Chase, K.A., O'Farrell, T.J., Murphy, C.M., Fals-Stewart, W. and Murphy, M. (2003) Factors associated with partner violence among female alcoholic patients and their male partners, *Journal of Studies on Alcohol*, 64: 137–49.

Check, J.V. and Malamuth, N. (1985) An empirical assessment of some feminist hypotheses about rape, *International Journal of Women's Studies*, 8(4): 414–23.

Cheng, K.M., Burns, J.T. and McKinney, F. (1983) Forced copulation in captive mallards III, sperm competition, *The Auk*, 100: 302–10.

Chermack, S.T., Fuller, B.E. and Blow, F.C. (2000) Predictors of expressed partner and non-partner violence among patients in substance abuse treatment, *Drug and Alcohol Dependence*, 58: 43–54.

Cho, A.J., Kim, S.K. and Kim, Y.K. (2000) *Study on the Prevalence of Elder Abuse in Korea*. Korea: Institute for Health and Social Affairs.

Clough, R. (1999) Scandalous care: interpreting public enquiry reports of scandals in residential care. *Journal of Elder Abuse and Neglect*, 10(1/2): 13–27.

Coker, A.L., Sanderson, M., Fadden, M.K. and Pirisi, L. (2000a) Intimate partner violence and cervical neoplasia, *Journal of Women's Health and Gender-Based Medicine*, 9(9): 1015–23.

Coker, A.L., Smith, P.H., Bethea, L., King, M.R. and McKeown, R.E. (2000b) Physical health consequences of physical and psychological intimate partner violence, *Archives of Family Medicine*, 9: 451–6.

Coker, A.L., Smith, P.H., McKeown, R.E. and King, M.J. (2000c) Frequency and correlates of intimate partner violence by type: physical, sexual, and psychological battering, *American Journal of Public Health*, 90(4): 553–9.

Coker, A.L., Davis, K.E., Arias, I., Desai, S., Sanderson, M. and Brandt, H.M. (2002a) Physical and mental health effects of intimate partner violence for men and women, *American Journal of Preventive Medicine,* 23: 260–8.

Coker, A., Bethea, L., Smith, P., Fadden, M. and Brandt, H. (2002b) Missed opportunities: intimate partner violence in family practice settings, *Preventive Medicine,* 34(4): 445–54.

Coker, A.L., Watkins, K.W., Smith, P.H. and Brandt, H.M. (2003) Social or emotional support reduces the impact of partner violence on health: application of structural equation modeling, *Preventive Medicine,* 37(3): 259–67.

Coker, A.L., Smith, P.H. and Fadden, M.K. (2005) Intimate partner violence and disabilities among women attending family practice clinics, *Journal of Women's Health,* 14(9): 829–38.

Cokkinides, V.E., Coker, A.L., Sanderson, M., Addy, C. and Bethea, L. (1999) Physical violence during pregnancy: maternal complications and birth outcomes, *Obstetrics and Gynecology,* 93: 661–6.

Collins, J.J., Kroutil, L.A., Roland, E.J. and Moore-Gurrera, M. (1997) Recent developments in alcoholism, in M. Galanter (ed.) *Alcoholism and Violence,* pp. 387–405. New York: Plenum Press.

Connell, R.W. (1995) *Masculinities.* Berkeley, CA: University of California Press.

Connors, G.J., Maisto, S.A. and Donovan, D.M. (1996) Section I – theoretical perspectives on relapse: conceptualizations of relapse, a summary of psychological and psychobiological models, *Addiction, 91 (Suppl.),* S–13.

Court of Appeal UK (2000) *re L, V M and H,* 19 June, *Family Law,* 615: 623–4.

Craig, M.E. (1990) Coercive sexuality in dating relationships: a situational model, *Clinical Psychology Review,* 10: 395–423.

Cranwell, M.R., Kolodinsky, J.M., Anderson, K. and Schmidt, F.E. (2004) Evaluating a domestic violence task force: methods to strengthen a community collaboration, *Journal of Extension,* 42(6).

Cronin, C. (1995) Adolescent Reports of Parental Spousal Violence In Military and Civilian Families. *Journal of Interpersonal Violence* 10(1): 117–22.

Crowell, N.A. and Burgess, A.W. (1996). *Understanding Violence Against Women.* Washington, DC: National Academy Press.

Culbertson, K.A. and Dehle, C. (2001) Impact of sexual assault as a function of perpetrator type, *Journal of Interpersonal Violence,* 16(10): 992–1007.

Cwik, M.S. (1995) Couples at risk? A feminist exploration of why spousal abuse may develop within orthodox Jewish marriages, *Family Therapy,* 22(3): 165–83.

Daly, M. and Wilson, M. (1988) *Homicide.* Hawthorne, NY: Aldine de Gruyter.

Daniels, J.W. and Murphy, C.M. (1997) Stages and processes of change in batterers' treatment, *Cognitive and Behavioral Practice*, 4: 123–45.

Danielson, K., Moffitt, T., Caspi, A. and Silva, P. (1998) Comorbidity between abuse of an adult and DSM-III-R mental disorders: evidence from an epidemiological study, *American Journal of Psychiatry*, 155(1): 131–3.

Dansky, B.S., Roitzsch, J.C., Brady, K.T. and Saladin, M.E. (1997) Posttraumatic stress disorder and substance abuse: use of research in a clinical setting, *Journal of Traumatic Stress*, 10: 141–8.

Dasgupta, S.D. (1999) Just like men? A critical view of violence by women, in M.F. Shepard and E.L. Pence (eds) *Coordinating Community Responses to Domestic Violence: Lessons from Duluth and Beyond*, pp. 195–222. Thousand Oaks, CA: Sage.

Dasgupta, S.D. (2002) A framework for understanding women's use of nonlethal violence in intimate heterosexual relationships, *Violence Against Women*, 8: 1364–89.

Davis, R.E. and Harsh, K.E. (2001) Confronting barriers to universal screening for domestic violence, *Journal of Professional Nursing*, 17(6): 313–20.

Davison, J. (1997) Domestic violence: the nursing response, *Community Health*, 12(9): 632–3.

De Zulueta, F. (2003) Psychological causes of family violence, in S. Amiel and I. Heath (eds) *Family Violence in Primary Care*. Oxford: Oxford University Press.

Dearwater, S., Coben, J. and Nah, G. (1998) Prevalence of domestic violence in women treated at community hospital emergency department, *Journal of the American Medical Association*, 480: 433–8.

DeKeseredy, W.S. (2000) Current controversies on defining nonlethal violence against women in intimate heterosexual relationships: empirical implications, *Violence Against Women*, 6: 728–46.

DeKeseredy, W.S. and Schwartz, M.D. (1998a) *Measuring the Extent of Woman Abuse in Intimate Heterosexual Relationships: A Critique of the Conflict Tactics Scales*. Retrieved 7 May 2002, from www.vawnet.org/vnl/library/general/AR_ctscrit.html.

DeKeseredy, W.S. and Schwartz, M. (1998b) *Woman Abuse on Campus: Results from the Canadian National Survey*. Thousand Oaks, CA: Sage.

DeKeseredy, W.S. and Schwartz, M. (eds) (1998c) *Rethinking Violence Against Women*. Thousand Oaks, CA: Sage.

Del Vecchio, T. and O'Leary, K. D. (2004) Effectiveness of anger treatments for specific anger problems: a meta-analytic review. *Clinical Psychology Review*, 24: 15–34.

Dewey, J. (1997) *How We Think*. Mineola, NY: Dover Publications Inc.

DiClemente, C.C. and Hughes, S.O. (1990) Stages of change profiles in outpatient alcoholism treatment, *Journal of Substance Abuse*, 2: 217–35.

Dienemann, J., Campbell, J., Wiederhorn, N., Laughon, K. and Jordan, E. (2003) A critical pathway for intimate partner violence across the continuum of care, *Journal of Obstetric, Gynecologic, and Neonatal Nursing*, 32(5): 594–603.

Dixson, A.F. (1998) *Primate Sexuality*. Oxford: Oxford University Press.

Dobash, R.E. and Dobash, R.P. (1979) *Violence Against Wives: A Case Against the Patriarchy*. New York: Free Press.

Dobash, R.P. and Dobash, R.E. (2004) Women's violence to men in intimate relationships, *British Journal of Criminology*, 44(3): 324–49.

Dobash, R.P., Dobash, R.E., Cavanagh, K. and Lewis, R. (1998) Separate and intersecting realities: a comparison of men's and women's accounts of violence against women, *Violence Against Women*, 4: 382–414.

DoH (Department of Health) (2000) *Domestic Violence: A Resource Manual for Health Care Professionals*. London: Department of Health.

DoH (Department of Health) (2005) *Responding to Domestic Violence: A Handbook for Health Professionals*. London: Department of Health.

Domjan, M. (2003) *The Principles of Learning and Behavior*, 5th edn. Belmont, CA: Thomson/Wadsworth.

Donnelly, D.A. (1993) Sexually inactive marriages, *The Journal of Sex Research*, 30: 171–9.

Douglass, R.L., Hickey, T. and Noel, C. (1980). *A Study of Maltreatment of the Elderly and Other Vulnerable Adults*. Ann Arbor, MI: University of Michigan, Institute of Gerontology.

Doyle, R. (1996) *The Woman Who Walked Into Doors*. London: Jonathan Cape.

Dugan, L. (2003) Domestic violence legislation: exploring its impact on the likelihood of domestic violence, police involvement, and arrest, *Criminology and Public Policy*, 2(2): 283–309.

Dugan, L. and Castro, J.L. (2005) Comparing predictors of violent victimization for NCVS women with those for incarcerated women, in K. Heimer and C. Kruttschnitt (eds) *Gender and Crime: Patterns in Victimization and Offending*, pp. 171–94. New York: New York University Press.

Dugan, L., Nagin, D.S. and Rosenfeld, R. (1999) Explaining the decline in intimate partner homicide: the effects of changing domesticity, women's status, and domestic violence resources, *Homicide Studies*, 3: 187–214.

Dugan, L., Nagin, D.S. and Rosenfeld, R. (2003) Exposure reduction or retaliation? The effects of domestic violence legislation on intimate-partner homicide, *Law and Society Review*, 37(1): 169–98.

Dunford, F.W. (2000) The San Diego Navy Experiment: an assessment of interventions for men who assault their wives, *Journal of Consulting and Clinical Psychology*, 68: 468–76.

Dunkle, K.L., Jewkes, R.K., Brown, H.C., Gray, G.E., McIntyre, J.A. and Harlow, S.D. (2004) Gender-based violence, relationship power and risk of prevalent HIV infection among women attending antenatal clinics in Soweto, South Africa, *The Lancet,* 363: 1415–21.

Dunn, C., Deroo, L. and Rivara, F.P. (2001) The use of brief interventions adapted from motivational interviewing across behavioral domains: a systematic review, *Addiction,* 96: 1725–42.

Dutton, D.G. (1996) *The Abusive Personality.* New York: Guilford Press.

Dutton, D.G. and Corvo, K. (2006) Transforming a flawed policy: a call to revive psychology and science in domestic violence research and practice, *Aggression and Violent Behavior,* 11(5): 457–83.

Dutton, M.A. (1996) Battered women's strategic response to violence: the role of context, in J.L. Edleson and Z.C. Eisikovits (eds) *Future Interventions With Battered Women and Their Families*, pp. 105–24. Thousand Oaks, CA: Sage.

Dworkin, A. (1993) Living in Terror and Pain, Being a Battered Wife in P.B. Bart and E.G. Moran (eds) *Violence Against Women: The Bloody Footprints*, pp. 237–39. Newbury Park, CA: Sage Publications.

Easteal, P. (1994) Homicide-suicides between adult sexual intimates: an Australian study, *Suicide and Life-Threatening Behavior,* 24(2): 140–51.

Eastman, M. (1984) *Old Age Abuse.* Mitcham: Age Concern.

Easton, C. and Sinha, R. (2002) Treating the addicted male batterer: promising directions for dual-focused programming, in C. Wekerle and A.-M. Wall (eds) *The Violence and Addiction Equation: Theoretical and Clinical Issues in Substance Abuse and Relationship Violence.* New York: Brunner-Routledge.

Eaton, A. (2001) Assessing learning needs, in S. Hinchcliff (ed.) *The Practitioner as Teacher*, pp. 77–107. China: Bailiere Tindall.

Eby, K.K. and Campbell, J.C. (1995) Health effects of experiences of sexual violence for women with abusive partners, *Women's Health Care International,* 14: 563–76.

Edleson, J. and Syers, M. (1990) The relative effectiveness of group treatments for men who batter, *Social Work Research and Abstracts,* 26: 10–17.

Edleson, J. and Tolman, R. (1992) *Intervention for Men who Batter: An Ecological Approach.* Newbury Park, CA: Sage.

Ehrensaft, M.K. and Vivian, D. (1996) Spouses' reasons for not reporting existing marital aggression as a marital problem, *Journal of Family Psychology,* 10: 443–53.

Eifert, G.H., McKay, M. and Forsyth, J.P. (2006) *Act on Life not on Anger: The New Acceptance and Commitment Therapy Guide to Problem Anger.* Oakland, CA: New Harbinger.

El-Bassel, N., Gilbert, L., Witte, S., Wu, E., Gaeta, T., Schilling, R. and Wada, T. (2003) Intimate partner violence and substance abuse among minority women receiving care from an inner-city emergency department, *Women's Health Issues,* 13(1): 16–22.

El Kady, D., Gilbert, W.M., Xing, G. and Smith, L.H. (2005) Maternal and neonatal outcomes of assaults during pregnancy, *Obstetrics and Gynecology,* 105(2): 357–63.

Elliott, L., Nerney, M., Jones, T. and Friedmann, P. (2002) Barriers to screening for domestic violence, *Journal of General Internal Medicine,* 17(2): 112–16.

Ellis, D. and Stuckless, N. (1996) *Mediating and Negotiating Marital Conflicts.* Thousand Oaks, CA: Sage Publications.

Elsner, A. (2001) Protecting battered US women saves the lives of men, *Reuters Newswire.* Retrieved 5 January 2001,from www.eurowrc.org/01.eurowrc/ 04.eurowrc_en/43.en_ewrc.htm.

Erez, E. (2000) Immigration, culture conflict and domestic violence/woman battering, *Crime Prevention and Community Safety: An International Journal,* 2(1): 27–36.

Erez, E. (2002) Domestic violence and the criminal justice system: an overview, *Online Journal of Issues in Nursing,* 7(1): manuscript 3.

Erez, E. and Belknap, J. (1998a) In their own words: battered women's assessment of the criminal processing system's responses, *Violence and Victims,* 13(3): 251–68.

Erez, E. and Belknap, J. (1998b) Battered women and the criminal justice system: the perspectives of service providers, *European Journal of Criminal Policy and Research,* 6: 37–87.

Ernst, A. and Weiss, S.J. (2002) Intimate partner violence from the emergency medicine perspective, *Women and Health,* 35(2/3): 71–81.

Ernst, A., Weiss, S., Cham, E. and Marquez, M. (2002) Comparison of three instruments for assessing ongoing intimate partner violence, *Medical Science Monitor,* 8(3): CR197–201.

Fals-Stewart, W. (2003) The occurrence of partner violence on days of alcohol consumption: a longitudinal diary study, *Journal of Consulting and Clinical Psychology,* 71: 41–52.

Fals-Stewart, W., Kashdan, T.B., O'Farrell, T.J. and Birchler, G.R. (2002) Behavioral couples therapy for drug-abusing patients: effects on partner violence, *Journal of Substance Abuse Treatment,* 22: 87–96.

False Memory Syndrome Foundation (1994a) *False Memory Syndrome.* Brochure sent upon enquiry about the False Memory Syndrome Foundation.

False Memory Syndrome Foundation, (1994b) *Memorandum, September, 1994.* Follow-up letter after enquiry about the False Memory Syndrome Foundation.

False Memory Syndrome Foundation (1994c) *Frequently Asked Questions, March 1994.* Pamphlet sent upon enquiry about the False Memory Syndrome Foundation.

Family Violence Prevention Fund (2006) New system tracks homicides, suicides. Retrieved February 2007 from www.endabuse.org/newsflash/index.php3?Search=ArticleandNewsFlashID=8.

Fanslow, J.L. and Robinson, E. (2004) Violence against women in New Zealand: prevalence and health conseqences, *The New Zealand Medical Journal,* 117: 1–12.

Farr, K.A. (2002) Battered women who were 'being killed and survived it': straight talk from survivors, *Violence and Victims,* 17(3): 267–82.

Feder, L. and Forde, D.R. (2000) *A Test of the Efficacy of Court-Mandated Counseling for Domestic Violence Offenders: The Broward Experiment.* Washington, DC: National Institute of Justice.

Feld, S.L. and Straus, M.A. (1990) Escalation and desistance from wife assault in marriage, in M.A. Straus and R.J. Gelles (eds) *Physical Violence in American Families: Risk Factors and Adaptations in 8,145 Families,* pp. 489–505. New Brunswick, NJ: Transaction.

Feldhaus, K., Koziol-McLain, J., Amsbury, H., Norton, I., Lowenstein, S. and Abbott, J. (1997) Accuracy of 3 brief screening questions for detecting partner violence in the emergency department, *Journal of the American Medical Association,* 277(17): 1357–61.

Ferguson, D. and Beck, C. (1983) HALF – a tool to assess elder abuse within the family, *Geriatric Nursing,* 4: 301–4.

Ferraro, K.J. (1989) Policing woman battering, *Social Problems,* 36(1): 61–74.

Ferraro, K.J. (1993) Limitations of the medical model in the care of battered women, in P.B. Bart and E.G. Moran (eds) *Violence Against Women: The Bloody Footprints,* pp. 165–77. Newbury Park, CA: Sage.

Ferris, L. (1994) Canadian family physicians' and general practitioners' perceptions of their effectiveness in identifying and treating wife abuse, *Medical Care,* 32(12): 1163–72.

Fiebert, M. (1997) Annotated bibliography: references examining assaults by women on their spouses/partners, *Sexuality and Culture,* 1: 273–86.

Fincham, F.D. and Beach, S.R.H. (1999) Conflict in marriage: implications for working with couples, *Annual Review of Psychology,* 50: 47–77.

Figueredo, A.J. and McClosky, L.A. (1993) Sex, money, and paternity: the evolution of domestic violence, *Ethology and Sociobiology,* 14: 353–79.

Finkelhor, D. and Yllo, K. (1985) *License to Rape: Sexual Abuse of Wives.* New York: Free Press.

Finkler, K. (1997) Gender, domestic violence, and sickness in Mexico, *Social Science and Medicine,* 45: 1147–60.

Fischer, D.H. (1978) *Growing Old in America.* Oxford: Oxford University Press.

Fischer, K. and Rose, M. (1995) When 'enough is enough': battered women's decision making around court orders of protection, *Crime and Delinquency,* 41(4): 414–29.

Fisher, A.L. (1995) *A.L.J.R.* v. *H.C.G.R.,* Ontario Court of Justice (Provincial Division), Milton, Ontario, O.J. No. 4226, Para 17, Quicklaw version.

Fontes, L.A. (1993) Disclosures of sexual abuse by Puerto Rican children: oppression and cultural barriers, *Journal of Child Sexual Abuse,* 2: 21–35.

Fox, J.A. and Zawitz, M.W. (2007) Homicide trends in the United States. Washington, DC: US Department of Justice. Retrieved 8 November 2007 from www.ojp.usdoj.gov/bjs/homicide/homtrnd.htm.

Francis, E.A. (2001) Social work practice with African-descent immigrants, in F.G. Reamer (series ed.) and P.R. Balgopal (vol. ed.) *Foundations of Social Work Knowledge: Social Work Practice with Immigrants and Refugees,* pp. 127–66. New York: Columbia University Press.

Frank, E., Elon, L., Saltzman, L.E., Houry, D., McMahon, P. and Doyle, J. (2006) Clinical and personal intimate partner violence training experiences of US medical students. *Journal of Women's Health,* 15(9): 1071–9.

Fraser, R. (1998) *R.* v. *Ghanem,* 1998, ABPC 79, The Provincial Court of Alberta, Criminal Division, Calgary, Alberta. Alberta Reports.

Frieze, I.H. (1983) Investigating the causes and consequences of marital rape, *Signs: Journal of Women in Culture and Society,* 8: 532–53.

Frude, N. (1994) Marital violence: an interactional perspective, in J. Archer (ed.) *Male Violence* , pp. 153–69. London: Routledge.

Fulmer, T., Paveza, G., Abraham, I. and Fairchild, S. (2000). Elder neglect assessment in the emergency department, *Journal of Emergency Nursing,* 26(5): 436–43.

Gage, A.J. and Hutchinson, P.L. (2006) Power, control, and intimate partner sexual violence in Haiti, *Archives of Sexual Behavior,* 35: 11–24.

Gallup G.G., Burch, R.L., Zappieri, M.L., Parvez, R.A., Stockwell, M.L. and Davis, J.A. (2003) The human penis as a semen displacement device, *Evolution and Human Behavior,* 24: 277–89.

Gamache, D., Edleson, J. and Schock, M. (1988) Coordinated police, judicial, and social service response to woman battering: a multi-baseline evaluation across three communities, in G.T. Hotaling, D. Finkelhor, J. Kirkpatrick and M. Straus (eds) *Coping with Family Violence: Research and Policy Perspectives,* pp. 193–209. Newbury Park, CA: Sage.

Gangestad, S.W., Thornhill, R. and Garver, C.E. (2002) Changes in women's sexual interests and their partner's mate-retention tactics across the menstrual cycle: evidence for shifting conflicts of interest, *Proceedings of the Royal Society of London,* 269: 975–82.

Garcia-Moreno, C., Jansen, H.A., Ellsberg, M., Heise, L. and Watts, H.C. on behalf of the WHO Multi-country Study on Women's Health and Domestic Violence against Women Study Team. (2006) Prevalence of intimate partner violence: findings from the WHO multi-country study on women's health and domestic violence, *The Lancet*, 368: 1260–9.

Garimella, R., Plichta, S., Houseman, C. and Garzon, L. (2000) Physician beliefs about victims of spouse abuse and about the physician role, *Journal of Women's Health and Gender-Based Medicine*, 9(4): 405–11.

Gayford, J.J. (1975) Wife battering: a preliminary survey of 100 cases, *British Medical Journal*, 298: 194–7.

Gearhart, S.M. (1982) The future, if there is one, is female, in P. McAllister (ed.) *Reweaving the Web of Life: Feminism and Nonviolence*. New York: New Society Publishers.

Geffner, R., Mantooth, C., Franks, D. and Rao, L. (1989) A psychoeducational, conjoint therapy approach to reducing family violence, in P.L. Caesar and L.K. Hamberger (eds) *Treating Men Who Batter: Theory, Practice, and Programs*, pp. 103–33. New York: Springer.

Geffner, R., Campbell, J., Williams, O., LaViolette, A., Rosenbaum, A. and Stosny, S. (2006) *Power and Control Within the Family Violence Movements: A Roundtable Discussion*. Panel presentation at the 11th International Conference on Violence, Abuse, and Trauma, San Diego, CA, September.

Gelles, R. (2000) Domestic violence: not an even playing field, *The Safety Zone*. Retrieved 12 October 2000 from www.serve.com/zone/everyone/gelles/html.

Gelles, R. and Straus, M. (1979) Violence in the American family, *Journal of Social Issues*, 35(2): 15–39.

Gelles, R.J. and Straus, M.A. (1988) *Intimate Violence: The Causes and Consequences of Abuse in the American Family*. New York: Simon & Schuster.

Gelles, R. and Straus, M. (1999) Profiling violent families, in A. Skolnick and J. Skolnick (eds) *The Family in Transition*, pp. 414–31. New York: Longman.

Gerbert, B., Abercrombie, P., Caspers, N., Love, C. and Bronstone, A. (1999a) How health care providers help battered women: the survivor's perspective, *Women Health*, 29: 115–35.

Gerbert, B., Bronstone, A., Pantilat, S., McPhee, S., Allerton, M. and Moe, J. (1999b) When asked, patients tell: disclosure of sensitive health-risk behaviors, *Medical Care*, 37(1): 104–11.

Gerbert, B., Moe, J., Caspers, N., Salber, P., Feldman, M., Herzig, K. and Bronstone, A. (2002) Physicians' response to victims of domestic violence: towards a model of care, *Women and Health*, 35(2/3): 1–22.

Gielen, A.C. *et al.* (2000) Women's opinions about domestic violence screening and mandatory reporting, *American Journal of Preventative Medicine.* 19: 279–85.

Gillespie, R. (2000) When no means no: disbelief, disregard and deviance as discourses of voluntary childlessness, *Women's Studies International Forum,* 23: 223–34.

Gilligan, C. (1982) *In a Different Voice: Psychological Theory and Women's Development.* Boston, MA: Harvard University Press.

Gilligan, J. (2000) *Violence: Reflections on our Deadliest Epidemic.* London: Jessica Kingsley.

Glowa, P., Frasier, P. and Newton, W. (2002) Increasing physician comfort level in screening and counseling patients for intimate partner violence: hands-on practice, *Patient Education and Counseling,* 46(3): 213–20.

Goetz, A.T. and Shackelford, T.K. (2006) Sexual coercion and forced in-pair copulation as sperm competition tactics in humans, *Human Nature,* 17: 265–82.

Goetz, A.T., Shackelford, T.K., Weekes-Shackelford, V.A., Euler, H.A., Hoier, S., Schmitt, D.P. and LaMunyon, C.W. (2005) Mate retention, semen displacement, and human sperm competition: a preliminary investigation of tactics to prevent and correct female infidelity, *Personality and Individual Differences,* 38: 749–63.

Golding, J.M. (1999a) Intimate partner violence as a risk factor for mental disorders: a meta-analysis, *Journal of Family Violence,* 14: 99–132.

Golding, J.M. (1999b) Sexual assault history and headache: five general population studies. *Journal of Nervous and Mental disease,* 187(10): 624–9.

Goldkamp, J.S. (1996) *The Role of Drug and Alcohol Abuse in Domestic Violence and its Treatment: Dade County's Domestic Violence Court Experiment: Final Report.* Available from the Crime and Justice Research Institute, Philadelphia, PA.

Goldner, V. (1999) Morality and multiplicity: perspectives on the treatment of violence in intimate life, *Journal of Marital and Family Therapy,* 25(3): 325–36.

Gondolf, E.W. (1997) Patterns of reassault in batterer programs, *Violence and Victims,* 12: 373–87.

Gondolf, E.W. (1999) A comparison of four batterer intervention systems: do court referral, program length, and services matter? *Journal of Interpersonal Violence,* 14: 41–61.

Gondolf, E.W. (2000a) How batterer program participants avoid re-assault, *Violence Against Women,* 6: 1204–22.

Gondolf, E.W. (2000b) Re-assault 30 months after batterer program intake, *International Journal of Offender Therapy and Comparative Criminology,* 44: 111–28.

Gondolf, E.W. (2000c) Mandatory court review and batterer program compliance, *Journal of Interpersonal Violence,* 15(4): 428–37.

Gondolf, E.W. and White, R. (2000) Consumers' recommendations for batterers programs, *Violence Against Women,* 6: 196–215.

Gonzalez, D.M. (1997) Why females initiate violence: a study examining the reasons behind assaults on men. Unpublished masters thesis, California State University, Long Beach.

Goodwin, D. (1955) Some observations on the reproductive behavior of rooks, *British Birds,* 48: 97–107.

Goodwin, M.M., Gazmararian, J.A., Johnson, C.H., Gilbert, B.C. and Saltzman, L.E. (2000) Pregnancy intendedness and physical abuse around the time of pregnancy: findings from the pregnancy risk assessment monitoring system, 1996–1997, PRAMS Working Group, Pregnancy Risk Assessment Monitoring System, *Maternity and Child Health Journal,* 4: 85–92.

Gordon, M.M. (1978) *Human Nature, Class, and Ethnicity.* New York: Oxford University Press.

Gottman, J.M., Jacobson, N.S., Rushe, R.H., Shortt, J.W., Babcock, J., La Taillade, J.J. and Waltz, J. (1995) The relationship between heart rate reactivity, emotionally aggressive behavior, and general violence in batterers, *Journal of Family Psychology,* 9: 227–48.

Green, T. (1984) *Weeds Among the Wheat.* Notre Dame, IN: Ave Maria Press.

Guillet, J. (1970) *Discernment of Spirits.* Collegeville, MN: Liturgical Press.

Gutmanis, I., Beynon, C., Tutty, L., Wathen, C.N. and MacMillan, H.L. (2007) Factors influencing identification of and response to intimate partner violence: a survey of physicians and nurses, *BMC Public Health,* 24: 7–12.

Hadi, A. (2000) Prevalence and correlates of the risk of marital sexual violence in Bangladesh, *Journal of Interpersonal Violence,* 15: 787–805.

Haley, J. (1987) *Problem-solving Therapy,* 2nd edn. San Francisco: Jossey-Bass.

Halford, W.K., Sanders, M.R. and Behrens, B.C. (1994) Self-regulation in behavioral couples' therapy, *Behavior Therapy,* 25: 431–52.

Halpern, C.T., Young, M.L., Waller, M.W., Martin, S.L. and Kupper, L.L. (2004) Prevalence of partner violence in same-sex romantic and sexual relationships in a national sample of adolescents, *Journal of Adolescent Health,* 35(2): 124–31.

Hamlett, N. (1998) *Women Who Abuse in Intimate Relationships.* Domestic Abuse Project, Minneapolis, MN. Retrieved November 2007 from www.domesticabuseproject.org/services.asp.

Hansen, M. (1993) Feminism and family therapy: a review of feminist critiques of approaches to family violence, in M. Hansen and M. Harway (eds) *Battering and Family Therapy: A Feminist Perspective.,* pp. 69–81. Newbury Park, CA: Sage.

Hansen, M. and Harway, M. (eds) (1993) *Battering and Family Therapy: A Feminist Perspective*. Newbury Park, CA: Sage.

Harrykisson, S.D., Rickert, V.I. and Wiemann, C.M. (2002) Prevalance and patterns of intimate partner violence among adolescent mothers during the postpartum period, *Archives of Pediatric Adolescent Medicine,* 156: 325–30.

Hasday, J.E. (2000) Contest and consent: a legal history of marital rape, *California Law Review,* 88(5): 1373–498.

Haselton, M.G. and Nettle, D. (2006) The paranoid optimist: an integrative evolutionary model of cognitive biases, *Personality and Social Psychology Review,* 10: 47–66.

Hassouneh-Phillips, D. (2001) Polygamy and wife abuse: a qualitative study of Muslim women in America, *Health Care for Women International,* 22(8): 735–48.

Hassouneh-Phillips, D. (2003) Strength and vulnerability: spirituality in abused American Muslim women's lives, *Issues in Mental Health Nursing,* 24(6–7): 681–94.

Hathaway, J.E. *et al.* (2002) Listening to survivors' voices, *Violence Against Women,* 8(6): 687–719.

Healey, K. and Smith, C. (1998) Batterer programs: what criminal justice agencies need to know, *National Institute of Justice: Research in Action.* Washington, DC: National Institute of Justice.

Healey, K., Smith, C. and O'Sullivan, C. (1998) *Batterer Intervention: Program Approaches and Criminal Justice Strategies.* Washington, DC: USDOJ.

Heckert, D. and Gondolf, E.W. (2000) The effect of perceptions of sanctions on batterer program outcome, *Journal of Research on Crime and Delinquency,* 37: 369–91.

Hegarty, K.L. and Bush, R. (2002) Prevalence and associations of partner abuse in women attending general practice: a cross-sectional survey, *Australia New Zealand Journal of Public Health,* 26(5): 437–42.

Hegarty, K.L. and Roberts, G. (1998) How common is domestic violence against women? The definition of partner abuse in prevalence studies. *Australia and New Zealand Journal of Public Health,* 22(1): 49–54.

Henning, K. and Feder, L. (2004) A comparison of men and women arrested for domestic violence: who presents the greater threat? *Journal of Family Violence,* 19(2): 69–80.

Herman, D. (1984) The rape culture, in J. Freeman (ed.) *Women: A Feminist Perspective.* Palo Alto, CA: Mayfield.

Herman, J.L. (1992). *Trauma and Recovery.* New York: Basic Books.

Hester, M., Pearson, C. and Harwin N. (2000) *Making an Impact: Children and Domestic Violence – A Reader.* London: Jessica Kingsley.

Heyman, R.E. (2001) Observation of couple conflicts: clinical assessment applications, stubborn truths, and shaky foundations, *Psychological Assessment,* 13: 5–35.

Heyman, R.E. and Neidig, P.N. (1997) Physical aggression treatment in a couples format, in W.K. Halford and H.J. Markman. (eds) *Clinical Handbook of Couples Relationships and Couples Interventions,* pp. 589–617. New York: Wiley.

Heyman, R.E. and Neidig, P.H. (1999) A comparison of Spousal Aggression Prevalence Rates in U.S. Army and Civilian Representative Samples. *Journal of Consulting and Clinical Psychology* 67(2): 239–42.

Heyman, R.E. and Schlee, K.A. (2003) Stopping wife abuse via Physical Aggression Couples Treatment, in D.G. Dutton and D.J. Sonkin (eds) *Intimate Violence: Contemporary Treatment Innovations,* pp. 135–57. New York: Haworth Maltreatment and Trauma Press.

Heyman, R.E. and Slep, A.M.S. (2007) Therapeutic treatments for violence, in D.J. Flannery, A.T. Vazsonyi and I. Waldman (eds) *The Cambridge Handbook of Violent Behavior,* pp. 602–17. New York: Cambridge University Press.

Hildesheim, A. *et al.* (1997) Immune activation in cervical neoplasia: cross-sectional association between plasma soluble interleukin 2 receptor levels and disease, *Cancer Epidemiology Biomarkers and Prevention,* 13(6): 807–13.

Hirschel, D. and E. Buzawa (2002) Understanding the context of dual arrest with directions for future research, *Violence Against Women,* 8(12): 1449–73.

Hogben, M., Byrne, D. and Hamburger, M.E. (1995) Coercive heterosexual sexuality in dating relationships of college students: implications of differential male-female experiences, *Journal of Psychology and Human Sexuality,* 8(1–2): 69–78.

Holtzworth-Munroe, A. (2000) A typology of men who are violent toward their female partners: making sense of the heterogeneity in husband violence, *Current Directions in Psychological Science,* 33: 140–43.

Holtzworth-Munroe, A., Meehan, J.C., Herron, K., Rehman, U. and Stuart, G.L. (2000) Testing the Holtzworth-Munroe and Stuart (1994) batterer typology, *Journal of Consulting and Clinical Psychology,* 68: 1000–19.

Home Office (2000) *Criminal Statistics: England and Wales, 1999/00.* London: Government Statistical Service.

Home Office (2005a) *Crime in England and Wales: Homicide and Gun Crime.* London: Home Office.

Home Office (2005b) *Domestic Violence: National Plan for Domestic Violence.* London: Home Office.

Houle, C. (1972) *The Design of Education.* San Francisco: Jossey-Bass.

Houry, D., Kemball, R., Rhodes, K.V. and Kaslow, N.J. (2006) Intimate partner violence and mental health symptoms in African American female ED patients, *American Journal of Emergency Medicine,* 24(4): 444–50.

Howard, A., Riger, S. Campbell, R. and Wasco, S. (2003) Counseling services for battered women: a comparison of outcomes for physical and sexual assault survivors, *Journal of Interpersonal Violence,* 18(7): 717–34.

Hudson, M.F. (1991) Elder mistreatment: a taxonomy with definitions by Delphi, *Journal of Elder Abuse and Neglect,* 3(2): 1–20.

Hwalek, M. and Sengstock, M. (1986) Assessing the probability of abuse of the elderly: towards the development of a clinical screening instrument, *Journal of Applied Gerontology,* 5: 153–73.

Iecovich, E., Lankri, M. and Drori, D. (2004) Elder abuse and neglect – a pilot incidence study in Israel, *Journal of Elder Abuse and Neglect,* 16(3): 45–63.

Indridason, A. (2006) *Silence of the Grave.* London: Vintage.

Jackson, S., Feder, L., Forde, D., Davis, R., Maxwell, C. and Taylor, B. (2003) *Batterer Intervention Programs: Where Do We Go From Here?* Washington, DC: United States Department of Justice.

Jacobson, N.S. and Margolin, G. (1979) *Marital Therapy: Strategies Based on Social Learning and Behavior Exchange Principles.* New York: Brunner/Mazel.

Jacobson, N.S., Gottman, J.M., Gortner, E., Berns, S. and Shortt, J.W. (1996) Psychological factors in the longitudinal course of battering: when do the couples split up? When does the abuse decrease? *Violence and Victims,* 11(4): 371–92.

Jacoby, M., Gorenflo, D., Wunderlich, C. and Eyler, A.E. (1999) Rapid repeat pregnancy and experiences of interpersonal violence among low-income adolescents, *Journal of Interpersonal Violence,* 16(4): 318–21.

Jarvis, P. (1995) *Adult and Continuing Education.* London: Routledge.

Johnson, D.W. and Johnson, F.P. (2003) *Joining Together Group Theory and Group Skills.* London: Pearson Education.

Johnson, H. (2003) The cessation of assault on wives, *Journal of Comparative Studies,* 34(1): 75–94.

Johnson, J.K., Haider, F., Ellis, K., Hay, D.M. and Lindow, S.W. (2003) The prevalence of domestic violence in pregnant women. *BJOG: An International Journal of Obstetrics and Gynaecology,* 110: 272–5.

Johnson, M.P. (1995) Patriarchal terrorism and common couple violence: two forms of violence against women, *Journal of Marriage and the Family,* 57: 283–94.

Johnson, M.P. (2000) Conflict and control: symmetry and asymmetry in intimate partner violence, in A. Booth and A. C. Crouter (eds) *Couples in Conflict,* pp. 178–204. Mahwah, NJ: Lawrence Erlbaum.

Johnson, M.P. (in press) Domestic violence: the intersection of gender and control, in LL. O'Toole, J.R. Schiffman and M. Kitner (eds) *Gender Violence: An Interdisciplinary Perspective,* 2nd edn. New York: New York University Press.

Johnson, M.P. and Ferraro, K. (2000) Research on domestic violence in the 1990s: making distinctions, *Journal of Marriage and the Family*, 62: 948–63.

Johnson, M.P. and Leone, J.M. (2005) The differential effects of intimate terrorism and situational couple violence: findings from the National Violence Against Women Survey, *Journal of Family Issues*, 26: 322–49.

Johnson, T. (1986) Clinical issues in the definition of elder mistreatment, in K.A. Pillemer and R.S. Wolf (eds) *Elder Abuse: Conflict in the Family*, pp.167–96. Dover, MA: Auburn House.

Jones, A., Campbell, J., Schollenberger, J., Gielen, A., Dienemann, J., Kub, J., O'Campo, P. and Wynne, E. (1999) Annual and lifetime prevalence of partner abuse in sample of female HMO enrollees, *Women's Health Issues*, 9(6): 295–305.

Kalichman, S.C., Williams, E.A., Cherry, C., Belcher, L. and Nachimson, D. (1998) Sexual coercion, domestic violence, and negotiating condom use among low-income African American women, *Journal of Women's Health*, 7: 371–8.

Kaufman, G. (2001) *Individual Therapy for Batterers*. Atlanta, GA: Men Stopping Violence.

Kaufman Kantor, G. and Jasinski, J. (1998) *Dynamics of Partner Violence and Types of Abuse and Abusers*. United States Air Force, NNFR research report. Retrieved 12 May 2002 from www.nnfr.org/research/pv/pv_ch1.html.

Kawamoto, W.T. (2001) Community mental health and family issues in sociohistorical context: the confederated tribes of Coos, Lower Umpqua, and Siuslaw Indians, *American Behavioral Scientist*, 44: 1482–91.

Kebede, M. (2001) The rehabilitation of violence and the violence of rehabilitation: Fanon and colonialism, *Journal of Black Studies*, 31(5): 539–62.

Keeling, J. (2002) Support and education: the role of the domestic violence co-ordinator, *Nursing Times*, 98(48): 34–5.

Keeling, J. and Birch, L. (2002) Domestic violence in nursing curricula, *Nursing Times*, 98(48): 36–7.

Keeling, J. and Birch, L. (2004) Asking pregnant women about domestic abuse, *British Journal of Midwifery*, 12(12): 746–9.

Kendall-Tackett, K.A. (2004) *Health Consequences of Abuse in the Family: A Clinical Guide for Evidence-Based Practice*. Washington, DC: American Psychological Association.

Kennerley, R.J. (2000) The ability of a motivational pre-group session to enhance readiness for change in men who have engaged in domestic violence, *Dissertation Abstracts International*, 60.

Kernsmith, P. (2005a) Exerting power or striking back: a gendered comparison of motivations for domestic violence perpetration, *Violence and Victims*, 20(2): 173–85.

Kernsmith, P. (2005b) Treatment of perpetrators of domestic violence: gender differences in the applicability of the theory of planned behavior change, *Sex Roles,* 52(11/12): 757–70.

Kilgallon, S.J. and Simmons, L.W. (2005) Image content influences men's semen quality, *Biology Letters,* 1: 253–5.

Kilpatrick, D.G., Acierno, R., Resnick, H.S., Saunders, B.E. and Best, C.L. (1997) A 2-year longitudinal analysis of the relationships between violent assault and substance use in women, *Journal of Consulting and Clinical Psychology,* 65: 834–47.

Kim, U. (1994) Individualism and collectivism: conceptual clarification and elaboration, in U. Kim, H.C. Triandis, C. Kagitcibasi, S. Choi and G. Yoon, (eds) *Individualism and Collectivism: Theory, Method, and Applications: Cross-cultural Research and Methodology Series,* 18(19–40). Thousand Oaks, CA: Sage.

Kimmel, M. (1994) Masculinity as homophobia: fear, shame and silence in the construction of gender identity, in H. Brod and M. Kaufman (eds) *Theorizing Masculinities,* pp. 119–41. Thousand Oaks, CA: Sage Publications.

Kimmel, M. (1996) *Manhood in America: A Cultural History.* New York: The Free Press.

Kimmel, M. (2000) *The Gendered Society.* New York: Oxford University Press.

Kimmel, M. (2001) The myth of gender symmetry in domestic violence, *The Irish Times,* 5 December: 16.

Kimmel, M. (2002a) Beyond the myths on domestic violence, *The Irish Times,* 26 January: 16.

Kimmel, M. (2002b) 'Gender symmetry' in domestic violence: a substantive and methodological research review, *Violence Against Women,* 8(11): 1332–63.

Kivel, P. (1992) *Men's Work: How to Stop the Violence that Tears our Lives Apart.* Center City, MN: Hazelden.

Kivela, S.L., Kongas-Saviaro, P., Kesti, E., Pahkala, K. and Ijas, M.L. (1992) Abuse in old age: epidemiological data from Finland, *Journal of Elder Abuse and Neglect,* 4(3): 1–18.

Kohlberg, L. (1969) Stage and sequence: the cognitive developmental approach to socialisation, in D. Goslin (ed.) *Handbook of Socialisation Theory and Research,* pp. 347–80. Chicago: Rand McNally.

Kolbo, J., Blakeley, E.H. and Engelman, D.,(1996) Children who witness domestic violence: a review of the empirical literature, *Journal of Interpersonal Violence,* 11(2): 281–93.

Kosberg, J.E., Lowenstein, A., Garcia, J.L. and Biggs, S. (2003) Study of elder abuse within diverse cultures, *Journal of Elder Abuse and Neglect,* 15(3/4): 71–89.

Koss, M., Koss, P. and Woodruff, W. (1991) Deleterious effects of criminal victimization on women's health and medical utilization, *Archives of Internal Medicine,* 151(2): 342–7.

Kraemer, S. (1988) Splitting and stupidity in child sexual abuse, *Psychoanalytic Psychotherapy,* 3(3): 247–57.

Krasnoff, M. and Moscati, R. (2002) Domestic violence screening and referral can be effective, *Annals of Emergency Medicine,* 40(5): 485–92.

Kubany, E.S., Haynes, S.N., Leisen, M.B., Owens, J.A., Kaplan, A. and Burns, K. (2000) Development and preliminary validation of the Traumatic Life Events Questionnaire, *Psychological Assessment,* 12: 210–24.

Kurst-Swanger, K. and Petcosky, J. (2003) *Violence in the Home: Multidisciplinary Perspectives.* New York: Oxford University Press.

Kurz, D. (1993) Physical assaults by husbands: a major social problem, in R.J. Gelles and D.R. Loseke (eds) *Current Controversies on Family Violence,* pp. 88–103. Thousand Oaks, CA: Sage.

Lachs, M.S. and Pillemer, K. (2004) Elder abuse, *The Lancet,* 364: 1263–72.

Lachs, M.S., Berkman, L., Fulmer, T. and Horowitz, R. (1994) A prospective community-based pilot study of risk factors for the investigation of elder mistreatment, *Journal of the American Geriatrics Society,* 42(2): 169–73.

Lalumière, M.L., Harris, G.T., Quinsey, V.L. and Rice, M.E. (2005) *The Causes of Rape: Understanding Individual Differences in Male Propensity for Sexual Aggression.* Washington, DC: APA Press.

Langan, P.A. and Innes, C.A. (1986) *Preventing Domestic Violence Against Women.* Washington, DC: Bureau of Justice Statistics.

Laroche, M., Kim, C., Hui, M.K. and Tomiuk, MA. (1998) Test of nonlinear relationship between linguistic acculturation and ethnic identification, *Journal of Cross-Cultural Psychology,* 29: 418–33.

LaTaillade, J.J., Epstein, N.B. and Werlinich, C.A. (2006) A conjoint treatment of intimate partner violence: a cognitive behavioral approach, *Journal of Cognitive Psychotherapy,* 20: 393–410.

Lehmann, P. and Rabenstein, S. (2002) Children exposed to domestic violence: the role of impact, assessment, and treatment, in A.R. Roberts (ed.) *Handbook of Domestic Violence Intervention Strategies: Policies, Programs and Legal Remedies,* pp. 343–64. New York: Oxford University Press.

Leonard, K.E. (1993) Drinking patterns and intoxication in marital violence: review, critique, and future directions for research, in US Department of Health and Human Services *Research Monograph 24: Alcohol and Interpersonal Violence: Fostering Multidisciplinary Perspectives* (NIH Publication No. 93–3496, pp. 253–80). Rockville, MD: National Institutes of Health.

Leserman, J., Li, Z., Drossman, D.A. and Hu, J.B. (1998) Selected symptoms associated with sexual and physical abuse history among female patients with gastrointestional disorders: the impact on subsequent health care visits, *Psychological Medicine*, 28: 417–25.

Letourneau, E.J., Holmes, M. and Chasedunn-Roark, J. (1999) Gynecologic health consequences to victims of interpersonal violence, *Women's Health Issues*, 9: 115–20.

Liebschutz, J.M., Feinman, G., Sullivan, L., Stein, M. and Samet, J. (2000) Physical and sexual abuse in women infected with the human immunodeficiency virus: increased illness and health care utilization, *Archives of Internal Medicine*, 160: 1659–4.

Lipsky, S., Caetano, R., Field, C.A. and Bazargan, S. (2005a) The role of alcohol use and depression in intimate partner violence among black and Hispanic patients in an urban emergency department, *American Journal of Drug and Alcohol Abuse*, 31(2): 225–42.

Lipsky, S., Caetano, R., Field, C.A. and Larkin, G.L. (2005b) Is there a relationship between victim and partner alcohol use during an intimate partner violence event? Findings from an urban emergency department study of abused women, *Journal of Studies on Alcohol*, 66: 407–12.

Lipstadt, D. L. (1994) *Denying the Holocaust: The Growing Assault on Truth and Memory*. New York: Plume.

Long, H.B. (1983) *Adult Learning*. New York: Cambridge Book Company.

Lo Vecchio, F., Bhatia, A. and Sciallo, D. (1998) Screening for domestic violence in the emergency department, *European Journal of Emergency Department*, 5(4): 441–4.

Lovendski, J. and Randall, V. (1993) *Contemporary Feminist Politics: Women and Power*. Oxford: Oxford University Press.

Lown, A.E. and Vega, W.A. (2001) Alcohol abuse or dependence among Mexican American women who report violence, *Alcohol Clin Exp Research*, 25(10): 1479–86.

Loy, E, Machen, L., Beaulieu, M. and Greif, G.L. (2005) Common themes in clinical work with women who are domestically violent, *The American Journal of Family Therapy*, 33: 33–44.

MacKinnon, C. (1983) Feminism, Marxism, method and the state: toward feminist jurisprudence, *Signs*, 8(4): 635–58.

Mackintosh, N.J. and Colman, A.M. (1995) *Learning and Skills. Essential Psychology*. New York: Logman.

MacMillan, H., Wathen, C., Jamieson, E., Boyle, M., McNutt, L. and Worster, A. (2006) Approaches to screening for intimate partner violence in health care settings: a randomized trial, *Journal of the American Medical Association*, 296(5): 530–6.

Madaripur Legal Aid Association (1996) Khukumoni and Masud, in F.E. Jandt and P.B. Pedersen (eds) *Constructive Conflict Management: Asia-Pacific Cases*, pp. 82–7. Thousand Oaks, CA: Sage.

Maden, A. (1997) *Guide to Assessment of Students' Progress and Achievements*. London: DfEE.

Mahoney, P. (1999) High rape chronicity and low rates of help-seeking among wife rape survivors in a nonclinical sample: implications for research and practice, *Violence Against Women*, 5(9): 993–1016.

Mandel, D. (2006) *Highlights From 'A National Study of Batterers' Perceptions of their Children's Exposure to the Violence and Abuse'*. www.endingviolence.com.

Margolin, G. and Burman, B. (1993) Wife abuse versus marital violence: different terminologies, explanations, and solutions, *Clinical Psychology Review*, 13: 59–73.

Markman, H.J., Renick, M.J., Floyd, F.J., Stanley, S.M. and Clements, M. (1993) Preventing marital distress through communication and conflict management training: a 4- and 5-year follow-up, *Journal of Consulting and Clinical Psychology*, 61: 70–7.

Marsh,I. (1986) *Sociology in Focus: Crime*. London: Longman.

Martin, D. (1995) Letter from a battered wife in P.A. Weiss and M. Friedman (eds) *Feminism and Community*, pp. 45–9. Philadelphia, PA: Temple University Press.

Martin, S.L., Beaumont, J.L. and Kupper, L.L. (2003) Substance use before and during pregnancy: links to intimate partner violence, *American Journal of Drug and Alcohol Abuse*, 29(3): 599–617.

Marzuk, P., Tardiff, K. and Hirsch, C. (1992) The epidemiology of murder-suicide, *Journal of the American Medical Association*, 267(23): 3179–83.

Mason,T. and Chandley,M. (1999) *Managing Violence and Aggression: A Manual for Nurses and Health Care Workers*. Edinburgh: Churchill Livingstone.

Masuda, K. (1975) Bride's progress: how a Yome becomes a Shutome, *Journal of Asian and African Studies*, 10: 10–9.

McCaroll, J.E., Newby, J.H., Thayer, L.E., Norwood, A.E., Fullerton, C.S. and Ursano, R.J. (1999) Reports of Spouse Abuse in the U.S. Army Central Registry (1989–1997) *Military Medicine* 164(2): 77–84.

McCauley *et al.* (1995) The 'battering syndrome': prevalence and clinical characteristics of domestic violence in primary care internal medicine practices, *Annals of Internal Medicine*, 123: 737–46.

McCloskey, L.A., Lichter, E., Williams, C., Gerber, M., Wittenberg, E. and Ganz, M. (2006) Assessing intimate partner violence in health care settings leads to women's receipt of interventions and improved health, *Public Health Reports*, 121(July–August): 435–44.

McClusky, L.J. (1999) Domestic violence among Belizean Maya, *Humanity and Society*, 23: 319–38.

McCullough, J. P. (2000) *Treatment for Chronic Depression: Cognitive Behavioral Analysis System of Psychotherapy*. New York: Guilford Press.

McFarlane, J. and Soeken, K. (1999) Weight change of infants, age birth to 12 months, born to abused women, *Pediatric Nursing,* 25: 19–23.

McFarlane, J., Parker, B., Soeken, K. and Bullock, L. (1992) Assessing for abuse during pregnancy. Severity and frequency of injuries and associated entry into prenatal care, *Journal of the American Medical Association,* 267(23): 3176–8.

McFarlane, J., Campbell, J. C., Sharps, P. W. and Watson, K. (2002) Abuse during pregnancy and femicide: urgent implications for women's health. *Obstet.Gynecol.,* 100: 27–36.

McGuigan, W.M. *et al.* (2000) Domestic violence, parents' view of their infant and risk for child abuse, *Journal of Family Psychology,* 14(4): 613–24.

McKinney, F., Derrickson, S.R. and Mineau, P. (1983) Forced copulation in waterfowl, *Behavior,* 86: 250–94.

McLeer, S., Anwar, R., Herman, S. and Maquiling, K. (1989) Education is not enough: a systems failure in protecting battered women, *Annals of Emergency Medicine,* 18(6): 651–3.

McMahon, M. and Pence, E. (1996) Physical aggression in intimate relationships can be treated within a marital context under certain circumstances: comment, *Journal of Interpersonal Violence,* 11: 452–55.

McNutt, L., Carlson, B., Rose, I. and Robinson, D. (2002) Partner violence intervention in the busy primary care environment, *American Journal of Preventive Medicine,* 22(2): 84–91.

Medley, A., Garcia-Moreno, C., McGill, S. and Maman, S. (2004) Rates, barriers and outcomes of HIV serostatus disclosure among women in developing countries: implications for prevention of mother-to-child transmission programmes, *Bulletin of World Health Organization,* 82(4): 299–307.

Mehta, S. (1998) Relationship between acculturation and mental health for Asian Indian immigrants in the United States, *Genetic, Social, and General Psychology Monographs,* 124(1): 61–78.

Mezey, G. and Bewley, S. (1997) Domestic violence and pregnancy, *British Journal of Obstetrics and Gynaecology,* 104: 528–31.

Mezey, G.C., Bewley, S., Bacchus, L. and Haworth, A. (2001) *An Exploration of the Prevalence, Nature and Effects of Domestic Violence in Pregnancy,* Violence Research Program. Surrey: University of London.

Mihalic, S.W. and Elliott, D. (1997) A social learning theory model of marital violence, *Journal of Family Violence,* 12: 21–47.

Miller, B.A., Wilsnack, S.C. and Cunradi, C.B. (2000) Family violence and victimization: treatment issues for women with alcohol problems, *Alcoholism: Clinical and Experimental Research,* 24: 1288–97.

Miller, S. (2005) *Victims as Offenders: The Paradox of Women's Violence in Relationships.* New Brunswick, NJ: Rutgers University Press.

Miller, J. (1993) *The Passion of Foucault.* London: Flamingo Press.

Miller, W.R. and Rollnick, S. (2002) *Motivational Interviewing: Preparing People for Change*, 2nd edn. New York: Guilford Press.

Miller, W.R, Benefield, R.G. and Tonigan, J.S. (1993) Enhancing motivation for change in problem drinking: a controlled comparison of two therapist styles, *Journal of Consulting and Clinical Psychology,* 61: 455–61.

Minuchin, S. (1974) *Families and Family Therapy.* Cambridge, MA: Harvard University Press.

Mirrlees-Black, C. (1999) *Domestic Violence: Findings from a new British Crime Survey Self-completion Questionnaire.* Home Office Research Study 191. London: Home Office. Retrieved 1 December 2006 from www.homeoffice.gov.uk/rds/pdfs/hors191.pdf.

Mitchell, W.L. (1994) Women's hierarchies of age and suffering in an Andean community, *Journal of Cross-Cultural Gerontology,* 9: 179–91.

Moffitt, T.E., Caspi, A., Rutter, M. and Silva, P.A. (2001) *Sex Differences in Antisocial Behaviour.* Cambridge: Cambridge University Press.

Monson, C.M. and Langhinrichsen-Rohling, J. (1998) Sexual and nonsexual marital aggression: legal considerations, epidemiology, and an integrated typology of perpetrators, *Aggression and Violent Behavior,* 3(4): 369–89.

Morse, B.J. (1995) Beyond the Conflict Tactics Scale: assessing gender differences in partner violence, *Violence and Victims,* 10(4): 251–72.

Muehlenhard, C.L. and Falcon, P.L. (1990) Men's heterosocial skill and attitudes toward women as predictors of verbal sexual coercion and forceful rape, *Sex Roles,* 23(5–6): 241–59.

Mullerman, R., Lenaghan, P.A. and Pakieser, R.A. (1996) Battered women: injury locations and types, *Annals of Emergency Medicine,* 28: 486–92.

Mulroney, J. (2003) *Australian Statistics on Domestic Violence.* Australian Domestic and Family Violence Clearinghouse. Retrieved 1 December 2006 from www.austdvclearinghouse.unsw.edu.au/topics/topics_pdf_files/Statistics_final.pdf.

Murdoch, M. and Nichol, K.L. (1995) Woman Veterans' Experiences with Domestic Violence and with Sexual Harassment while in the Military: *Archives of Family Medicine* 4: 411–18.

Murphy, C.C., Schei, B., Myhr, T.L., and Du Mont, J. (2001) Abuse: a risk factor for low birth weight? A systematic review and meta-analysis, *Canadian Medical Association Journal,* 164: 1567–72.

Murphy, C.M. and O'Farrell, T.J. (1997) Couple communication patterns of maritally aggressive and nonaggressive male alcoholics, *Journal of Studies on Alcohol,* 58: 83–90.

Nahmiash, D. and Reis, M. (2000) Most successful intervention strategies for abused older adults, *Journal of Elder Abuse and Neglect*, 12(3/4): 53–70.

Nakazawa, S. (1996) Lives and consciousness of foreign wives from Asia in Japanese rural villages: Chinese/Taiwanese, Korean and Filipina brides in Mogami District, Yamagata Prefecture, *Japanese Journal of Family Sociology*, 8: 81–96.

National Center on Elder Abuse (1998, September) *The National Elder Abuse Incidence Study*. Washington, DC: Author.

National Center on Elder Abuse (2006) Frequently asked questions. Retrieved 12 November 2006 from www.elderabusecenter.org/default.cfm?p=faqs.cfm#one.

National Institute on Alcohol Abuse and Alcoholism (2003) *Assessing Alcohol Problems: A Guide for Clinicians and Researchers* (NIH Publication No. 03–3745). Washington, DC: US Department of Health and Human Services.

National Research Council (1996) *Understanding Violence Against Women*. Washington, DC: National Academies Press.

National Research Council (2003) *Elder Mistreatment: Abuse, Neglect, and Exploitation in an Aging America*. Washington, DC: National Academies Press.

NationMaster.com (2007) Crime statistics: murder by country. Retrieved February 2007 from www.nationmaster.com/graph/cri_mur_percap-crime-murders-per-capita.

NCH Action for Children (1994) *The Hidden Victims: Children and Domestic Violence*. London: NCH Action for Children.

Neidig, P.H. and Friedman, D. (1984) *Spouse Abuse: A Treatment Program for Couples*. Champaign, IL: Research Press.

Nelson, H., Nygren, P., McInerney, Y. and Klein, J. (2004) Screening women and elderly adults for family and intimate partner violence: a review of the evidence for the US Preventive Services Task Force, *Annals of Internal Medicine*, 140(5): 387–404.

New York Office for the Prevention of Domestic Violence (1998) *Model Domestic Violence Policy for Counties*. New York: NYS Office for the Prevention of Domestic Violence.

New York Office for the Prevention of Domestic Violence (2001) *Family Protection and the Domestic Violence Intervention Act of 1994: Evaluation of the Mandatory Arrest Provisions*. New York: NYS Office for the Prevention of Domestic Violence.

New York Office for the Prevention of Domestic Violence (2004) Court response to batterer program noncompliance: a national perspective. Unpublished concept paper available at www.nymbp.org..

New York Office for the Prevention of Domestic Violence (2006) *New York State's Response to Domestic Violence: Systems and Services Making a Difference*. New York: NYS Office for the Prevention of Domestic Violence.

Nicklin, P. and Kenworthy, N. (1996) *Teaching and Assessing in Nursing Practice: An Experiential Approach*. London: Bailliere Tindall.

Nicolaidis, C. and Touhouliotis, V. (2006) Addressing intimate partner violence in primary care: lessons from chronic illness management, *Violence and Victims,* 21(1): 101–15.

Nicolaidis, C., Curry, M. and Gerrity, M. (2005) Measuring the impact of the Voices of Survivors program on health care workers' attitudes toward survivors of intimate partner violence, *Journal of General Internal Medicine,* 20(8): 731–7.

Nixon, R.D., Resick, P.A. and Nishith, P. (2004) An exploration of comorbid depression among female victims of intimate partner violence with posttraumatic stress disorder, *Journal of Affective Disorders,* 82(2): 315–20.

NMC (2004) *Standards of Proficiency for Pre-registration Nursing Education*. London: Nursing and Midwifery Council. Retrieved 2 March, 2007, from www.nmc-uk.org.

Norton, L., Peipert, J., Zierler, S., Lima, B. and Hume, L. (1995) Battering in pregnancy: an assessment of two screening methods, *Obstetrics and Gynecology,* 85(3): 321–5.

Nurius, P.S., Macy, R.J., Bhuyan, R., Holt, V.L., Kernic, M.A. and Rivara, F.P. (2003) Contextualizing depression and physical functioning in battered women, *Journal of Interpersonal Violence,* 18: 1411–31.

O'Campo, P. *et al.* (2006) Depression, PTSD and comorbidity related to intimate partner violence in civilian and military women, *Brief Treatment and Crisis Intervention,* 6(2): 99–110.

O'Farrell, T.J. and Murphy, C.M. (1995) Marital violence before and after alcoholism treatment, *Journal of Consulting and Clinical Psychology,* 63: 256–62.

O'Farrell, T.J., Van Hutton, V. and Murphy, C.M. (1999) Domestic violence after alcoholism treatment: a two-year longitudinal study, *Journal of Studies on Alcohol,* 60: 317–21.

O'Farrell, T.J, Murphy, C.M., Stephan, S.H., Fals-Stewart, W. and Murphy, M. (2004) Partner violence before and after couples-based alcoholism treatment for male alcoholic patients: the role of treatment involvement and abstinence, *Journal of Consulting and Clinical Psychology,* 72: 202–17.

Official Report of Debates (2000) Legislative Assembly of Ontario, Standing Committee on Justice and Social Policy, *Domestic Violence Act, 2000*, 31 October, pp. J-537–42.

Ogg, J. (1993) Researching elder abuse in Britain, *Journal of Elder Abuse and Neglect,* 5(2): 37–54.

Ohbuchi, K., Fukushima, O. and Tedeschi, J.T. (1999) Cultural values in conflict management: goal orientation, goal attainment, and tactical decision, *Journal of Cross-Cultural Psychology*, 30(1): 51–71

Olatubosun, A. (2001) Addressing the phenomenon of child marriage in Nigeria, *Ife Psychologia: An International Journal*, 9: 159–69.

O'Leary, K.D. (1993) Through a psychological lens: personality traits, personality disorders, and levels of violence, in R.J. Gelles and D. Loseke (eds) *Current Controversies on Family Violence*, pp. 7–29. Newbury Park, CA: Sage.

O'Leary, K.D. (1996) Physical aggression in intimate relationships can be treated within a marital context under certain circumstances, *Journal of Interpersonal Violence*, 11: 450–2.

O'Leary, K.D. (1999) Developmental and affective issues in assessing and treating partner aggression, *Clinical Psychology: Science and Practice*, 6: 400–14.

O'Leary, K.D. (2000) Are women really more aggressive than men in intimate relationships? *Psychological Bulletin*, 126: 685–9.

O'Leary, K.D., Vivian, D. and Malone, J. (1992) Assessment of physical aggression in marriage: the need for a multimodal method, *Behavioral Assessment*, 14: 5–14.

O'Leary, K.D., Barling, J., Arias, I., Rosenblum, A., Malone J. and Tyree. A. (1989) Prevalence and stability of physical aggression between spouses: a longitudinal analysis, *Journal of Consulting and Clinical Psychology*, 57: 263–8.

O'Leary, K.D., Malone, J. and Tyree, A. (1994) Physical aggression in early marriage: prerelationship and relationship effects, *Journal of Consulting and Clinical Psychology*, 62: 594–602.

O'Leary, K.D., Heyman, R.E. and Jongsma, A.E. (1998) *The Couples Therapy Treatment Planner*. New York: Wiley.

O'Leary, K.D., Heyman, R.E. and Neidig, P.H. (1999) Treatment of wife abuse: a comparison of gender-specific and couples approaches, *Behavior Therapy*, 30: 475–505.

O'Leary, K.D., Slep, A.M.S. and O'Leary, S.G. (2007) Multivariate models of men's and women's partner aggression, manuscript submitted for publication.

O'Neill, O. (2002) *Autonomy and Trust in Bioethics*. Cambridge: Cambridge University Press.

Osthoff, S. (2002) But, Gertrude, I beg to differ, a hit is not a hit is not a hit, *Violence Against Women*, 8: 1521–44.

Pagelow, M. (1988) Marital rape, in V.B.V. Hasselt, R. Morrison, A. Bellack and M. Hersen (eds) *Handbook of Family Violence*, pp. 207–32. New York: Plenum.

Palermo, G.B. (1994) Murder-suicide – an extended suicide, *International Journal of Offender Therapy and Comparative Criminology*, 8(3): 205–16.

Pallitto, C. and O'Campo, P. (2005) Community level effects of gender inequality on intimate partner violence and unintended pregnancy in Colombia: testing the feminist perspective, *Socology of Science and Medicine*, 60: 2205–16.

Parker, G. A. (1970) Sperm competition and its evolutionary consequences in the insects, *Biological Reviews,* 45: 525–67.

Patterson, G.R. (1982) *Coercive Family Processes.* Eugene, OR: Castilla Press.

Pawson, R., Greenhalgh, T., Harvey, G. and Walshe, K. (2005) Realist review – a new method of systematic review designed for complex policy interventions, *Journal of Health Services Research Polic,* 10(Suppl. 1): 21–34.

Pence, E. and Paymar, M. (1986) *Power and Control: Tactics of Men who Batter.* Duluth, MN: Minnesota Program Development Inc.

Pence, E. and Paymar, M. (1993) Education Groups for Men Who Batter: The Duluth Model. New York: Springer.

Peters, J. (2003) The domestic violence myth acceptance scale: development and psychometric testing of a new instrument. Available at http://library.umaine.edu/theses/pdf/PetersJ2003.pdf.

Peters, J. (in press) Measuring myths about domestic violence: development and initial validation of the domestic violence myth acceptance scale, *Journal of Aggression, Maltreatment & Trauma.* Pre-press copy available at www.umaine.edu/sws/rsrchProjects.htm.

Peters, J. and Goodman, L. (1997). Holocaust denial and the False Memory Syndrome movement: an examination of the techniques of denial. Paper presented at the International Society for the Study of Dissociation, Orlando, FL.

Piaget, J. and Inhelder, B. (1969) *The Psychology of the Child.* New York: Basic Books.

Pico-Alfonso, M.A., Garcia-Linares, M.I., Celda-Navarro, N., Blasco-Ros, C., Echeburua, E. and Martinez, M. (2006) The impact of physical, psychological, and sexual intimate male partner violence on women's mental health: depressive symptoms, posttraumatic stress disorder, state anxiety, and suicide, *Journal of Women's Health (Larchmt),* 15(5): 599–611.

Pillemer, K. and Finkelhor, D. (1988) The prevalence of elder abuse: a random sample survey, *The Gerontologist,* 28: 51–7.

Pizzey, E. (1998) 'When did you last beat your wife?' *The Observer,* 5 July: 24.

Pizzey, E. and Forbes, A. (1974) *Scream Quietly or the Neighbours Will Hear.* Harmondsworth: Penguin.

Platek, S.M. and Shackelford, T.K. (eds) (2006) *Female Infidelity and Paternal Uncertainty.* New York: Cambridge University Press.

Plichta, S.B. (1992) The effects of women abuse on health care utilization and health status: a literature review, *The Jacobs Institute of Women's Health,* 2: 154–63.

Plichta, S.B. and Falik, M. (2001) Prevalence of violence and its implications for women's health, *Womens Health Issues,* 11(3): 244–58.

Podneiks, E. (1992) National survey on abuse of the elderly in Canada, *Journal of Elder Abuse and Neglect*, 4(1/2): 5–58.

Podneiks, E. (ed.) (2006) World elder abuse awareness day: 'Many voices, one song', *INPEA Bulletin*: 1–10.

Podneiks, E., Anetzberger, G. and Teaster, P.B. (2006) International Network for the Prevention of Elder Abuse: preliminary findings from a world wide environmental scan. Paper presented at the Annual Scientific Meeting of the Gerontological Society of America, Dallas, TX.

Pound, N. (2002) Male interest in visual cues of sperm competition risk, *Evolution and Human Behavior*, 23: 443–66.

Project MATCH Research Group (1997) Project MATCH secondary a priori hypotheses, *Addiction*, 92: 1671–98.

Quinn, F.M. (2000) *Principles and Practice of Nurse Education*. Cheltenham: Stanley Thornes Ltd.

Rabin, B., Markus, E. and Voghera, N. (1999) A comparative study of Jewish and Arab battered women presenting in the emergency room of a general hospital, *Social Work in Health Care*, 29: 69–84.

Raj, A., Silverman, J.G. and Amaro, H. (2004) Abused women report greater male partner risk and gender-based risk for HIV: findings from a community-based study with Hispanic women, *AIDS Care*, 16(4): 519–29.

Ramsay, J., Richardson, J., Carter, Y.H., Davidson, L.L. and Feder, G. (2002) Should health professionals screen women for domestic violence? Systematic review, *British Medical Journal*, 325: 314.

Rand, M.R. and Saltzman, L.E. (2003) The nature and extent of recurring intimate partner violence against women in the United States, *Journal of Comparative Family Studies*, 34(1): 137–49.

Rathus, J.H. and Feindler, E.L. (2004) *Assessment of Partner Violence: A Handbook for Researchers and Practitioners*. Washington, DC: American Psychological Association.

RCN (Royal College of Nursing) (2004) Domestic violence demands greater training and multi-agency response, warns nursing research. Retrieved 20 March 2007 from www.rcn.org.uk.

Reece, I. and Walker, S. (2003) *Teaching Training and Learning: A Practical Guide*. Sunderland: Business Education Publishers.

Regan, L. and Kelly, L. (2003) Rape: still a forgotten issue. Rape Crisis Network Europe. Retrieved April 2007 from www.rcne.com/downloads/RepsPubs/Attritn.pdf.

Reinharz, S. (1986) Loving and hating one's elders: twin themes in legend and literature, in K.A. Pillemer and R.S. Wolf (eds) *Elder Abuse: Conflict in the Family*, pp. 25–48. Dover, MA: Auburn House.

Reis, M. and Nahmiash, D. (1998) Validation of the Indicators of Abuse (IOA) screen, *The Gerontologist,* 38(4): 471–80.

Rennison, C.M. (2003) *Intimate Partner Violence (1993–2001).* Bureau of Justice

Statistics. Washington, DC: US Department of Justice.

Renzetti, C.M. (1997) Violence in lesbian and gay relationships, in L.L. O'Toole and J.R. Schiffman (eds) *Gender Violence: Interdisciplinary Perspectives,* pp. 285–93. New York: New York University Press.

Rhodes, K., Lauderdale, D., Stocking, C., Howes, D., Roizen, M. and Levinson, W. (2001) Better health while you wait: a controlled trial of a computer based intervention for screening and health promotion in the emergency department, *Annals of Emergency Medicine,* 37(3): 284–91.

Richardson, J., Coid, J., Petruckevitch, A., Chung, W., Moorey, S. and Feder, G.F. (2002) Identifying domestic violence: cross sectional study in primary care, *British Medical Journal,* 324(7332): 274–7.

Richie, B.E., (1996) *Compelled to Crime: The Gender Entrapment of Battered Black Women.* London: Routledge.

Riger, S., Ahrens, C. and Blickenstaff, A. (2000) Measuring interference with employment and education reported by women with abusive partners: preliminary data, *Violence and Victims,* 15(2): 161–73.

Roberts, A.R. (2002) Duration and severity of woman battering: a conceptual model/continuum, in A. Roberts (ed.) *Handbook of Domestic Violence Intervention Strategies,* pp. 64–79. New York: Oxford University Press.

Roberts, A.R. (2007) Overview and new directions, in A.R.Roberts (ed.) *Battered*

Women and their Families: Intervention Strategies and Treatment Programs, 3rd edn, pp. 3–31. New York: Springer.

Roberts, G., Williams, G., Lawrence, J. and Raphael, B. (1998) How does domestic violence affect women's mental health? *Women's Health Issues,* 28(1): 117–29.

Rodriguez, M., Quiroga, S. and Bauer, H. (1996) Breaking the silence: battered women's perspectives on medical care, *Archives of Family Medicine,* 5(3): 153–8.

Rodriguez, M., Bauer, H., McLoughlin, E. and Grumbach, K. (1999) Screening and intervention for intimate partner abuse, *Journal of the American Medical Association,* 282(5): 468–74.

Rodriguez, M., McLoughlin, E., Nah, G. and Campbell, J. (2001a) Mandatory reporting of domestic violence injuries to the police: what do emergency department patients think? *Journal of the American Medical Association,* 286(5): 580–3.

Rodriguez, M., Sheldon, W., Bauer, H. and Perez-Stable, E. (2001b) The factors associated with disclosure of intimate partner abuse to clinicians, *Journal of Family Practice,* 50(4): 338–44.

Rogers, C. (1983) *Freedom to Learn for the 80s*. Columbus, OH: Charles E. Merrill.

Rosen, K.H., Matheson, J.L., Stith, S.M., McCollum, E.E. and Locke, L.D. (2003) Negotiated time-out: a de-escalation tool for couples, *Journal of Marital and Family Therapy*, 29: 291–98.

Rosenbaum, M. (1990) The role of depression in couples involved in murder-suicide and homicide, *American Journal of Psychiatry*, 147(8): 1036–9.

Ross, J. and Walther, V.E.I. (2004) Screening Risks for Intimate Partner Violence and Primary Care Settings: Implications for Future Abuse. *Social Work in Health Care* 38(4): 1–23.

Royal College of Psychiatrists (2002) Domestic violence, *Council Report CR102*. London: Rpyal College of Psychiatrists.

Russell, D.E.H. (1982) *Rape in Marriage*. New York: Macmillan.

Russell, D.E.H. (1990) *Rape in Marriage*, 2nd edn. Bloomington, IN: Indiana University Press.

Rychtarik, R.G. and McGillicuddy, N.B. (2005) Coping skills training and 12-step facilitation for women whose partner has alcoholism: effects on depression, the partner's drinking, and partner physical violence, *Journal of Consulting and Clinical Psychology*, 73: 249–61.

Saenger, G. (1963) Male and female relations in the American comic strip, in D.M. White and R.H. Abel (eds) *The Funnies, an American Idiom*, pp. 219–31). Glencoe, NY: The Free Press.

Sagarin, B.J., Becker, D.V., Guadagno, R.E., Nicastle, L.D. and Millevoi, A. (2003) Sex differences (and similarities) in jealousy: the moderating influence of infidelity experience and sexual orientation of the infidelity, *Evolution and Human Behavior*, 24: 17–23.

Saltzman, L.E., Fanslow, J.L., McMahon, P.M. and Shelley, G.A. (1999) *Intimate Partner Violence Surveillance: Uniform Definitions and Recommended Data Elements, Version 1.0*. Atlanta, GA: National Center for Injury Prevention and Control, Centers for Disease Control and Prevention.

Saunders, D.G. (1988) Wife abuse, husband abuse, or mutual combat? A feminist perspective on the empirical findings, in K. Yllo and M. Bograd (eds) *Feminist Perspectives on Wife Abuse*, pp. 90–113. Newbury Park, CA: Sage.

Saunders, D.G. (1996) Feminist-cognitive-behavioral and process-psychodynamic treatments for men who batter: interaction of abuser traits and treatment models, *Violence and Victims*, 11: 393–414.

Schafer, J., Caetano, R. and Clark, C. (1998) Rates of intimate partner violence in the United States, *American Journal of Public Health*, 88: 1702–4.

Schmitt, D.P. and Buss, D.M. (2001) Human mate poaching: tactics and temptations for infiltrating existing mateships, *Journal of Personality and Social Psychology*, 80: 894–917.

Schorr, L.B. (1998) *Common Purpose: Strengthening Families and Neighborhoods to Rebuild America*. New York: Anchor Books.

Schuck, A.M. and Widom, C.S. (2001) Childhood victimization and alcohol symptoms in females: causal inferences and hypothesized mediators, *Child Abuse and Neglect*, 25(8): 1069–92.

Schumacher, J.A., Feldbau-Kohn, S.R., Slep, A.M.S. and Heyman, R.E. (2001) Risk factors for male-to-female partner physical abuse, *Aggression and Violent Behavior*, 6: 269–352.

Schumacher, J.A., Fals-Stewart, W. and Leonard, K.E. (2003) Domestic violence treatment referrals for men seeking alcohol treatment, *Journal of Substance Abuse Treatment*, 24: 279–83.

Schützwohl, A. and Koch, S. (2004) Sex differences in jealousy: the recall of cues to sexual and emotional infidelity in personally more and less threatening context conditions, *Evolution and Human Behavior*, 25: 249–57.

Scott, K.A. and Wolfe, D.A. (2000) Change among batterers: examining men's success stories, *Journal of Interpersonal Violence*, 15(8): 827–42.

Scuka, R. (2006) *Checklist for Differentiating Two Different Forms of Interpersonal Violence*. Retrieved 19 March 2007 from www.nire.org.

Seattle Weekly (2005) Home front casualties, 31 August. Retrieved November 2007 from www.veteransforCommonSense.org.

Second World Assembly on Ageing (2002) *Madrid International Plan of Action on Ageing in Brief*. New York: United Nations Department of Economic and Social Affairs.

Serovich, J.M. (2001) A test of two HIV disclosure theories, *AIDS Education and Prevention*, 13: 355–64.

Shackelford, T.K. and Buss, D.M. (1997) Cues to infidelity, *Personality and Social Psychology Bulletin*, 23: 1034–45.

Shackelford, T.K. and Goetz, A.T. (2006) Comparative psychology of sperm competition. *Journal of Comparative Psychology*, 120: 139–46.

Shackelford, T.K. and Goetz, A.T. (2007) Adaptation to sperm competition in humans, *Current Directions in Psychological Science*, 16: 47–50.

Shackelford, T.K., LeBlanc, G.J., Weekes-Shackelford, V.A., Bleske-Rechek, A.L., Euler, H.A. and Hoier, S. (2002) Psychological adaptation to human sperm competition, *Evolution and Human Behavior*, 23: 123–38.

Shackelford, T.K., Buss, D.M. and Weekes-Shackelford, V.A. (2003) Wife killings committed in the context of a 'lovers' triangle', *Basic and Applied Social Psychology*, 25: 137–43.

Shackelford, T.K., Goetz, A.T., Buss, D.M., Euler, H.A. and Hoier, S. (2005) When we hurt the ones we love: predicting violence against women from men's mate retention tactics, *Personal Relationships,* 12: 447–63.

Sharon, N. and Zoabi, S. (1997) Elder abuse in a land of tradition: the case of Israel's Arabs, *Journal of Elder Abuse and Neglect,* 8(4): 43–58.

Sharps, P.W. and Campbell, J.C. (1999) Health consequences for victims of violence in intimate relationships, in X.B.Arriaga and S. Oskamp (eds) *Violence in Intimate Relationships,* pp. 163–80. Thousand Oaks, CA: Sage.

Sharps, P.W., Koziol-McLain, J., Campbell, J.C., McFarlane, J., Sachs, C.J. and Xu, X. (2001a) Health care provider's missed opportunities for preventing femicide, *Preventative Medicine,* 33: 373–80.

Sharps, P.W., Campbell, J.C., Campbell, D.W., Gary, F.A. and Webster, D. (2001b) The role of alcohol use in intimate partner femicide, *The American Journal on Addictions,* 10: 122–35.

Shepard, M., *et al.* (1999) Public health nurses' responses to domestic violence: a report from the enhanced domestic abuse intervention project, *Public Health Nursing,* 16: 359.

Sherin, K., Sinacore, J., X-Q, L., Zitter, R. and Shakil, A. (1998) HITS: a short domestic violence screening tool for use in a family practice setting, *Family Medicine,* 30(7): 508–12.

Sherman, L.W. and Berk, R.A. (1984) The specific deterrent effects of arrest for domestic assault, *American Sociological Review,* 49: 261–72.

Sherman, P.W. and Alcock, J. (1994) The utility of the proximate-ultimate dichotomy in ethology. *Ethology,* 96: 58–62.

Shields, J. P. (2006) *I Tried to Stop Them: Children's Exposure to Domestic Violence in San Francisco.* San Francisco: CA.ETR Associates.

Shields, N.M. and Hanneke, C.R. (1983) Battered wives' reactions to marital rape, in R. Gelles, G. Hotaling, M. Straus and D. Finkelhor (eds) *The Dark Side of Families,* pp. 131–48. Beverly Hills, CA: Sage.

Short, L., Johnson, D. and Osattin, A. (1998) Recommended components of health care provider training programs on intimate partner violence, *American Journal of Preventive Medicine,* 14(4): 283–8.

Short, L.M., Surprenant, Z.J. and Harris, J.M. Jr. (2006) A community-based trial of an online intimate partner violence CME program, *American Journal of Preventive Medicine,* 30(2): 181–5.

Simic, A. (1983) Machismo and cryptomatriarchy: power, affect, and authority in the contemporary Yugoslav family, *Ethos,* 11: 66–86.

Slep, A.M.S. and O'Leary, S.G. (2005) Parent and partner violence in families with young children: rates, patterns, and connections, *Journal of Consulting and Clinical Psychology*, 73: 435–44.

Slobodian, L. (2000) Researcher claims men, women, equal abusers, *Calgary Herald*, 6 November.

Smith, R.L. (1984) Human sperm competition, in R.L. Smith (ed.) *Sperm Competition and the Evolution of Animal Mating Systems*, pp. 601–60. New York: Academic Press.

Smuts, B. (1996) Male aggression against women: an evolutionary perspective, in D.M. Buss and N.M. Malamuth (eds) Sex, Power, Conflict: Evolutionary and Feminist Perspectives, pp. 231–68. New York: Oxford University Press.

Sorenson, S.B. (1996) Violence against women: examining ethnic differences and commonalities, *Evaluation Review*, 20: 123–45.

Spanier, G.B. (1976) Measuring dyadic adjustment: new scales for assessing the quality of marriage and similar dyads, *Journal of Marriage and the Family*, 38: 15–28.

Spitzberg, B.H. (1999) An analysis of empirical estimates of sexual aggression victimization and perpetration, *Violence and Victims*, 14(3): 241–60.

Stark, E., Flitcraft, A. and Frazier, W. (1979) Medicine and Patriarchal Violence: The Social Construction of a 'Private' Event *International Journal of Health Services* 9(3): 461–93.

Stark, E. and Flitcraft, A. (1988) Women and children at risk: a feminist perspective on child abuse, *International Journal of Health Services*, 18: 97–118.

Stark, E. and Flitcraft, A. (1996) *Women At Risk: Domestic Violence and Women's Health*. Thousand Oaks, CA: Sage.

Starratt, V.G., Goetz, A.T., Shackelford, T.K., McKibbin, W.F. and Stewart-Williams, S. (2007) Men's partner-directed insults and sexual coercion in intimate relationships, *Acta Sinica Psychologica*.

Statistics Canada (1998) *Family Violence in Canada: A Statistical Profile 1998*.Ottawa: Statistics Canada.

Statistics Canada (2005) *Family Violence in Canada: A Statistical Profile 2005*. Ottawa: Statistics Canada.

Stearns, P.J. (1986) Old age family conflict: the perspective of the past, in K.A. Pillemer and R.S. Wolf (eds) *Elder Abuse: Conflict in the Family*, pp. 3–24. Dover, MA: Auburn House.

Steigel, L.A. and Klem, E.M.V. (2006) *Analysis of 2005 State Legislation Amending Adult Protective Services Laws*. Washington, DC: American Bar Association.

Stein, K.F. (2006) What does the elder abuse field need? *The Gerontologist*, 46(5): 701–3.

Stein, M.B. and Kenney, C.J. (2001) Major depressive and post-traumatic stress disorder comorbidity in female victims of intimate partner violence, *Affective Disorders*, 66: 133–8.

Steinmetz, S.K. (1978a) Overlooked aspects of family violence: battered husbands, battered siblings, and battered elderly. Testimony presented to the US House of Representatives Committee on Science and Technology, Washington, DC. 15 February.

Steinmetz, S.K. (1978b) The battered husband syndrome, *Victimology*, 2: 499–509.

Steinmetz, S.K. (1988) *Dutybound: Elder Abuse and Family Care*. Newbury Park, CA: Sage.

Stenning, D.J. (1958) Household viability among the pastoral Fulani, in J. Goody (ed.) *The Developmental Cycle in Domestic Groups*. Cambridge, MA: Cambridge University Press.

Stermac, L., Del Bove, G. and Addison, M. (2001) Violence, injury, and presentation patterns in spousal sexual assaults, *Violence Against Women*, 7(11): 1218–33.

Stets, J.E. and Straus, M.A. (1990) Gender differences in reporting marital violence and its medical and psychological consequences, in M.A. Straus and R.J. Gelles (eds) *Physical Violence in American families*, pp. 151–65. New Brunswick, NJ: Transaction Publishers.

Stinson, C.K. and Robinson, R. (2006) Intimate partner violence: continuing education for registered nurses, *Journal of Continuing Education in Nursing*, 37(2): 58–62.

Stith, S.M., Rosen, K.H. and McCollum, E.E. (2002) Developing a manualized couples treatment for domestic violence: overcoming challenges, *Journal of Marital and Family Therapy*, 28: 21–5.

Stith, S.M., Rosen, K.H., McCollum, E.E. and Thomsen, C.J. (2004) Treating intimate partner violence within intact couple relationships: outcomes of multi-couple versus individual couple therapy, *Journal of Marital and Family Therapy*, 30: 305–18.

Stosny, S. (1995) *Treating Attachment Abuse: A Compassionate Approach*. New York: Springer.

Strathclyde Regional Council (1995) *Male Violence Against Women with Disability: A Report for the Zero Tolerance Campaign*. Glasgow: Strathclyde Regional Council.

Straton, J. (1994) The myth of the 'battered husband syndrome', *Masculinities*, 2: 79–82.

Straus, M. (1990a) Measuring intrafamily conflict and violence: The Conflict Tactic (CT) Scales, in M.A. Straus and R.J. Gelles (eds) *Physical Violence in American Families*, pp. 29–47. New Brunswick, NJ: Transaction Publishers.

Straus, M. (1990b) The conflict tactics scales and its critics: an evaluation and new data on validity and reliability, in M.A. Straus and R.J. Gelles (eds) *Physical Violence in American families*, pp. 151–65. New Brunswick, NJ: Transaction Publishers.

Straus, M. (1993) Physical assaults by wives: a major social problem, in R.J. Gelles and D.R. Loseke (eds) *Current Controversies on Family Violence*. Newbury Park, CA: Sage.

Straus, M. (1997) Physical assaults by women partners: a major social problem, in M.R. Walsh (ed.) *Gender: Ongoing Debates*, pp. 204–21. New Haven, CT: Yale University Press.

Straus, M. (2005) Women's violence toward men is a serious social problem, in R. Gelles and D.R. Loseke (eds) *Current Controversies in Family Violence*. New York: Sage.

Straus, M. and Gelles, R. (1986) Societal change and family violence from 1975 to 1985 as revealed by two national surveys, *Journal of Marriage and the Family*, 48: 445–79.

Straus, M. and Gelles, R. (1990a) *Physical Violence in American Families*. New Brunswick, NJ: Transaction Publishers.

Straus, M.A.and Gelles, R.J. (1990b) How violent are American families? Estimates from the National Family Violence Resurvey and other studies, in M.A. Straus and R.J. Gelles (eds) *Physical Violence in American Families*, 113–31. New Brunswick, NJ: Transaction Publishers.

Straus, M.A. and Gelles, R.J. (1990c) Societal change and change in family violence from 1975 to 1985 as revealed by two national surveys, in M.A. Straus and R.J. Gelles (eds) *Physical Violence in American Families*, pp. 113–31. New Brunswick, NJ: Transaction Publishers.

Straus, M. Gelles, R.J., and Steinmetz , S.K. (1980) *Behind Closed Doors: Violence in American Families*. New York: Doubleday.

Straus, M, Hamby, S.L., Boney-McCoy, S.B. and Sugarman, D.B. (1996) The revised Conflict Tactics Scale (CTS2), *Journal of Family Issues*, 17: 283–316.

Street, A.E., Gibson, L.E. and Holohan, D.R. (2005) Impact of childhood traumatic events, trauma-related guilt, and avoidant coping strategies on PTSD symptoms in female survivors of domestic violence, *Journal of Trauma Stress*, 18(3): 245–52.

Struckman-Johnson, C. and Struckman-Johnson, D. (1994) Men pressured and forced into sexual experience, *Archives of Sexual Behavior*, 23(1): 93–114.

Stuart, G.L., Moore, T.M., Kahler, C.W. and Ramsey, S.E. (2003) Substance abuse and relationship violence among men court-referred to batterers' intervention programs, *Substance Abuse*, 24: 107–22.

Stuart, G.L., Meehan, J.C., Moore, T.M., Morean, M., Hellmuth, J. and Follansbee, K. (2006) Examining a conceptual framework of intimate partner violence in men and women arrested for domestic violence, *Journal of Studies on Alcohol*, 67: 102–12.

Substance Abuse and Mental Health Services Administration (2004) *Results from the 2003 National Survey on Drug Use and Health: National Findings* (Office of Applied Studies, NSDUH Series H-25, DHHS Publication No. SMA 04–3964). Rockville, MD: Substance Abuse and Mental Health Services Administration.

Sugarman, D.B. and Hotaling, G.T. (1989) Dating violence: prevalence, context, and risk markers, in M.A. Pirog-Good and J.E Stets (eds) *Violence in Dating Relationships: Emerging Social Issues*, pp. 91–107. New York: Praeger.

Sullivan, C.M. and Davidson II, W.S. (1991) The Provision of Advocacy Services to Women Leaving Abusive Partners; An Examination of the Short-Term Effects. *American Journal of Community Psychology* 19(6): 953–60.

Sullivan, C.M., Basta, J. Tan, C. and Davidson II, W.S. (1992) After the Crisis: A Needs Assessment of Women Leaving a Domestic Violence Shelter. *Violence and Victims* 7(3): 267–75.

Sullivan, C.M. Campbell, R., Angelique, H., Eby, K.K. and Davidson II, W.S. (1994) An Advocacy Intervention Program for Women with Abusive Partners: Six Month Follow-up. *American Journal of Community Psychology* 22(1): 101–22.

Sullivan, C. and Bybee, D. (1999) Reducing violence using community-based advocacy for women with abusive partners, *Journal of Consulting Clinical Psychology*, 67(1): 43–53.

Sullivan, C.M. (2006) Interventions to address intimate partner violence: the current state of the field, in J. Lutzker (ed.) *Preventing Violence: Research and Evidence-Based Intervention Strategies*, pp. 195–212. Washington, DC: American Psychological Association.

Sullivan, T.P., Meese, K.J., Swan, S.C., Mazure, C.M. and Snow, D.L. (2005) Precursors and correlates of women's violence: child abuse, traumatization, victimization of violence. Findings from the National Violence Against Women Survey, *Psychology of Women Quarterly*, 29: 290–301.

Sully, P. (2002) Commitment to partnership: interdisciplinary initiatives in developing expert practice in the care of survivors of violence, *Nurse Education in Practice*, 2: 92–8.

Sully, P. *et al.* (2005) Domestic violence policing and health care: collaboration and practice, *Primary Health Care Research and Development*, 6: 31–6.

Sutherland, C., Bybee, D. and Sullivan, C. (1998) The long term effects of battering on women, *Women's Health Issues*, 4(1): 41–70.

Sutton, A. and Hughes, L. (2005) The psychotherapy of parenthood: towards a formulation and valuation of concurrent work with parents, *Journal of Child Psychotherapy*, 31(2): 169–88.

Swan, S.C. and Snow, D.L. (2002) A typology of women's use of violence in intimate relationships, *Violence against Women*, 8(3): 286–319.

Swan, S.C. and Snow, D.L. (2003) Behavioral and psychological differences among abused women who use violence in intimate relationships, *Violence Against Women*, 9: 75–109.

Syers, M. and Edleson, J.L. (1992) The combined effects of coordinated criminal justice intervention in women abuse, *Journal of Interpersonal Violence,* 7: 490–502.

Taket, A., Wathen, C. and MacMillan, H. (2004) Should health professionals screen all women for domestic violence? *PLoS Medicine,* 1(1): e4–9.

Tatara, T. (1996) *Elder Abuse: Questions and Answers.* Washington, DC: National Center on Elder Abuse.

Teaster, P.B. and Nerenberg, L. (2004) *A National Look at Elder Abuse Multidisciplinary Teams.* Washington, DC: National Committee for the Prevention of Elder Abuse.

Teaster, P.B., Duggan, T.A., Mendiondo, M.S. and Otto, J.M. (2005) *The 2004 Survey of State Adult Protective Services: Abuse of Adults 60 Years of Age and Older.* Washington, DC: National Center on Elder Abuse.

Tendler, S. (1999) Men suffer equally from violence in the home, *London Times,* 22 January: 23

Testa, M., Livingston, J.A. and Leonard, K.E. (2003) Women's substance use and experiences of intimate partner violence: a longitudinal investigation among a community sample, *Addictive Behaviors,* 28(9): 1649–64.

Thomas, C. (2000) Is domestic violence screening helpful? *Journal of the American Medical Association,* 284(5): 551–3.

Thompson, R.S., Bonomi, A.E., Anderson, M., Reid, R.J., Dimer, J.A., Carrell, D. and Rivara, F.P. (2006) Intimate partner violence: prevalence, types, and chronicity in adult women, *American Journal of Preventive Medicine,* 30(6): 447–57.

Thornhill, R. and Palmer, C. T. (2000) *A Natural History of Rape.* Cambridge, MA: MIT Press.

Thornhill, R. and Thornhill, N.W. (1992) The evolutionary psychology of men's coercive sexuality, *Behavioral and Brain Sciences,* 15: 363–421.

Thornton, B. (1984). Defensive attribution of responsibility: evidence for an arousal-based motivational bias, *Journal of Personality and Social Psychology,* 46(4): 721–34.

Ting-Toomey, S. (1988) Intercultural conflict styles: a face negotiation theory, in Y. Kim and W. Gudykunst (eds) *Theories in Intercultural Communication,* pp. 213–38. Newbury Park, CA: Sage.

Titus, K. (1996) When physicians ask, women tell about domestic abuse and violence, *Journal of the American Medical Association,* 275(24): 1863–5.

Tiwari, A., Leung, W., Leung, T., Humphreys, J., Parker, B. and Ho, P.C. (2005) A randomised controlled trial of empowerment training for Chinese abused pregnant women in Hong Kong, *An International Journal of Obstetrics and Gynaecology,* 112(9): 1249–56.

Tjaden, P. and Thoennes, N. (1997) *Stalking in America: Findings from the National Violence Against Women Survey* (NIJ Grant No. 93-IJ-CX-0012). Washington, DC: National Institutes of Justice/Centers for Disease Control.

Tjaden, P. and Thoennes, N. (1998) *Prevalence, Incidence, and Consequences of Violence Against Women: Findings from the National Violence Against Women Survey.* Washington, DC: National Institute of Justice and Centers for Disease Control and Prevention.

Tjaden, P. and Thoennes, N. (2000a) *Extent, Nature, and Consequences of Intimate Partner Violence.* Washington, DC: National Institute of Justice and Centers for Disease Control and Prevention.

Tjaden, P.and Thoennes, N. (2000b) Prevalence and consequences of male-to-female and female-to-male intimate partner violence as measured by the National Violence Against Women Survey, *Violence Against Women,* 6: 142–61.

Tolman, R. (1989) The development of a measure of psychological maltreatment of women by their male partners, *Violence and Victims,* 7: 159–77.

Tolman, R.M. (1999) The validation of the psychological maltreatment of women inventory, *Violence and Victims,* 14: 25–37.

Tolman, R.M. and Edleson, J.L. (1995) Intervention for men who batter: a research review, in S.M. Stith and M.A. Straus (eds) *Understanding Partner Violence: Prevalence, Causes, Consequences, and Solutions,* pp. 163–73. Minneapolis, MN: National Council on Family Relations.

Tolman R.M., Edleson, J.L. and Fendrich, M. (1996) The applicability of the theory of planned behavior to abusive men's cessation of violent behavior, *Violence and Victims,* 11(4): 341–54.

Tornstam, L. (1989) Abuse of the elderly in Denmark and Sweden: results from a population study, *Journal of Elder Abuse and Neglect,* 1(1): 35–44.

Tran, C.G. and DesJardins, K. (2000) Domestic violence in Vietnamese refugee and Korean immigrant communities, in J.L. Chin (ed.) *Relationship Among Asian American Women: Psychology of Women,* pp. 71–96. Washington, DC: American Psychological Association.

Triandis, H.C. (1995) *Individualism and Collectivism.* Boulder, CO: Westview Press.

Triandis, H.C. and Suh, E.M. (2002) Cultural influences on personality, *Annual Review of Psychology,* 53(1): 133–60.

Tutty, L. (1996) Post-shelter services: the efficacy of follow-up programs for abused women, Research on Social Work Practice, 6(4): 425–41.

Tutty, L.M., Babins-Wagner, R. and Rothery, M.A. (in press) Group treatment for aggressive women: an initial evaluation, *Journal of Family Violence.*

Tyree, A. and Malone, J. (1991) How can it be that wives hit husbands as much as husbands hit wives and none of us knew it? Paper presented at the annual meeting of the American Sociological Association. Cincinnati, OH, August.

United Nations (2002) *Abuse of Older Persons: Recognizing and Responding to Abuse of Older Persons in a Global Context, Report to the Secretary-General.* New York: United Nations.

UNFPA (2000) *Chapter 3: Ending Violence Against Women and Girls. State of the World Population.* Retrieved 1 December 2006 from www.unfpa.org/swp/2000/english/ ch03.html.

United States Department of Justice (Bureau of Justice Statistics) (2005) *Family Violence Statistics: Including Statistics on Strangers and Acquaintances.* Retrieved 19 November 2006 from www.ojp.usdoj.gov/bjs/pub/pdf/fvs.pdf.

Uys, L. and Gwele, N. (2005) *Curriculum Development in Nursing: Process and Innovations.* London: Routledge.

Valera, F., Hoi, H. and Kristin, A. (2003) Male shrikes punish unfaithful females, *Behavioral Ecology,* 14: 403–8.

Van Wormer, K. and Bartollas, C. (2007) *Women and the Criminal Justice System,* 2nd edn. Boston, MA: Allyn & Bacon.

Varvarro, F.F. and Lasko, D.L. (1993) Physical abuse as cause of injury in women: information for orthopaedic nurses. *Orthopaedic Nursing,* 12: 37–41.

Violence Policy Center (VPC) (2006) *American Roulette: Murder-Suicide in the United States.* Retrieved February 2007 from www.vpc.org/studies/amroul2006.pdf.

Vitanza, S., Vogel, L.C. and Marshall, L.L. (1995) Distress and symptoms of posttraumatic stress disorder in abused women, *Violence Victims,* 10(1): 23–34.

Vivian, D. and Heyman, R.E. (1996) Is there a place for conjoint treatment of couple violence? *In Session,* 2: 25–48.

von Bertalanffy, L. (1976) *General System Theory: Foundations, Development, Applications,* revised edn. New York: George Braziller.

Waalen, J., Goodwin, M., Spitz, A., Petersen, R. and Saltzman, L. (2000) Screening for intimate violence by health care providers – barriers and interventions, *American Journal of Preventive Medicine,* 19(4): 230–7.

Walby, S. (1999) Comparing methodologies used to study violence against women: men and violence against women. Proceedings from a seminar at the Council of Europe. Strasbourg, France, October.

Waldo, M. (1988) Relationship enhancement counselling groups for wife abusers, *Journal of Mental Health Counseling,* 10: 37–45.

Walker, L.E. (1984) *The Battered Woman Syndrome.* New York: Springer.

Walster, E. (1966) Assignment of responsibility for an accident, *Journal of Personality and Social Psychology,* 3(1): 73–9.

Walton-Moss, B.J., Manganello, J., Frye, V. and Campbell, J.C. (2005) Risk factors for intimate partner violence and associated injury among urban women, *Journal of Community Health*, 30: 377–89.

Wang, H. (1990) Toward a description of the organization of Korean speech levels, *International Journal of the Sociology of Language*, 82: 25–39.

Ward, C.A. (1995) *Attitudes Toward Rape: Feminist and Social Psychological Perspectives*. London: Sage.

Warshaw, C. (1989) Limitations of the medical model in the care of battered women. *Gender & Society*, 3: 506–17.

Warshaw, C. (1993) Limitations of the Medical Model in the Care of Battered Women in P.B. Bart and E.G. Moran (eds) *Violence Against Women: The Bloody Footprints*, pp 134–45. Newbury Park, CA: Sage Publications.

Warshaw, C. and Ganley, A. (1996) *Improving the Health Care Response to Domestic Violence: A Resource Manual for Health Care Providers*, 2nd edn. San Francisco: The Family Violence Prevention Fund.

Wathen, C. and MacMillan, H. (2003) Canadian Task Force on Preventive Health Care. Prevention of violence against women: recommendation statement from the Canadian Task Force on Preventive Health Care, *Canadian Medical Association Journal*, 169(6): 582–4.

Watlington,C.G. (2003) The roles of women's verbal and physical aggression as predictors of treatment outcome for their male partners involved in domestic violence treatment. Unpublished masters thesis, University of Maryland, Baltimore County.

Watts, C., Keogh, E., Ndlovu, M. and Kwaramba, R. (1998) Withholding of sex and forced sex: dimensions of violence against Zimbabwean women, *Reproductive Health Matters*, 6: 57–65.

Weaver, H. (2001) Indigenous identity, *American Indian Quarterly*, 25: 240–55.

Weil, S. (2005) The Iliad, or the poem of force, in S. Weil and R. Bespaloff (eds) *War and the Iliad*. New York: New York Review of Books.

Weiss, R.L. and Cerreto, M. (1980) The Marital Status Inventory: development of a measure of dissolution potential, *American Journal of Family Therapy*, 8: 80–6.

Weiss, R.L. and Heyman, R.E. (1997) Couple interaction, in W.K. Halford and H.J. Markman (eds) *Clinical Handbook of Marriage and Couples Intervention*, pp. 13–41. New York: Wiley.

Weiss, R.L., Hops, H. and Patterson, G.R. (1973) A framework for conceptualizing marital conflict: a technology for altering it, some data for evaluating it, in L.D. Handy and E.L. Mash (eds) *Behavior Change: Methodology Concepts and Practice*, pp. 309–42. Champaign, IL: Research Press.

Weisner, C.M. (1990) Coercion in alcohol treatment, in Institute of Medicine, *Broadening the Base of Treatment for Alcohol Problems*, pp. 589–609. Washington, DC: National Academy Press.

White, G.L. (1981) Some correlates of romantic jealousy, *Journal of Personality*, 49: 129–47.

Wiederman, M.W. and Allgeier, E.R. (1993) Gender differences in sexual jealousy: adaptionist or social learning explanation? *Ethology and Sociobiology*, 14: 115–40.

Williams, C.L. and Berry, J.W. (1991) Primary prevention of acculturative stress among refugees: application of psychological theory and practice, *American Psychologist*, 46: 632–41.

Wilson, B. (1990) 'Will women judges really make a difference?' Fourth Annual Barbara Betcherman Lecture, Osgoode Hall Law School, 8 February.

Wilson, M. and Daly, M. (1992) The man who mistook his wife for a chattel, in J.H. Barkow, L. Cosmides and J. Tooby (eds) *The Adapted Mind*, pp. 289–322). New York: Oxford University Press.

Wilson, M. and Daly, M. (1996) Male sexual proprietariness and violence against women, *Current Directions in Psychological Science*, 5: 2–7.

Wilson, M., Daly, M. and Daniele, A. (1995a) Familicide: the killing of spouse and children, *Aggressive Behavior*, 21: 275–91.

Wilson, M., Johnson, H. and Daly M. (1995b) Lethal and nonlethal violence against wives, *Canadian Journal of Criminology*, 37: 331–61.

Wingood, G.M., DiClemente, R.J. and Raj, A. (2000) Adverse consequences of intimate partner abuse among women in non-urban domestic violence shelters, *American Journal of Preventive Medicine*, 19(4): 270–75.

Winnicott D.W. (1956) The antisocial tendency, in C. Winnicott, R. Shepherd and M. Davis (eds) *Deprivation and Delinquency*. London: Tavistock.

Wolf, R.S. (1988) Elder abuse: ten years later, *Journal of the American Geriatrics Society*, 36(8): 758–62.

Wolfe, D.A., Wekerle, C., Scott, S., Straatman, A., Grasley, C. and Reitzel-Jaffe, D. (2003) Dating violence prevention with at-risk youth: a controlled outcome evaluation, *Journal of Consulting and Clinical Psychology*, 71: 279–91.

Women's Aid Federation of England (1992) *Domestic Violence: Memorandum of Evidence*. Memorandum 22, in Home Affairs Committee. London: HMSO.

WONCA Europe (2002) *The European Definition of General Practice/Family Medicine*. Retrieved 1 February 2007 from www.woncaeurope.org.

Wong, S.L.F. *et al.* (2006) Increased awareness of intimate partner abuse after training: a randomised controlled trial, *British Journal of General Practice*, 56: 249–57.

Woods, A.B., Page, G.G., O'Campo, P., Pugh, L.C., Ford, D. and Campbell, J.C. (2005) The mediation effect of posttraumatic stress disorder symptoms on the relationship of intimate partner violence and IFN levels, *American Journal of Community Psychology,* 36: 159–75.

Woods, S. (2000) Prevalence and patterns of post traumatic stress disorder in abused and post-abused women, *Issues in Mental Health Nursing,* 21(3): 309–24.

World Health Organization (1996) *Multiaxial Classification of Child and Adolescent Psychiatric Disorders: The ICD-10 Classification of Mental and Behavioural Disorders in Children and Adolescents.* Cambridge: Cambridge University Press.

World Health Organization (2002) Abuse of the elderly, in E.Krug *et al.* (eds) *World Report on Violence and Health.* Geneva: World Health Organization.

Wu, E., El-Bassel, N., Witte, S.S., Gilbert, L. and Chang, M. (2003) Intimate partner violence and HIV risk among urban minority women in primary health care settings, *AIDS and Behavior,* 7(3): 291–301.

Wyckoff, G.J., Wang, W., and Wu, C. (2000) Rapid evolution of male reproductive genes in the descent of man, *Nature,* 403: 304–8.

Yllo, K. and Straus, M. A. (1990) Patriarchy and violence against wives: the impact of structural and normative factors, in M.A. Straus and R.J. Gelles (eds.) *Physical Violence in American Families,* pp. 383–99. New Brunswick, NJ: Transaction Publishers.

Yoshioka, M.R. (2001a) Attitudes toward marital violence: an examination of four Asian communities, *Violence Against Women,* 7(8): 900–26.

Yoshioka, M.R. (2001b) A typology of abuse among battered South Asian women. Paper presented at the Annual Convention of the American Psychological Association, San Francisco.

Yoshioka, M.R, Gilbert, L. and El-Bassel, N. (2003) Social support and disclosure of abuse: a comparison of African American, Hispanic, and South Asian battered women, *Journal of Family Violence,* 18(3): 171–80.

Zink, T. and Sill, M. (2004) Intimate partner violence and job instability, *Journal of the American Medical Women's Association,* 59(1): 32–5.

Zink, T., Elder, N., Jacobson, J. and Klostermann, B. (2004) Medical management of intimate partner violence considering the stages of change: precontemplation and contemplation, *Annals of Family Medicine,* 2(3): 231–9.

Index